Current Topics in Intensive Care
Number 4

CURRENT TOPICS IN INTENSIVE CARE

Current Topics in Intensive Care
Number 4

edited by

H. Burchardi
Zentrum Anaesthesiologie,
Rettungs und Intensivmedizin,
Georg August Universität,
Göttingen, Germany

W.B. SAUNDERS COMPANY LTD
London · Philadelphia · Toronto
Sydney · Tokyo

W.B. Saunders Company Ltd 24–28 Oval Road
London NW1 7DX

The Curtis Center
Independence Square West
Philadelphia, PA 19106–3399, USA

Harcourt Brace & Company
55 Horner Avenue
Toronto, Ontario, M8Z 4X6, Canada

Harcourt Brace & Company, Australia
30–52 Smidmore Street
Marrickville
NSW 2204, Australia

Harcourt Brace & Company, Japan
Ichibancho Central Building
22–1 Ichibancho
Chiyoda-ku, Tokyo 102, Japan

A catalogue record for this book is available from the British Library

ISBN 0–7020–2161–X

Typeset by Blackpool Typesetting Services Ltd, Blackpool
Printed and bound in Great Britain by Biddles Ltd, Guildford and Kings Lynn

Contents

Contributors

Simon Atkinson, Senior Registrar, Department of General Surgery, Royal Perth Hospital, Wellington Street, Perth, WA 6000, Australia.

Dr Rinaldo Bellomo, Department of Anaesthesia and Intensive Care, Austin Hospital, Studley Road, Heidelberg 3084, Melbourne, Victoria, Australia.

Dr Frederick R. Bode, Associate Professor of Clinical Medicine, University of Missouri – Columbia, Division of Pulmonary and Critical Care Medicine, One Hospital Drive, Columbia, MO 65212, USA.

Professor Hilmar Burchardi, Professor of Medicine, Zentrum Anaesthesiologie, Rettungs- und Intensivmedizin, University Hospital, Robert-Koch-Strasse 40, D-37070 Göttingen, Germany.

Professor R. Phillip Dellinger, Professor of Medicine, Chief of Pulmonary and Critical Care Medicine, University of Missouri – Columbia and Harry S. Truman Memorial Veterans' Hospital, One Hospital Drive, MA419, Columbia, MO 65212, USA.

Professor Erwin Deutsch, Professor of Law, Department for Medical Law, University of Göttingen, Platz der Göttinger Sieben 6, D-37073 Göttingen, Germany.

Dr Geoff Dobb, Specialist in Intensive Care, Intensive Care Unit, Royal Perth Hospital, Perth, WA 6001, Australia.

Professor Tom S.J. Elliott, Professor and Consultant Microbiologist, Clinical Microbiology and Infection Control, The Queen Elizabeth Hospital, Edgbaston, Birmingham B15 2TH, UK.

Dr Rolf W. Günther, Professor and Chairman, Department of Diagnostic Radiology, University of Technology Aachen, Pauwelsstrasse 30, W-52057 Aachen, Germany.

Katherine Hall, Clinical Lecturer, University of Otago, Bioethics Research Centre, Medical Centre, Dunedin, New Zealand.

Dr Andreas Meier-Hellmann, Department of Anaesthesia and Critical Care Medicine, Friedrich Schiller University Jena, Bachstrasse 18, D-07743 Jena, Germany.

Dr T.J.J. Inglis, Medical Microbiologist, Western Australian Centre for Pathology and Medical Research, Queen Elizabeth Medical Centre, Locked Bag 2009, Nedlands, WA 6009, Australia.

Professor Jeff Lipman, Senior Staff Specialist, Intensive Care Unit, Royal Brisbane Hospital and Associate Professor, Division of Anaesthesiology and Intensive Care, University of Queensland, Australia.

Dr Jörg M. Neuerburg, Department of Diagnostic Radiology, University of Technology Aachen, Pauwelsstrasse 30, W-52057 Aachen, Germany.

Dr Gilbert R. Park, Director, Intensive Care Unit, Addenbrookes Hospital, Hills Road, Cambridge CB2 2QQ, UK.

Dr Jörg Rathgeber, Zentrum Anaesthesiologie, Rettungs- und Intensivmedizin, University Hospital, Robert-Koch-Strasse 40, D-37070 Göttingen, Germany.

Professor Konrad Reinhart, Professor of Medicine, Department of Anaesthesia and Critical Care Medicine, Friedrich Schiller University Jena, Bachstrasse 18, D-07743 Jena, Germany.

Dr Claudio Ronco, Divisione di Nefrologia, Ospedale San Bortolo, Via Ridolfi 8, 36100 Vicenza, Italy.

Dr James A. Russell, St Paul's Hospital, Department of Intensive Care, 1081 Burrard Street, Vancouver, British Columbia, Canada.

Dr Dan Schuller, Assistant Professor of Medicine, Washington University School of Medicine at Washington University Medical Center, Division of Pulmonary and Critical Care Medicine, Box 8052, 660 South Euclid Avenue, St Louis, MO 63110-1093, USA.

Professor Daniel P. Schuster, Professor of Medicine and Radiology, Washington University School of Medicine at Washington University Medical Center, Division of Pulmonary and Critical Care Medicine, Box 8052, 660 South Euclid Avenue, St Louis, MO 63110-1093, USA.

Dr Richard Straube, Director, Clinical Investigations, Ohmeda PPD, 110 Allen Road, P.O. Box 804, Liberty Corner, NJ 07938, USA.

Dr Janice L. Zimmerman, Associate Professor of Medicine, Baylor College of Medicine, Director, Medicine Emergency Center, Ben Taub General Hospital, 1504 Taub Loop, Houston, TX 77030, USA.

Contents of previous volumes
No 1

Contents of previous volumes No 2

Contents of previous volumes
No 3

Preface

For the fourth volume of *Current Topics in Intensive Care* we have again chosen subjects of interest to clinicians involved in intensive care medicine. Of course, topics like sepsis, acute renal failure and mechanical ventilation, are always of interest to those involved in critical care medicine and various aspects of these areas continue to be represented in this series. Other subjects of current importance have been chosen from the rapidly increasing spectrum of relevant interdisciplinary subject areas. In some cases a commentary has been provided to offer a different perspective, or highlight areas of controversy.

Fluid strategy in the treatment of acute respiratory distress syndrome (ARDS) is a topic that has stimulated controversy for many years. Opinions vary between two extremes; on the one hand Dr Russell discusses the concept of aiming for supranormal oxygen delivery by generous fluid supply and vasoactive medical support while, on the other hand Drs Schuller and Schuster present the case for keeping the lung dry in order to improve pulmonary gas exchange. Recently, a different strategy has been introduced in ARDS therapy, that of using nitric oxide inhalation for selective pulmonary vasodilation. Results are still contradictory and therefore Dr Dellinger's review of the current state of debate is extremely helpful.

Infection and sepsis are still a challenge for the intensivist and the increasing frequency of multiple antibiotic resistance, outlined in Dr Inglis's chapter, is frightening. New concepts of preventing catheter-associated infection described by Dr Elliott may help to restrict nosocomial infection. In sepsis, the wide choice of inotropic drugs makes the critical overview produced by Drs Meier-Hellmann and Reinhart of great practical use, and points to opportunities for further research. Dr Dobb meanwhile illuminates the role of gastrointestinal function in the process of sepsis.

Continuous renal replacement techniques are the subject of current debate. Bellomo and Ronco's recommendation that they should be utilized early on rather than only in the case of manifest acute renal organ failure may stimulate further discussion in this area. New modes of mechanical ventilation have opened a debate described by myself and Dr Rathgeber, on the possibility of improving the strategy of analgosedation in ventilated patients. Partial ventilatory support may offer the opportunity to adapt the level of sedation to meet the real needs, and thus, to promote communication and patient cooperation.

Pulmonary embolism, an important topic all too often disregarded by intensivists, is covered here by Dr Bode who gives an overview of pathophysiology and general treatment and Drs Neuerburg and Günther who describe interventional measures by vena cava filtering. Last, but not least, the ethical and legal aspects for research in critically ill patients are reviewed by Dr Deutsch who describes the main principles and international differences in regulations and legal conditions. As it is impossible to obtain informed consent from unconscious, critically ill patients research in this area is difficult and, in some countries, virtually unobtainable – a problem of great relevance in intensive care medicine.

I would like to thank all the authors who have contributed chapters of high scientific quality to this volume. I also very much appreciate the help of my co-editors as well as the professional assistance of Maria Khan and Linda Clark at W.B. Saunders.

I hope that once more we have been able to select a varied bouquet of contributors and topics which will stimulate our readers' interest and their knowledge.

H. Burchardi

1.1

Fluid Strategy in ARDS: The Concept of 'Keeping the Lung Dry'

Dan Schuller, Daniel P. Schuster

INTRODUCTION

Pulmonary edema remains one of the most common causes for admission to medical intensive care units (ICUs) with respiratory failure. Of the patients admitted with cardiogenic pulmonary edema, approximately one-half will require intubation and mechanical ventilation, despite initial medical therapy. Of patients with noncardiogenic pulmonary edema, acute respiratory distress syndrome (ARDS) continues to be the major cause of morbidity and mortality. However, recent evidence suggests that the mortality has fallen significantly over the last decade, particularly among the subset of patients with sepsis-related ARDS (Kollef and Schuster, 1995; Milberg *et al.*, 1995; Schuster, 1995a; Anzueto *et al.*, 1996; Hudson, 1995).

In clinical practice, the optimal management of any critically ill patient always involves therapies aimed at controlling the source of the acute insult while providing the 'best supportive care' to maintain organ function and homeostasis. Although it is difficult to quantify the relative benefit of each one of the 'routine' supportive measures used in the ICU (optimal treatment of infections, shift from parenteral to enteral nutrition, suctioning of respiratory secretions, stress ulcer and deep venous thrombosis prophylaxis, etc.), few would argue that it is precisely the effectiveness of these measures that frequently determines outcome. In the case of ARDS, no specific therapy has improved survival in any large randomized, prospective study (Zapol *et al.*, 1979; Bernard *et al.*, 1987; Bone *et al.*, 1987, 1989; Holzapfel *et al.*, 1987; Luce *et al.*, 1988; Morris *et al.*, 1988; Jepsen *et al.*, 1992; Milberg *et al.*, 1995; Anzueto *et al.*, 1996). Therefore, the reason for the improvement in survival, if real, can only be attributed to better overall supportive care.

Among the supportive therapies in ARDS, fluid management has been the focus of debate for some time. The controversy surrounding fluid management in ARDS is not only related to its impact on outcome, but also on which clinical end-points to follow and which strategy to use in order to achieve the desired goal. In a hypotensive patient with respiratory failure, clinicians often try to balance the potential benefits of intravascular volume expansion on reversing shock and improving organ perfusion against the potential deleterious effect of causing or worsening pulmonary edema. Even if one decides to pursue a negative fluid balance strategy, it is often difficult to achieve this goal in individual patients because of the demands associated with nutrition, antibiotics, etc.

Based on our current understanding of edema pathogenesis, as well as experimental and clinical data currently available, we believe that a negative fluid balance in pulmonary edema patients can, on average, have a salutary impact on outcome. Although definitive studies remain to be performed, we strongly favor implementing strategies that attempt to achieve the 'lowest possible wedge' compatible with adequate cardiac output and organ perfusion. However, keeping the lung 'dry' is often a difficult task to achieve. Therefore, we favor using protocols that target therapy to individual measurable end-points, instead of routine orders that often fail to achieve the desired therapeutic goal.

THEORY AND PHYSIOLOGICAL RATIONALE

The theoretical basis for attempting to achieve a negative fluid balance in pulmonary edema by restricting fluids or administering diuretics is centered around the familiar Starling equation, which can be modified to emphasize the influence of lymphatic flow (and other mechanisms for resolution) on the accumulation of fluid in the extravascular compartment:

$$\text{EVLW} = K_{fc}[(P_c - P_i) - \sigma(\pi_c - \pi_i)] - \text{Lymph flow}$$

where EVLW is extravascular lung water, K_{fc} is the hydraulic coefficient, P_c and P_i are the capillary and interstitial hydrostatic pressure, respectively, σ is a mathematical factor for vascular permeability to protein, and π_c and π_i are the capillary and interstitial oncotic pressure, respectively. It is important to keep in mind, however, that this equation is a model of fluid accumulation in the interstitium. In the lung, the onset of *alveolar edema* is a function of a different set of less well understood factors that result in the all-or-none development of alveolar edema (Matthay, 1985). The capacity of the perivascular interstitium depends on: (a) the degree of lung inflation, which can increase the capacity 20-fold; (b) the presence or absence of ventilation; (c) the time for accumulation of fluid; (d) the integrity of the alveolar epithelium; and (e) the interstitial compliance and pressure gradients which favor filtration and clearance toward the hilum (Zwinkler *et al.*, 1994). The distribution and clearance of fluid from the airspace in the edematous lung depends on factors such as the compliance of the interstitium and the active sodium transport by the lung epithelium (Zwinkler *et al.*, 1994). Furthermore, it is now clear that anatomic or functional heterogeneities act in addition to hydrostatic forces to influence patterns of edema formation (Bachofen *et al.*, 1993a,b; Crapo, 1993).

Although interstitial edema is presumably a necessary antecedent to the development of alveolar edema, it is not at all clear that, once alveolar edema has developed, further accumulation of that edema is accurately described by the Starling equation. Furthermore, the factors controlling the resolution of alveolar edema are almost certainly different than the factors that control its onset (Matthay and Wiener-Kronish, 1990).

Whenever the permeability of the alveolocapillary membrane increases (increased K_{fc}, decreased σ), various 'safety factors' which minimize the accumulation of extravascular water (e.g. the dilution of extravascular proteins and the reduction in extravascular oncotic pressures as edema develops) become less efficient (Matthay, 1985). As a result, lung edema develops at a lower pulmonary capillary pressure for two reasons: decreased membrane integrity, and reduced effects of these safety factors. Also, when membrane permeability is abnormal, the rate of increase in edema is greater for any given change in pulmonary capillary pressure than when membrane function is normal. Thus, the theoretical benefit of reducing pulmonary capillary pressures is enhanced, not reduced, when membrane permeability is increased.

EXPERIMENTAL EVIDENCE IN ANIMALS

The theoretical sensitivity of the lung to hydrostatic stress when membrane permeability is abnormal has been demonstrated experimentally in numerous acute lung injury models (Chernicki and Wood, 1979; Huchon *et al.*, 1981; Prewitt *et al.*, 1981; Winn *et al.*, 1984; Molloy *et al.*, 1985; Sivak *et al.*, 1986; Sznajder *et al.*, 1986; Allen *et al.*, 1987; Long *et al.*, 1988; Berner *et al.*, 1989; Zucker *et al.*, 1989; Townsley *et al.*, 1990). For instance, after oleic acid administration, Prewitt *et al.* (1981) showed that decreasing left atrial pressures by only 4 mmHg (either by controlled hemorrhage or nitroprusside) resulted in a 25–32% reduction in extravascular lung water accumulation during the first 4 hours of injury. Likewise, using an in situ, perfused, dog-lung preparation,

Huchon *et al.* (1981) showed that significantly more edema accumulated after the same dose of injurious agent in animals maintained with 'high' left atrial pressures (~18 mmHg) than in those animals with pressures kept at 0 mmHg. Using positron emission tomography to measure lung water concentrations before and after oleic acid injury, as well as the pulmonary transcapillary escape rate for gallium-68 labeled transferrin (an index of vascular permeability), Schuster and Haller (1990) showed that changes in lung water accumulation correlated well ($r^2 = 0.73$) with hydrostatic pressure and pulmonary transcapillary escape rate combined, but not with either variable alone. However, the influence of the hydrostatic pressure was the more important variable.

The most common method of reducing hydrostatic pressure clinically is to administer a diuretic, such as furosemide. This maneuver is associated with reductions in extravascular lung water after experimental lung injury (Chernicki and Wood, 1979; Sivak *et al.*, 1986). However, Ali *et al.* (1983) speculated that furosemide might have vasoactive effects that reduced shunt and extravascular lung water in injured regions. In subsequent studies (Ali and Wood, 1984), this same group showed in a lobar model of oleic acid injury that furosemide decreased shunt even though perfusion to the injured lobe increased, while extravascular lung water was unchanged compared with a control group. These data suggested that furosemide caused the preferential perfusion of nonflooded lung units. Ali and Wood (1984) showed, using an isolated, perfused lung model that furosemide caused a parallel downward shift in the pulmonary arterial pressure–cardiac output relationship, resulting in a lower 'effective downstream pressure', while for any given driving pressure blood flow to the isolated lobe increased. These effects were inversely proportional to the amount of edema present. They are consistent with vasodilation of a portion of the pulmonary vascular bed acting as a Starling resistor. Stevens *et al.* (1992) also confirmed that furosemide vasodilates pulmonary vessels, in addition to a bronchodilating effect. Rusch *et al.* (1986) found that 24 hours after oleic acid edema, furosemide failed to improve either oxygenation or extravascular lung water, unlike its apparent salutary effect in the first few hours after oleic acid injury.

Other maneuvers that reduce either the perfusion or the hydrostatic pressure to injured lung regions, such as regional hypoxic ventilation, stellate ganglion ablation, or an α-adrenergic blockade, are also associated with reduced extravascular lung water accumulation (Dauber and Weil, 1983; Bishop *et al.*, 1986; Cheney *et al.*, 1987; Leeman *et al.*, 1989). Conversely, interventions that increase perfusion or hydrostatic pressure are associated with increased extravascular lung water, even when occlusion pressure is kept constant (Hasinoff *et al.*, 1988).

All these experimental studies (Chernicki and Wood, 1979; Huchon *et al.*, 1981; Prewitt *et al.*, 1981; Dauber and Weil, 1983; Winn *et al.*, 1984; Molloy *et al.*, 1985; Bishop *et al.*, 1986; Sivak *et al.*, 1986; Sznajder *et al.*, 1986; Allen *et al.*, 1987; Cheney *et al.*, 1987; Takeda *et al.*, 1987; Hasinoff *et al.*, 1988; Long *et al.*, 1988; Berner *et al.*, 1989; Leeman *et al.*, 1989; Zucker *et al.*, 1989; Schuster and Haller, 1990; Townsley *et al.*, 1990; Schuster, 1994) lead to the conclusion that reduced capillary pressures and/or reduced perfusion to acutely injured lung units results in reduced extravascular lung water accumulation.

CLINICAL STUDIES

The above theory and experimental studies are also supported by clinical data. Although, until recently, such studies were either small or observational in design, larger prospective and retrospective studies in medical and surgical ICUs have now provided additional evidence that a positive fluid balance is associated with worse outcome and therapeutic efforts to achieve a negative fluid balance are associated with improved outcome (Tables 1.1.1 and 1.1.2) (Bone, 1978; Costello *et al.*, 1987; Eisenberg *et al.*, 1987; Simmons *et al.*, 1987; Humphrey *et al.*, 1990; Lowell *et al.*, 1990; Schuller *et al.*, 1991; Mitchell *et al.*, 1992).

In these studies, there is often a poor correlation between overall net intake versus output and the resolution of extravascular lung water. Actually, this is not surprising as net intake–output represents the relative fluid balance from all body compartments and not just the lung. Fluid balance can be expected to affect pulmonary microvascular hydrostatic pressures (but not necessarily in a 1 : 1 ratio). As embodied in the Starling equation, many other factors also affect extravascular lung water, and, in any given patient, these other factors may overwhelm the potential beneficial effect of reducing hydrostatic pressures on extravascular lung water accumulation. It is perhaps more correct to think of fluid balance as an important permissive factor, which can favorably affect extravascular lung water if hydrostatic pressures are reduced, and then only if other factors (e.g. magnitude of damage to the alveolocapillary membrane) are not greater in importance.

The association between improved outcome and fluid balance in pulmonary edema may be related to factors other than extravascular lung water reduction, including decreased gut edema with reduced bacterial translocation, improved gas exchange for reasons other than extravascular lung water reduction per se, or unknown reasons. Improved resolution of extravascular lung water itself might reduce

Table 1.1.1 Nonrandomized studies supporting the concept of 'keeping the lung dry'*

Study	Question addressed	Design and methods	Patient population	Results	Conclusion	Comments and criticism
Bone (1978)	Effect of diuretics, dialysis and PEEP on compliance, oxygenation, and urinary output	Not controlled; prospective series of patients with ARDS. Evaluation of response to therapeutic intervention	12 patients with ARDS	8 patients responded to diuretics; 2 patients responded to dialysis by improving static compliance, oxygenation, and urinary output	Improvement in pulmonary mechanics and gas exchange without impact on mortality (67%)	Small study (type-2 error)
Costello et al. (1987)	Effect of edema reduction on PEEP requirements, PCWP, and outcome	Comparative study of aggressive diuretic therapy in ARDS with high-dose furosemide	15 ARDS patients who underwent aggressive diuresis compared to 10 ARDS patients with conventional fluid management	Aggressive diuresis group associated with a 4 ± 2 kg weight loss, lower PEEP, lower PCWP, and 20% mortality compared to a 5 ± 4 kg weight gain and 60% mortality	Aggressive fluid management associated with improved clinical outcome and no evidence of renal or other end-organ failure	Preliminary report (abstract)
Simmons et al. (1987)	Effect of fluid balance on survival in ARDS	Prospective data collection without standardization of fluid therapy. Comparison by survival	113 ARDS patients from medical (55%) and surgical (45%) ICUs	Survivors lost weight and had significantly lower intake–output	Weight loss and negative fluid balance in ARDS associated with improved survival	Retrospective analysis. Lacking baseline data and severity of illness scores

Study	Aim	Method	Patients	Results	Conclusion	Comments
Lowell *et al.* (1990)	Effects of postoperative weight gain on outcome	Comparison of outcome and APACHE-II scores according to weight changes	48 consecutive patients admitted to the surgical ICU	29 patients (60%) gained up to 10% weight and had a 10% mortality; 16 patients (33%) with 11–20% weight gain had a 19% mortality, all 3 patients (6%) with >20% weight gain expired	Significant morbidity associated with postoperative fluid overload	Retrospective analysis. Not interventional trial
Humphrey *et al.* (1990)	Evaluate whether a management strategy of lowering PCWP is associated with improved outcome	Retrospective analysis of survival and ICU length of stay according to changes in PCWP	40 ARDS patients; 16 (40%) had a reduction of PCWP of ≥25% (group 1); 24 (60%) without PCWP reduction of at least 25% (group 2)	75% vs 29% survival in favor of group 1 ($p = 0.02$). Also, shorter ICU length of stay	Treatment of low pressure pulmonary edema with reduction of PCWP is associated with increased survival	Retrospective study; groups unequal at baseline. Lack of fluid balance data. Not clear that groups were treated differently
Schuller *et al.* (1991)	Evaluate the impact of fluid balance in patients with pulmonary edema sorted by survival and 'treatment received'	Retrospective analysis of the randomized controlled trial using EVLW measurements	89 patients with pulmonary edema (EVLW >7 ml/kg)	Survivors ($n = 51$) had no significant fluid gain compared to non-survivors ($n = 38$). Patients who gained <1 l by 36 h had better survival and shorter ventilator, ICU, and hospital days	Supports the concept that a positive fluid balance is at least partially responsible for poor outcome	'Treatment received' analysis; fluid balance was an independent predictor of survival even accounting for baseline differences (Cox proportional-hazard analysis)

* Modified from *Current Opinion in Critical Care* (1996) **2**: 1–7, with permission of the authors and Rapid Science Publishers.
ARDS, Acute respiratory distress syndrome; EVLW, extravascular lung water; ICU, intensive care unit; PCWP, pulmonary capillary wedge pressure; PEEP, positive end-expiratory pressure.

Table 1.1.2 Prospective, randomized studies supporting the concept of 'keeping the lung dry'*

Study	Question addressed	Design and methods	Patient population	Results	Conclusion	Comments and criticism
Eisenberg *et al.* (1987)	Evaluate safety and tolerance of a strategy of fluid restriction in critically ill patients based on EVLW measurements	Safety and feasibility study comparing EVLW vs PCWP end-points	25 patients randomized to EVLW protocol management; 23 patients routine management. Similar baseline characteristics	Hemodynamic management based on EVLW was associated with less fluid administration, and improved outcome (in ARDS)	Protocol of fluid restriction guided by EVLW safe and hastens the resolution of pulmonary edema	Small sample size to detect difference in mortality
Mitchell *et al.* (1992)	Evaluate whether a fluid management strategy that emphasized diuresis and fluid restriction can affect the resolution of EVLW and outcome implications	Randomized, controlled, prospective trial of fluid management based on direct measurements of EVLW vs PCWP management	89 patients with pulmonary edema out of 101 patients who required PAC; 52 patients, EVLW group, 49 patients, PCWP group	Patients managed in the EVLW group had no fluid gain and significantly reduced time on ventilator and in the ICU ($p < 0.05$)	A lower positive fluid balance in patients with pulmonary edema, regardless of cause, is associated with reduced EVLW, ventilator and ICU days	'Intention-to-treat' analysis. Small sample size to detect difference in mortality. Applicability of EVLW measurement remains problematic
Schuller and Lynch (1994)	Evaluate the relative benefit of two different diuretic strategies in the ICU	Prospective, randomized study comparing 'bolus' vs 'continuous' furosemide infusions using a weight-based algorithm	27 pulmonary edema patients: 15 randomized to 'bolus' diuresis; 12 randomized to 'continuous' infusion	Patients in the 'bolus' group received smaller cumulative furosemide dosages than those in 'continuous' group. Net hourly diuresis 185 ± 143 vs 169 ± 93 ml/h ($p = $ NS)	Both protocols proved safe and equally effective in achieving negative fluid balance	Preliminary, abstract form. Potential type-2 error

* From *Current Opinion in Critical Care* (1996) **2**: 1–7, with permission of the authors and Rapid Science Publishers.
ARDS, Acute respiratory distress syndrome; EVLW, extravascular lung water; ICU, intensive care unit; PAC, pulmonary artery catheter; PCWP, pulmonary capillary wedge pressure.

the number of ventilator days, thereby reducing the risks of infection, barotrauma, and oxygen toxicity associated with prolonged mechanical ventilation.

THE BOTTOM LINE

The theoretical, experimental, and clinical data, then, are all very consistent: EVLW accumulation is less and resolution is greater when clinical strategies are used that achieve wedge pressure reduction or diuresis/fluid restriction in patients with pulmonary edema (Schuster, 1993, 1995b; Schuller and Schuster, 1996). In patients with ARDS, these strategies are associated with less time on mechanical ventilation and in the ICU (Schuller *et al.*, 1991; Mitchell *et al.*, 1992). Unfortunately, no study has yet been large enough to demonstrate a statistically significant impact on mortality. Multiple editorials have called for larger randomized studies to finally resolve this controversy (Hyers, 1990; Sznajder, 1990; Hudson, 1992).

A WORD OF CAUTION

A strategy of relative or absolute fluid restriction for ARDS patients can certainly be misunderstood and abused. Fluid restriction and/or wedge pressure reduction in frankly hypovolemic patients is a prescription for clinical disaster, with vital organ hypoperfusion the expected adverse result. Careful clinical and even invasive monitoring of organ function and hemodynamics, and the willingness to adjust therapy as necessary to maintain adequate perfusion, must be part of the therapeutic plan. With this caveat in mind, currently available data suggest that diuresis/fluid restriction in euvolemic (and certainly in hypervolemic) ARDS patients can be accomplished without clinically important deterioration in either cardiac or renal function. Unanswered is whether perfusion, when treated, should be principally maintained by adjustments in volume status or by the use of inotropes and vasodilators. Likewise, the end-point for determining 'adequate' perfusion, as judged primarily from hemodynamic data, is unknown. Clinical trials of different end-points, with different therapeutic strategies, are needed.

HOW TO KEEP THE LUNG DRY

Since there are no specific measures to correct the permeability abnormality or the inflammatory reaction in ARDS, clinical management primarily involves supporting organ function while the lung injury itself resolves. The most common method of attempting to limit EVLW accumulation is by actively reducing intravascular hydrostatic pressure with the utilization of rapidly acting diuretics like furosemide. However, unless therapy is targeted to specific titratable end-points, it is often difficult to control fluid balance in patients with severe pulmonary edema and multi-organ failure. Schuller and Lynch (1994) recently examined the safety, efficacy, and relative benefit of two different protocol-guided strategies of fluid management and diuretic use in the ICU, based on either a continuous furosemide infusion, or more conventional intermittent bolus furosemide infusions (Table 1.1.3). Although each protocol was equally efficacious, input–output and total diuretic dose were lower, and ICU and hospital lengths of stay were longer in a separate group of patients who were not managed by either standardized protocol (Schuller, unpublished data). As it turned out, the benefits observed in the protocol-guided fluid manage-

Table 1.1.3 Diuresis and fluid management algorithms

1. Minimize sodium and fluid intake:
    (a) oral fluid restriction to 500–750 ml/day,
    (b) maximally concentrate all intravenous medications,
    (c) decrease maintenance intravenous fluid rate to 'keep vein open' (10 ml/h), and
    (d) substitute dextrose 5% for 0.9% sodium chloride

2. Bolus loading dose of furosemide (40–80 mg i.v. push)

3. Maintenance diuretic regimen titrated to net hourly diuresis:
    (a) *Continuous furosemide infusion*
    Furosemide 250 mg in 250 cm^3 dextrose 5%. Start drip at rate of 0.10 mg/kg/h, and increase hourly by 0.10 mg/kg until the net (input–output) hourly diuresis is at least 1 ml/kg, or a therapeutic end-point has been reached. Maximal infusion rate not to exceed 0.75 mg/kg/h.
    (b) *Bolus furosemide infusion*
    Assessment of diuretic response to loading bolus with subsequent dosing as follows:
    - *If* net hourly diuresis >1 ml/kg/h *and* therapeutic end-point accomplished, *then* no further diuretics for the next 6–12 hours; reassess
    - *If* net hourly diuresis >1 ml/kg/h *but* therapeutic end-point not accomplished, *then repeat* previous dosage of furosemide in 4–6 hours; reassess
    - *If* net hourly diuresis ≤1 ml/kg/h *and* therapeutic end-point not accomplished, *then* double previous dosage of furosemide and give within 1–2 hours; reassess

ment groups were related to the larger cumulative dose of furosemide administered. However, two additional factors that were different from 'routine' fluid management included: (a) measures to minimize fluid intake, and (b) the substitution of the regular nursing flow sheets for study flow sheets that require the hourly recording of inputs, outputs, net hourly input–output, the total cumulative fluid balance since diuretics were initiated, and the dosage of furosemide given. As a whole, these deviations from the 'routine' care not only provide a more aggressive use of diuretics, but also shift the responsibility of diuretic titration from physicians to nurses, and increases everyone's awareness of a patient's fluid balance.

As with other studies, this study (Schuller and Lynch, 1994) then seems to support the conclusion that outcome is often favorably affected when a carefully conceived protocol is effectively implemented (Hull *et al.*, 1992; Mitchell *et al.*, 1992; Morris, 1992; Tuchschmidt *et al.*, 1992; Barnea and Sheffer, 1993; Raschke *et al.*, 1993; Morris *et al.*, 1994; Reinersten, 1994). It is at least possible, then, that the favorable effects demonstrated in studies of fluid balance in severe pulmonary edema are due to constraints placed on individual physician practices when patients are studied as part of a therapeutic 'protocol'.

Potential additional interventions that may help to achieve a negative fluid balance in selected patients include: (a) use of combination diuretic therapy (e.g. chlorothiazide or metolazone with furosemide) (Oster *et al.*, 1983; Ellison, 1994), (b) low-dose dopamine (e.g. 2–3 µcg/kg/min) (Duke and Bersten, 1992; Duke *et al.*, 1994; Flancbaum *et al.*, 1994; de Lasson *et al.*, 1995), and (c) extracorporeal fluid removal techniques (e.g. slow continuous ultrafiltration) (Laurer *et al.*, 1983; Barzilay *et al.*, 1989; Agostoni *et al.*, 1993; Vincent and Tielmans, 1995). However, these approaches require further evaluation.

CONCLUSIONS

The determination of optimal fluid balance in ARDS has always posed a clinical dilemma. As with most controversies, a balanced view probably represents the most prudent course of action. Theory and experimental and currently available clinical data are all consistent with the concept that clinical strategies designed to reduce the accumulation or hasten the resolution of pulmonary edema are associated with improved outcome, especially when implemented during the first few days of ARDS. At later stages, especially when fibrosis has developed, such strategies are less likely to be efficacious, particularly if the mechanism of benefit is a reduction in extravascular lung water. At any time, it is important to monitor patients carefully for potentially deleterious effects of excessive intravascular volume reduction.

Until we have a breakthrough in the prevention and therapy of ARDS, we must continue to improve and optimize our supportive care. The current state of knowledge indicates that supportive management strategies which attempt to keep the lowest possible wedge pressure consistent with adequate organ perfusion, are associated with a better patient outcome. To this end, protocol-guided diuretic management can be readily and safely implemented in the ICU.

REFERENCES

Agostoni, P.G., Marenzi, G.C., Pepi, M., *et al.* (1993) Isolated ultrafiltration in moderate congestive heart failure. *J Am Coll Cardiol* **21**: 424–431.

Ali, J., Wood, L.D.H. (1984) Pulmonary vascular effects of furosemide on gas exchange in pulmonary edema. *J Appl Physiol* **57**: 160–167.

Ali, J., Unruh, H., Skoog, C., *et al.* (1983) The effect of lung edema on pulmonary vasoactivity of furosemide. *J Surg Res* **35**: 383–390.

Allen S.J., Drake, R.E., Katz, J., *et al.* (1987) Lowered pulmonary arterial pressure prevents edema after endotoxin in sheep. *J Appl Physiol* **63**: 1008-1011.

Anzueto, A., Baughman, R.P., Guntupalli, K.K., Weg, J.G., Wiedeman, H.P., *et al.* (1996) Aerosolized surfactant in adults with sepsis-induced acute respiratory distress syndrome. *N Engl J Med* **334**: 1417–1421.

Bachofen, H., Schurch, S., Michel, R.P., Weibel, E.R. (1993a) Experimental hydrostatic pulmonary edema in rabbit lungs. I. Morphology. *Am Rev Respir Dis* **147**: 989–996.

Bachofen, H., Schurch, S., Weibel, E.R. (1993b) Experimental hydrostatic pulmonary edema in rabbit lungs. II. Barrier lesions. *Am Rev Respir Dis* **147**: 997–1004.

Barnea, O., Sheffer, N. (1993) A computer model for analysis of fluid resuscitation. *Comput Biol Med* **23**: 443–454.

Barzilay, E., Kessler, D., Berlot, G., *et al.* (1989) Use of extracorporeal supportive technique as additional treatment for septic-induced multiple organ failure patients. *Crit Care Med* **17**: 634–637.

Bernard, G.R., Luce, J.M., Sprung, C.L., *et al.* (1987) High dose corticosteroids in patients with the adult respiratory distress syndrome. *N Engl J Med* **317**: 1565–70.

Berner, M.E., Teague, W.G., Scheerer, R.G., *et al.* (1989) Furosemide reduces lung fluid filtration in lambs with lung microvascular injury from air emboli. *J Appl Physiol* **67**: 1990–1996.

Bishop, M.J., Boatman, E.S., Webster, R., *et al.* (1986) Effects of lobar pulmonary blood flow on the evolution of oleic acid lung injury in dogs. *J Surg Res* **41**: 394–400.

Bone, R.C. (1978) Treatment of adult respiratory distress syndrome with diuretics, dialysis, and positive end-expiratory pressure. *Crit Care Med* **6**: 136–139.

Bone, R.C., Fisher, C.J., Clemmer, T.P., Slotman, G.J., Metz, C.A. (1987) Early methylprednisolone in preventing parenchymal lung injury and improving mortality in patients with septic shock. *Chest* **92**: 1032–1046.

Bone, R.C., Slotman, G., Maunder, R., Silverman, H., Hyers, H.M., Kerstein, M.D. (1989) Randomized double-blind, multicenter study of prostaglandin E_1 in patients without the adult respiratory distress syndrome. *Chest* **96**: 114–119.

Cheney, F.W., Bishop, M.J., Chi, E.Y., *et al.* (1987) Effect of regional alveolar hypoxia on permeability pulmonary edema formation in dogs. *J Appl Physiol* **62**: 1690–1697.

Chernicki, J.A.W., Wood, L.D.H. (1979) Effect of furosemide in canine low-pressure pulmonary edema. *J Clinic Invest* **64**: 1494–1504.

Costello, J.L., Dorinksy, P.M., Gadek, J.E. (1987) Edema reduction improves clinical abnormalities in ARDS: a clinical trial of aggressive diuretic therapy. *Am Rev Respir Dis* **135**: A9 [abstract].

Crapo, J.D. (1993) New concepts in the formation of pulmonary edema. *Am Rev Respir Dis* **147**: 790–792.

Dauber, I.M., Weil, J.V. (1983) Lung injury edema in dogs. Influence of sympathetic ablation. *J Clin Invest* **72**: 1977–1986.

de Lasson, L., Hansen, H.E., Juhl, B., Paaske, W.P., Pedersen, E.B. (1995) A randomized, clinical study of the effect of low-dose dopamine on central and renal haemodynamics in infrarenal aortic surgery. *Eur J Vasc Endovasc Surg* **10**: 82–90.

Duke, G.J., Bersten, A.D. (1992) Dopamine and renal salvage in the critically ill patient. *Anaesth Intensive Care* **20**: 277–287.

Duke, G.J,, Briedis, J.H., Weaver, R.A. (1994) Renal support in critically ill patients: low-dose dopamine or low-dose dubutamine? *Crit Care Med* **22**: 1919–1925.

Eisenberg, P.R., Hansbrough, J.R., Anderson, D., *et al.* (1987) A prospective study of lung water measurements during patient management in an intensive care unit. *Am Rev Respir Dis* **136**: 662–668.

Ellison, D.H. (1994) Diuretic drugs and the treatment of edema: From clinic to bench and back again. *Am J Kidney Dis* **23**: 623–643.

Flancbaum, L., Choban, P.S., Dasta, J.F. (1994) Quantitative effects of low-dose dopamine or urine output in oliguric surgical intensive care unit patients. *Crit Care Med* **22**: 61–68.

Hasinoff, I., Ducas, J., Prewitt, R.M. (1988) Increased cardiac output increases lung water in canine permeability pulmonary edema. *J Crit Care* **3**: 225–231.

Holzapfel, L., Robert, D., Perrin, F., Gaussorgues, P., Giudicelli, D.P. (1987) Comparison of high frequency jet ventilation to conventional ventilation in adults with respiratory distress syndrome. *Intensive Care Med* **13**: 100–105.

Huchon, G.J., Hopewell, P.C., Murray, J.F. (1981) Interactions between permeability and hydrostatic pressure in perfused dogs' lungs. *J Appl Physiol* **50**: 905–911.

Hudson, L.D. (1992) Fluid management strategy in acute lung injury. *Am Rev Respir Dis* **145**: 988–989.

Hudson, L.D. (1995) New therapies for ARDS. *Chest* **108**: 79S–91S [review].

Hull, R.D., Raskob, G.E., Rosenbloom, D., *et al.* (1992) Optimal therapeutic level of heparin therapy in patients with venous thrombosis. *Arch Intern Med* **152**: 1589–1595.

Humphrey, H., Hall, J., Sznajder, I., *et al.* (1990) Improved survival in ARDS patients associated with a reduction in pulmonary capillary wedge pressure. *Chest* **97**: 1176–1180.

Hyers, T.M. (1990) ARDS: the therapeutic dilemma. *Chest* **97**: 1025.

Jepsen, S., Herlevsen, P., Bud, M.I., Knudsen, P., Klaussen, N.O. (1992) Antioxidant treatment with *N*-acetylcysteine during adult respiratory distress syndrome. A prospective, randomized, placebo-controlled study. *Crit Care Med* **20**: 918–923.

Kollef, M.H., Schuster, D.P. (1995) The acute respiratory distress syndrome. *N Engl J Med* **332**: 27–37 [review].

Laurer, A., Saccaggi, A., Ronco, C. (1983) Continuous arteriovenous hemofiltration in the critically ill patient. *Ann Intern Med* **99**: 255.

Leeman, M., Closset, J., Vachiery, J., *et al.* (1989) Sino-aortic deafferentation reduces intrapulmonary shunt in dogs with oleic acid lung injury. *J Appl Physiol* **67**: 833–838.

Long, R., Breen, P.H., Mayers, I., *et al.* (1988) Treatment of canine aspiration pneumonitis: fluid volume reduction vs. fluid volume expansion. *J Appl Physiol* **65**: 1736–1744.

Lowell, J.A., Schifferdecker, C., Discoll, D.F., *et al.* (1990) Postoperative fluid overload: not a benign problem. *Crit Care Med* **18**: 728–733.

Luce, J.M., Montgomery, A.B., Marks, J.D., Turner, J., Metz, C.A., Murray, J.F. (1988) Ineffectiveness of high-dose methylprednisolone in preventing parenchymal lung injury and improving mortality in patients with septic shock. *Am Rev Respir Dis* **138**: 62–68.

Matthay, M.A. (1985) Pathophysiology of pulmonary edema. *Clin Chest* **6**: 301–312.

Matthay, M.A., Wiener-Kronish, J.P. (1990) Intact epithelial barrier function is critical for the resolution of alveolar edema in humans. *Am Rev Respir Dis* **142**: 1250–1257.

Milberg, J.A., Davis, D.R., Steinberg, K.P., Hudson, L.D. (1995) Improved survival of patients with acute respiratory distress syndrome. *JAMA* **273**: 306–309.

Mitchell, J.P., Schuller, D., Calandrino, F.S., *et al.* (1992) Improved outcome based on fluid management in critically ill patients requiring pulmonary artery catheterization. *Am Rev Respir Dis* **145**: 990–998.

Molloy, W.D., Lee, K.Y., Girling, L., *et al.* (1985) Treatment of canine permeability pulmonary edema: short-term effects of dobutamine, furosemide, and hydralazine. *Circulation* **72**: 1365–1371.

Morris, A.H. (1992) Evaluation of new therapy: Extracorporeal CO_2 removal, protocol control of intensive care unit care, and the human laboratory. *J Crit Care* **7**: 280–286.

Morris, A.H., Menlove, R.L., Rollins, R.J., Wallace, C.J., Beck, E. (1988) A controlled clinical trial of a new 3-step therapy that includes extracorporeal CO_2 removal for ARDS. *Trans Am Soc Artif* **11**: 48–53.

Morris, A.H., Wallace, C.J., Menlove, R.L., *et al.* (1994) Randomized clinical trial of pressure-controlled inverse ratio ventilation and extracorporeal CO_2 removal for adult respiratory distress syndrome. *Am J Respir Crit Care Med* **149**: 295–305.

Oster, Jr, Epstein, M., Smoler, S. (1983) Combined therapy with thiazide-type and loop diuretic agents for resistant sodium retention. *Ann Intern Med* **99**: 405–406.

Prewitt, R.M., McCarthy, J., Wood, L.D.H. (1981) Treatment of acute low pressure pulmonary edema in dogs. Relative effects of hydrostatic and oncotic pressure, nitroprusside, and positive end-expiratory pressure. *J Clin Invest* **67**: 409–418.

Raschke, R.A., Reilly, B.M., Guidry, J.R., Fontana, J.R., Srinivas, S. (1993) The weight-based heparin dosing nomogram compared with a 'standard care' nomogram. *Ann Intern Med* **119**: 874–881.

Reinersten, J.L. (1994) Algorithms, guidelines, and protocols: can they really improve what we do? *Transfusion* **34**: 281–282. [Excellent editorial that highlights the phases and importance of algorithm implementation.]

Rusch, V.W., Artman, L., Cheney, F.W. (1986) Effect of furosemide on fully established low pressure pulmonary edema. *J Surg Res* **41**: 141–145.

Schuller, D., Lynch, J.P. (1994) Prospective, randomized, comparative trial of continuous vs. bolus furosemide infusion in the intensive care unit. *Chest* **106**: 157S.

Schuller, D., Schuster, D.P. (1996) Fluid management in acute respiratory distress syndrome. *Current Opinion Crit Care* **2**: 1–7.

Schuller, D., Mitchell, J.P., Calandrino, F.S., *et al.* (1991) Fluid balance during pulmonary edema: is fluid gain a marker or a cause of poor outcome. *Chest* **100**: 1068–1075.

Schuster, D.P. (1993) The case for and against fluid restriction and occlusion pressure reduction in adult respiratory distress syndrome. *New Horizons* **1**: 478–488.

Schuster, D.P. (1994) ARDS: clinical lessons from the oleic acid model of acute lung injury. *Am J Respir Crit Care Med* **149**: 245–260.

Schuster, D.P. (1995a) What is acute lung injury? What is ARDS? *Chest* **107**: 1721–1726.

Schuster, D.P. (1995b) Fluid management in ARDS: 'Keep them dry' or does it matter? *Intensive Care Med* **21**: 101–103.

Schuster, D.P., Haller, J. (1990) A quantitative correlation of extravascular lung water accumulation with vascular permeability and hydrostatic pressure measurements. A positron emission tomography study. *J Crit Care* **5**: 161–168.

Simmons, R.S., Berdine, G.G., Seidenfeld, J.J., *et al.* (1987) Fluid balance and the adult respiratory distress syndrome. *Am Rev Respir Dis* **135**: 924–929.

Sivak, E.D., Tita, J., Meden, G., *et al.* (1986) Effects of furosemide versus isolated ultrafiltration on extravascular lung water in oleic acid-induced pulmonary edema. *Crit Care Med* **14**: 48–51.

Stevens, E.L., Uyehara, C.F.T., Southgate, W.M., *et al.* (1992) Furosemide differentially relaxes airway and vascular smooth muscle in fetal, newborn, and adult guinea pigs. *Am Rev Respir Dis* **146**: 1192–1197.

Sznajder, I. (1990) Beneficial effects of reducing pulmonary edema in patients with hypoxemic respiratory failure. *Chest* **100**: 890–891.

Sznajder, J.I., Zucker, A.R., Wood, L.D.H., *et al.* (1986) The effects of plasmapheresis and hemofiltration on canine acid aspiration pulmonary edema. *Am Rev Respir Dis* **134**: 222–228.

Takeda, K., Knapp, M.J., Wolfe, W.G., *et al.* (1987) Hypoxia enhances unilateral lung injury by increasing blood flow to the injured lung. *J Appl Physiol* **63**: 2516–2523.

Townsley, M.I., Lim, E.H., Sahawneh, T.M., *et al.* (1990) Interaction of chemical and high vascular pressure injury in isolated canine lung. *J Appl Physiol* **69**: 1647–1664.

Tuchschmidt, J., Fried, J., Astiz, M., Rackow, E. (1992) Elevation of cardiac output and oxygen delivery improves outcome in septic shock. *Chest* **102**: 216–220.

Vincent, J.L., Tielmans, G. (1995) Continuous hemofiltration in severe sepsis: is it beneficial? *J Crit Care* **10**: 27–32.

Winn, R., Strothert, J., Nadir, B., *et al.* (1984) Lung fluid balance, vascular permeability, and gas exchange after acid aspiration in awake goats. *J Appl Physiol* **56**: 979–985.

Zapol, W.M., Snider, M.T., Hill, J.D., *et al.* (1979) Extracorporeal membrane oxygenation in severe acute respiratory failure. *JAMA* **242**: 2193–2196.

Zucker, A.R., Sznajder, J.I., Becker, C.J., *et al.* (1989) The pathophysiology and treatment of canine kerosene pulmonary injury: effects of plasmapheresis and positive end-expiratory pressure. *J Crit Care* **4**: 184–193.

Zwinkler, M.P., Peters, T.M., Michel, R.P. (1994) Effects of pulmonary fibrosis on the distribution of edema. Computed tomographic scanning and morphology. *Am J Respir Crit Care Med* **149**: 1266–1275.

1.2

Fluid Strategy in ARDS: The Concept of Maintaining Peripheral Perfusion

James A. Russell

INTRODUCTION

The maintenance of peripheral perfusion is fundamental to critical care management and yet remains one of the most controversial subjects in the field. There is indeed continuing controversy regarding how much resuscitation is adequate, the level of perfusion that should be maintained and how adequate perfusion should be monitored. As a result, the clinician in the intensive care unit (ICU) faces dilemmas daily in the maintenance of peripheral perfusion in the critically ill patient. The major goal of this chapter is to address this controversy directly by reviewing the pertinent physiology and clinical studies, and then to make recommendations for a clinical approach to the maintenance of peripheral perfusion in the critically ill (Russell and Phang, 1994).

The maintenance of peripheral perfusion really means supplying the tissues with an adequate supply of oxygen relative to oxygen demand. Therefore, I will use the oxygen delivery/consumption relationship as a paradigm for the approach to maintaining peripheral perfusion in the critically ill.

This chapter addresses first the physiology of oxygen delivery (D_{O_2}) and consumption (V_{O_2}). Then, the pathologic dependence of oxygen consumption on delivery is presented. Next, I will review the studies that support the finding of pathologic dependence of oxygen consumption on delivery. These studies lead then naturally to a discussion of the problem of mathematical coupling of shared measurement error. This problem has been resolved by undertaking studies in which oxygen delivery and consumption were determined by independent methods. I then analyse the numerous randomized controlled trials (RCTs) of supernormal oxygen delivery. Finally, I present a clinical approach to the management of oxygen delivery, oxygen consumption and thus peripheral perfusion in the critically ill.

THE OXYGEN DELIVERY–CONSUMPTION RELATIONSHIP: PHYSIOLOGY

Oxygen must be supplied to the tissues continuously for the maintenance of aerobic metabolism because the human has trivial supplies of oxygen to draw on during conditions of oxygen deprivation. The supply of oxygen is used to maintain oxidative phosphorylation. If oxygen supply is decreased significantly, then oxygen consumption decreases, oxidative ATP synthesis ceases, and ATP must then be made by the much less efficient anaerobic pathways. Further decreases in oxygen supply cause cellular dysfunction and, ultimately, cell death.

The whole-body (global) oxygen delivery–consumption relationship is shown in Figure 1.2.1. Global oxygen delivery is the product of the cardiac output and the arterial oxygen content. As oxygen delivery decreases, oxygen consumption is maintained relatively constant (plateau phase) until the so-called critical oxygen delivery (critical DO_2) is reached. Below the critical DO_2, VO_2 falls as DO_2 falls; this is called the physiologic dependence of oxygen consumption on oxygen delivery. Arterial lactate levels begin to rise as DO_2 falls below the critical DO_2, because of the onset of anaerobic metabolism.

Oxygen consumption is maintained constant as DO_2 falls because of a progressive increase in the extraction of oxygen by the tissues. The extraction of O_2 may be expressed as the oxygen extraction ratio (O_2ER). The O_2ER is calculated as the arterial mixed venous O_2 content difference divided by the arterial O_2 content. Figure 1.2.1 shows the relationship between DO_2 and the O_2ER. The critical O_2ER is the O_2ER at the critical DO_2 point. Note that below the critical O_2ER the O_2ER continues to increase, but not sufficiently to maintain a constant VO_2.

The normal value of the critical DO_2 is 5–10 ml/kg/min, as determined from animal studies (Cain, 1977; Nelson *et al.*, 1987, 1988). The normal critical O_2ER of animals is 0.5–0.8 (Cain, 1977; Nelson *et al.*, 1987, 1988). Interestingly, until very recently, the normal critical DO_2 and O_2ER had not been determined in individual humans. Instead, the critical points were calculated from pooled data from studies of cardiac surgical patients (Shibutani *et al.*, 1983; Komatsu *et al.*, 1987). The pooled normal critical DO_2 was about 8 ml/kg/min. However, we have previously discussed in detail the potential errors that can occur when using pooled data (Russell and Phang, 1994). Therefore, we undertook a study designed to determine the critical DO_2 and O_2ER in individual critically ill humans (Figure 1.2.2) (Ronco *et al.*, 1993a). The study was approved by our institutional ethics review committees. Critically ill patients were studied when their attending physicians and families had agreed to stop life support. After informed consent had been

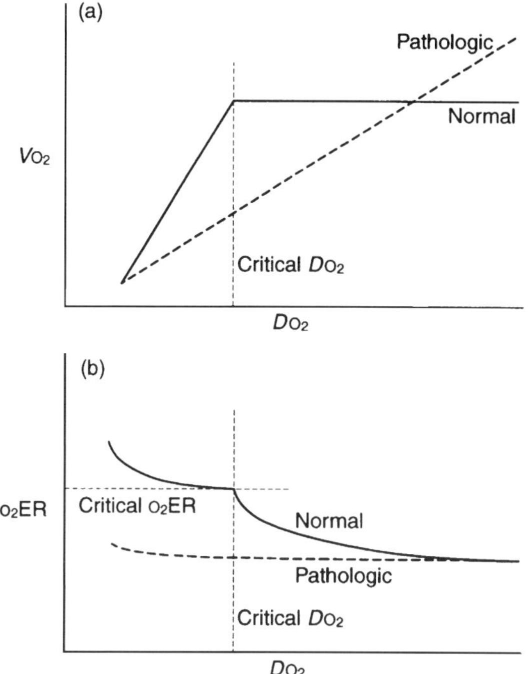

Figure 1.2.1. (a) The relationship between D_{O_2} and V_{O_2} in normal and pathologic conditions. Normally, as D_{O_2} decreases V_{O_2} is maintained relatively constant. Below the critical D_{O_2}, V_{O_2} decreases as D_{O_2} decreases: V_{O_2} is physiologically dependent on D_{O_2}. Compared with the physiological relationship between D_{O_2} and V_{O_2}, the pathologic dependence of V_{O_2} on D_{O_2} is characterized by a much wider range of dependence of V_{O_2} on D_{O_2} and by a higher critical D_{O_2}. (b) The relationship between D_{O_2} and the oxygen extraction ratio (O_2ER). Normally, as D_{O_2} decreases, the O_2ER increases to maintain V_{O_2} relatively constant. The critical O_2ER is the O_2ER at the critical D_{O_2}. Below the critical D_{O_2}, O_2ER continues to increase, but not sufficiently to maintain V_{O_2}. The pathologic dependence of V_{O_2} on D_{O_2} is characterized by a failure of the O_2ER to increase adequately (as D_{O_2} decreases) to maintain V_{O_2}. In pathologic conditions, there is often a small but inadequate increase in O_2ER as D_{O_2} decreases.

obtained from the families, life support was gradually withdrawn in a standardized protocol in each patient. Arterial lactate, D_{O_2} and V_{O_2} were determined throughout the period of withdrawal of life support at 5- to 20-minute intervals as we first withdrew vasopressors, then decreased the F_iO_2, and then discontinued mechanical ventilation. V_{O_2} was determined by indirect calorimetry. There were several important results obtained from this study. First, the critical D_{O_2} was 4.5 ml/kg/min, which is much lower than expected in the critically ill,

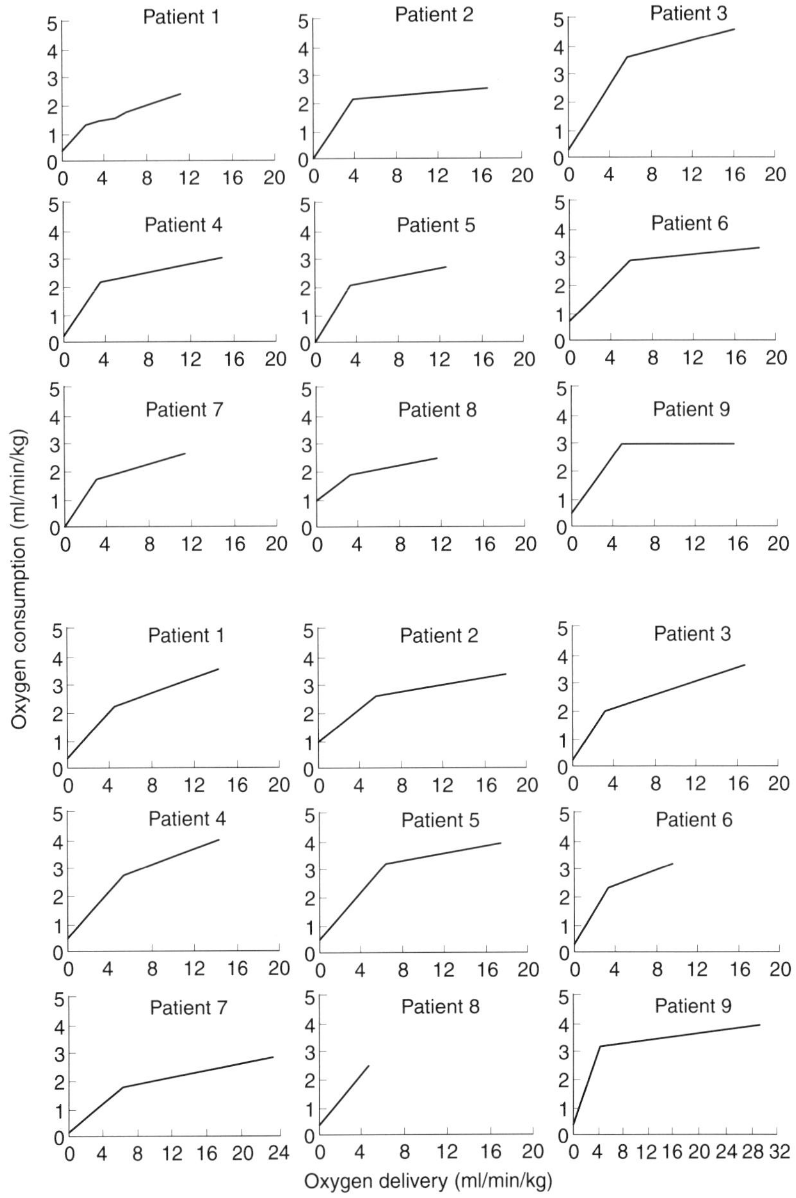

Figure 1.2.2. The D_{O_2}/V_{O_2} relationship in individual, critically ill patients. Oxygen delivery was decreased by withdrawal of vasoactive drugs, decreased F_iO_2, and discontinuation of mechanical ventilation. In all but one patient, the D_{O_2}/V_{O_2} relationship was biphasic. The critical D_{O_2} was 4.5 ml/kg/min, and did not differ between patients who had normal and patients who had increased lactate levels. (From Chittock *et al.*, 1996).

and the critical O_2ER was 0.6 higher than expected. Secondly, there were no differences between septic and non-septic patients in critical DO_2 or critical O_2ER values. Thirdly, there were no differences in critical DO_2 and O_2ER between patients who had normal and patients who had increased arterial lactate at the beginning of the protocol (Ronco *et al.*, 1993a). This study therefore suggests that the critical DO_2 and O_2ER of humans are about 5 ml/kg/min and 0.6, respectively.

THE PATHOLOGIC DEPENDENCE OF OXYGEN CONSUMPTION ON OXYGEN DELIVERY IN THE CRITICALLY ILL

The physiologic and the pathologic relationships of DO_2 and VO_2 are shown in Figure 1.2.1. The pathologic dependence of VO_2 on DO_2 is characterized by three differences from the physiologic relationship. First, VO_2 is dependent on DO_2 over a much wider range of DO_2 and at much higher values of DO_2. Thus, the critical DO_2 is higher in pathologic dependence of VO_2 on DO_2. Secondly, the critical O_2ER is lower in pathologic dependence of VO_2 on DO_2. This suggests that there is a decreased ability of the tissues to increase the extraction of oxygen as DO_2 is decreased. The third difference between these relationships is that the plateau phase of VO_2 is higher in the pathologic relationship than in the physiologic relationship, which is consistent with a state of increased oxygen demand.

Animal models of critical illness have shown a pathologic dependence of VO_2 on DO_2 and have identified physiologic mechanisms to explain the finding (Nelson *et al.*, 1987, 1988). Endotoxaemic and bacteraemic dogs have higher critical DO_2 and lower critical O_2ER values than do normal anaesthetized dogs. Failure to increase O_2 extraction as DO_2 decreases could be explained by a failure to redistribute blood flow and thus O_2 delivery between organs and within organs (Walley, 1996). Failure to redistribute the blood flow between and within organs could be caused by impaired vascular regulation, because the normal redistribution of blood flow requires intact vascular control by such mechanisms as the adrenergic nervous system. Furthermore, failure to redistribute the blood flow could be explained by microvascular obstruction by activated leukocytes and other cells.

However, what is the evidence for the pathologic dependence of VO_2 on DO_2 in clinical studies?

PATHOLOGIC DEPENDENCE OF OXYGEN CONSUMPTION ON OXYGEN DELIVERY: CLINICAL STUDIES

The clinical studies that showed the pathologic dependence of V_{O_2} on D_{O_2} were led by the pivotal study by Danek *et al.* (1980). They showed that V_{O_2} was dependent on D_{O_2} in patients who had acute respiratory distress syndrome (ARDS) but not in a control group of critically ill, mechanically ventilated patients who did not have ARDS. Their study design and methodology was similar to those used in many subsequent studies, and so will be reviewed here to illustrate the clinical studies that found a pathologic dependence of V_{O_2} on D_{O_2}.

Danek *et al.* (1980) made baseline determinations of V_{O_2} and D_{O_2} and then increased the peak end-expiratory pressure (PEEP) and re-measured V_{O_2} and D_{O_2} on PEEP. PEEP decreased cardiac output and D_{O_2}; V_{O_2} decreased in patients who had ARDS but not in the control group. Therefore, Danek *et al.* concluded that V_{O_2} was dependent on D_{O_2} in ARDS. They further described the phenomenon of the pathologic dependence of V_{O_2} on D_{O_2}, because V_{O_2} was found to be dependent on D_{O_2} at high levels of D_{O_2} (levels well above the normal critical D_{O_2} described in animal studies).

Subsequently, there was a flourish of very similar clinical studies which asked the question: 'Is V_{O_2} pathologically dependent on D_{O_2} in critical illness?' (Mohsenifar *et al.*, 1983; Kaufman *et al.*, 1984; Astiz *et al.*, 1987; Bihari *et al.*, 1987; Fenwick *et al.*, 1990; Vincent *et al.*, 1990). In these studies, D_{O_2} was altered by PEEP (Powers *et al.*, 1973), infusion of volume (Kaufman *et al.*, 1984; Astiz *et al.*, 1987), prostacyclin (a vasodilator) (Bihari *et al.*, 1987), blood transfusion (to increase the haemoglobin concentration and thus the D_{O_2}) (Fenwick *et al.*, 1990), and dobutamine (an inotrope that increases cardiac output and D_{O_2}) (Vincent *et al.*, 1990). In all these studies, which used widely varied techniques to change the D_{O_2}, the results obtained and conclusions drawn were remarkably similar: V_{O_2} was pathologically dependent on D_{O_2} in the majority of studies (Table 1.2.1).

It is now appropriate to review the methodology used in these studies, because there are several methodological problems that must be addressed as potential confounders in the interpretation of these studies (Russell, 1993; Russell and Phang, 1994). First, the O_2 demand of critically ill patients can vary considerably. As a result, increased oxygen demand can cause a secondary increase in D_{O_2} such as during exercise (Weissman *et al.*, 1986; Weissman and Kemper, 1991; Boyd *et al.*, 1992; Manthous *et al.*, 1995a, b). Several studies have clearly shown that the O_2 demand of critically ill patients varies with changes during routine ICU intervenions (Weissman *et al.*, 1986; Weissman and

Table 1.2.1 Representative studies of critically ill patients which used calculated oxygen consumption showing pathologic dependence of oxygen consumption on oxygen delivery

Study	No. of patients	D_{O_2} manipulation	Controls
Powers *et al.* (1973)	33	PEEP	None
Danek *et al.* (1980)	29	PEEP	Non-ARDS
Mohsenifar *et al.* (1983)	12	Random	None
Kaufman *et al.* (1984)	21	Random	CHF
Bihari *et al.* (1987)	27	Prostacyclin	Survivor vs non-survivors
Astiz *et al.* (1987)	10	Fluid	Septic shock
Fenwick *et al.* (1990)	32	Blood transfusion	Normal lactate vs high lactate
Vincent *et al.* (1990)	73	Dobutamine	Normal lactate vs high lactate
Total	237		

ARDS, acute respiratory distress syndrome; CHF, coronary heart failure; PEEP, positive end-expiratory pressure.

Kemper, 1991), with sedation (Boyd *et al.*, 1992), with changes in mechanical ventilation (Manthous *et al.*, 1995a) and by cooling of febrile patients (Manthous *et al.*, 1995b). During exercise, oxygen demand increases, oxygen consumption increases and oxygen delivery increases as a result of the increased O_2 demand. When the D_{O_2}/V_{O_2} relationship is examined, there is a linear relationship between D_{O_2} and V_{O_2} which can be misinterpreted as pathologic dependence of V_{O_2} on D_{O_2}. Some of the studies of V_{O_2} and D_{O_2} that showed pathologic dependence of these variables collected data over extended periods or care was not taken to control oxygen demand. Thus, the positive slope of a plot of V_{O_2} versus D_{O_2} may indicate an increase in D_{O_2} in response to an increase in oxygen demand rather than to a pathologic dependence of V_{O_2} on D_{O_2}.

The second problem in many of these studies that potentially confounds the interpretation of the results is the problem of mathematical coupling of shared measurement error. In many clinical studies of V_{O_2} and D_{O_2}, V_{O_2} and D_{O_2} were calculated from a common set of variables:

$$D_{O_2} = (Q \times Hg \times 1.34 \times S_aO_2) + (Q \times P_aO_2)$$

$$V_{O_2} = [Q \times Hg \times 1.34 \times (S_aO_2 - S_vO_2)] + [Q \times (P_aO_2 - P_vO_2)]$$

where Q is the cardiac output; S_aO_2 and S_vO_2 are the arterial and mixed venous oxygen saturations, respectively; Hg is the haemoglobin concentration; 1.34 is the binding constant of O_2 to haemoglobin; and P_aO_2 and P_vO_2 are the arterial and mixed venous oxygen tensions, respectively. Cardiac output is most commonly measured by the thermodilution method and Hg, S_aO_2, S_vO_2, and P_aO_2 and P_vO_2 are measured using commonly available blood gas analysers and oximeters. It is evident that the two equations share the following variables: Q, Hg, S_aO_2 and P_aO_2. Therefore, errors in the measurement of any one of these variables would cause errors in the calculation of DO_2 and VO_2. As a result, there is an artifactual relationship between DO_2 and VO_2 which is explained by the mathematical coupling of shared measurement error rather than by the presence or absence of a pathologic dependence of VO_2 on DO_2. Because the concept and the problem of mathematical coupling of shared measurement error is so important, it will now be reviewed separately.

MATHEMATICAL COUPLING OF SHARED MEASUREMENT ERROR IN STUDIES OF OXYGEN DELIVERY AND CONSUMPTION

Random error in the measurement of shared variables is a generic problem in research that was particularly important in the clinical studies of DO_2 and VO_2. A simple illustration is useful to explain the concepts underpinning the mathematical coupling of shared measurement error. Assume that one does a clinical study of DO_2 and VO_2 by making measurements of Q, S_aO_2, S_vO_2, Hg, P_aO_2, and P_vO_2, and then calculates DO_2 and VO_2. Let us also assume that all the measurements are exactly true values of each variable. The calculated DO_2 and VO_2 would then be the true DO_2 and VO_2, as shown in Figure 1.2.3. If one then makes a second set of measurements with no change in the patient's condition but there is an error, e.g. a 5% underestimation of the true cardiac output, then the calculated DO_2 and VO_2 would both be underestimated as shown by the lowest DO_2/VO_2 point in Figure 1.2.3. The 5% error in the measurement of the cardiac output is well within the coefficient of variation of cardiac output measurement, which has been reported as 3–15%. Then, if a third set of measurements is made, this time with a 5% overestimation of the true cardiac output, then the DO_2 and VO_2 will be overestimated as shown by the highest point in Figure 1.2.3. As a result, when one then analyses the DO_2/VO_2 relationship, it is found to be linear with a positive slope, which appears to show a dependence of VO_2 on DO_2. However, the linear relationship between DO_2 and VO_2 is in fact caused by the mathematical coupling of shared measurement error rather than any physiologic or pathologic relationship.

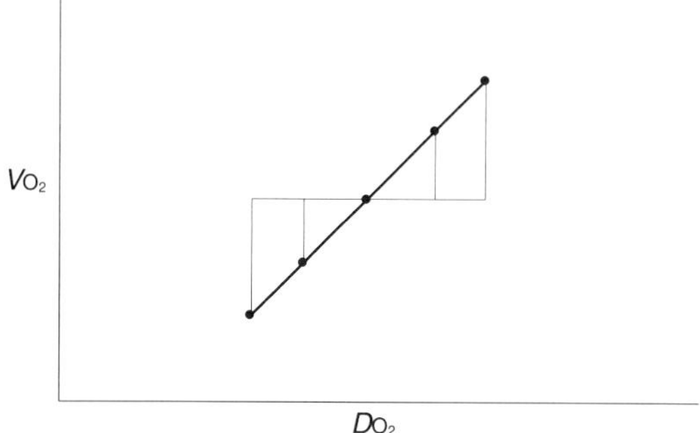

Figure 1.2.3. A simple illustration of the effects of the error in the measurement of a shared variable (e.g. cardiac output) on the relationship between DO_2 and VO_2. The central point reflects the true DO_2 and VO_2. The other points are obtained when there are overestimates or underestimates of the true values. See text for details.

Thus, clinical studies that use shared variables to calculate DO_2 and VO_2 could find a linear relationship between DO_2 and VO_2 because of mathematical coupling of shared measurement error.

If several thousand measurements of the component variables are made and the resulting DO_2 and VO_2 points plotted, then a positive slope would be obtained. This positive slope is called the *slope of measurement errors*. Thus, in this illustration, it can be seen that there is a point of truth surrounded by a cloud of uncertainty, i.e. the calculated DO_2 and VO_2 points that arise from the errors in the measurement of the shared variables. I will now briefly present some additional concepts that have been developed by statisticians to 'correct' for the effects of shared measurement error in order to make a better estimate of the true DO_2 and VO_2.

The elegant and fundamental work of Stratton *et al.* (1987) will be presented because they used mathematical principles to correct for the effects of the mathematical coupling of shared measurement error using data from clinical studies. This has been reviewed in more detail previously (Russell and Phang, 1994).

Several new key terms and concepts were developed by Stratton *et al.* First, they noted that if the VO_2 and DO_2 data from a clinical study were plotted to define a linear regression, then an *observed slope* can be calculated. The observed slope is a mathematical combination of the *true slope* and the slope of measurement errors. The true slope can never be measured because of the errors in the measurements of the component variables.

Because most clinicians are not familiar with these concepts and terms, it is useful to briefly summarize them here. The clinical DO_2 and

V_{O_2} data are plotted as an observed slope. The errors in the measurements of the shared variables define a positive slope, which is the slope of measurement errors. There is a true slope which cannot be determined because of the errors in the component measurements. The observed slope is therefore a combination of the true slope and the slope of the measurement errors.

To evaluate and solve the problem of mathematical coupling of shared measurement error, Stratton *et al.* (1987) used two methods: a mathematical simulation and a re-analysis of two previously published clinical studies of D_{O_2} and V_{O_2} (Powers *et al.*, 1973; Danek *et al.*, 1980). In the mathematical simulation, they simulated the usual experimental conditions and typical measurement errors for all shared variables in order to calculate the observed slope, the slope of measurement errors and the mathematically corrected 'true' slope. Their simulation showed that when the true slope was zero (i.e. no dependence of V_{O_2} on D_{O_2}), mathematical coupling of the shared measurement error could increase the risk of finding a false positive slope by up to five times. They also found that their proposed mathematical solution was very effective in correcting for the effect of mathematical coupling of shared measurement error.

The second method used by Stratton *et al.* involved using their mathematical solution to adjust for the mathematical coupling of shared measurement error in the real experimental data of two published studies (Powers *et al.*, 1973; Danek *et al.*, 1980). They found that the slopes of the measurement errors were much larger than the observed slopes; thus, mathematical coupling of shared measurement error had falsely increased the observed slope of V_{O_2} versus D_{O_2}. However, when Stratton and colleagues corrected for the effect of mathematical coupling of shared measurement error, the corrected (uncoupled or true) slopes were still statistically significantly greater than zero. Therefore, they concluded that, even after correction for mathematical coupling of the shared measurement error, there was true pathologic dependence of V_{O_2} on D_{O_2} in critical illness.

It is our belief that Stratton *et al.* did not exclude the possibility that the mathematical coupling of shared measurement error explained the dependence of V_{O_2} on D_{O_2}, because they had to use pooled patient data from the clinical studies. Pooling of patient data ignores the relationship between V_{O_2} and D_{O_2} in each individual patient. Thus, individual patients could show no relationship or even a negative relationship, but the pooled data could show a positive relationship. This effect of pooling patient data is shown in Figure 1.2.4; clearly, large errors can occur in any study when data are pooled.

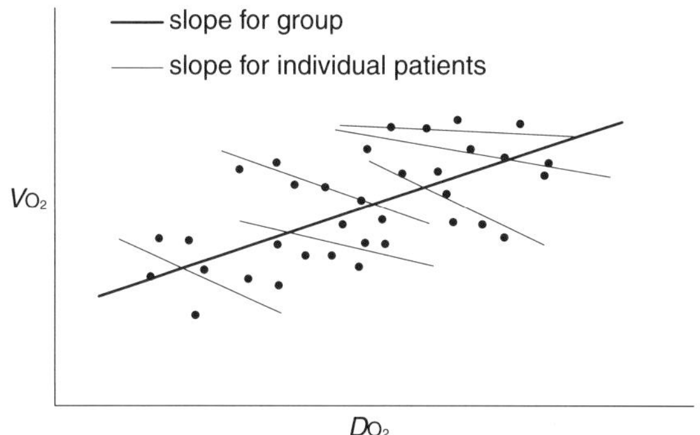

Figure 1.2.4. The effects of pooling of patient data. The relationship of V_{O_2} and D_{O_2} of each individual patient and pooled V_{O_2}/D_{O_2} data. The slope of individual patients are negative while the slope of the pooled data is positive. This shows the large errors that can occur when data are pooled. See text for details.

The reason why Stratton *et al.* pooled the patient data was that they had to in order to apply their mathematical solution, which requires at least three data points per patient (the published studies contained only two data points per patient).

To briefly summarize, the mathematical coupling of shared measurement error falsely increases the slope of V_{O_2} versus D_{O_2}, which can therefore give the appearance of a pathologic dependence of V_{O_2} on D_{O_2}. Stratton *et al.* showed that mathematical coupling did not fully explain the positive V_{O_2}/D_{O_2} relationship in two published studies, but they had to use pooled data, which itself introduces different errors into the analysis. Fortunately, Stratton *et al.* also suggested that the problem of mathematical coupling of shared measurement error could be avoided completely by determining V_{O_2} and D_{O_2} by independent methods that do not share variables in their determination.

STUDIES OF OXYGEN DELIVERY (D_{O_2}) AND OXYGEN CONSUMPTION (V_{O_2}) THAT USED INDEPENDENT METHODS TO DETERMINE D_{O_2} AND V_{O_2}

The mathematical coupling of shared measurement error can be avoided in studies of the relationship of V_{O_2} and D_{O_2} by determining the values by using mathematically independent techniques. In recent years, an increasing number of investigators have designed and successfully completed elegant studies of V_{O_2} and D_{O_2} in which the parameters were determined independently. More specifically, V_{O_2} has been measured by analysis of respiratory gases, and D_{O_2} has been calculated using thermodilution cardiac output and arterial oxygen content. In the analysis of respiratory gases using indirect calorimetry (Deltatrac Metabolic Cart) V_{O_2} is determined by measuring the difference between inspired and expired gas concentrations and by measuring the minute ventilation. More specifically, the inspired and expired concentrations of oxygen (F_iO_2 and F_EO_2) and carbon dioxide (F_iCO_2 and F_ECO_2) and the expired minute ventilation (V_E) are measured. Oxygen consumption is then calculated according to the following equation:

$$V_{O_2} = \frac{(1 - F_EO_2 - F_ECO_2)}{1 - F_iO_2} (F_iO_2 - F_EO_2) V_E$$

This technique of determining V_{O_2} is most accurate when the concentration of oxygen is low; the error increases as the F_iO_2 increases. In two validation studies it was found that the coefficient of variation of V_{O_2} measurement increased from 4% at an F_iO_2 of 0.4 to 7% at an F_iO_2 of 0.8 using a metabolic cart to measure gas concentrations in a lung model (Phang *et al.*, 1990; Ronco and Phang, 1991). Furthermore, the coefficient of variation of the V_{O_2} measurements in published studies of stable critically ill patients is approximately 5% (Russell *et al.*, 1990; Vermeij *et al.*, 1990, 1991; Ronco *et al.*, 1991, 1993a; Marik and Sibbald, 1993; Hanique *et al.*, 1994). Furthermore, patients who have an F_iO_2 of 0.8 or more were not included in any of our own studies.

In general, studies of D_{O_2}/V_{O_2} in which D_{O_2} and V_{O_2} are determined independently show that V_{O_2} is not pathologically dependent upon D_{O_2} when V_{O_2} is determined by independent techniques such as analysis of respiratory gases (Table 1.2.2). I will now describe a study by Ronco *et al.* (1991) in more detail to illustrate these points. Ronco *et al.* studied the relationship between D_{O_2} and V_{O_2} by increasing D_{O_2} using blood transfusion in a group of patients who had severe ARDS. The calculated V_{O_2} increased significantly when D_{O_2} was increased significantly following blood transfusion. In contrast, the simultaneously determined V_{O_2} using the metabolic cart did not change, despite a significant increase in D_{O_2}. If only V_{O_2} and D_{O_2} had been calculated, it would have been concluded that V_{O_2} is pathologically dependent on D_{O_2} in severe ARDS. However, it was in fact concluded that V_{O_2} was not dependent on D_{O_2} in severe ARDS, because there was concern about the problem of the mathematical coupling of shared

Table 1.2.2 Representative studies of critically ill patients in which oxygen consumption was measured: no pathologic dependence of oxygen consumption on oxygen delivery was shown

Study	No. of patients	Means of D_{O_2} manipulation	Controls
Lutch and Murray (1972)	19	PEEP	Normal, COPD, ALI
Annat *et al.* (1986)	8	PEEP + fluid	ARDS
Carlile and Gray (1989)	9	PEEP	ALI
Vermeij *et al.* (1990)	20	–	Abdominal surgery/ sepsis
Ronco *et al.* (1991)	14	RBCT	ARDS: normal lactate vs high lactate
Ronco *et al.* (1993b)	14	Dobutamine	Sepsis: normal lactate vs high lactate
Ronco *et al.* (1993a)	19	Life support discontinued	Dying patients: septic and non-septic
Manthous *et al.* (1993)	10	Dobutamine	Septic shock
Marik and Sibbald (1993)	23	RBCT	Sepsis
Phang *et al.* (1994)	17	Dobutamine	ARDS
Mira *et al.* (1994)	17	MAST + dobutamine	Sepsis: normal lactate vs high lactate
Total	170		

ALI, acute lung injury; ARDS, acute respiratory distress syndrome; COPD, chronic obstructive pulmonary disease; MAST, military anti-shock trousers; PEEP, positive end-expiratory pressure; RBCT, red blood cell transfusion.

measurement error and because the metabolic-cart-determined V_{O_2} did not change.

Some workers (e.g. Bredle and Reinhart, 1994) have questioned whether blood transfusion is a technique that increases D_{O_2} but does not adequately allow determination of whether V_{O_2} is pathologically dependent on D_{O_2} (Ronco *et al.*, 1993b; Phang *et al.*, 1994). Therefore, we have also used dobutamine to increase D_{O_2} in order to examine the relationship between V_{O_2} and D_{O_2}. In these studies we also found that the calculated V_{O_2} was dependent on D_{O_2}, but the independently determined V_{O_2} was not pathologically dependent on D_{O_2} (Ronco *et al.*, 1993b; Phang *et al.*, 1994). Patients who had increased concentration of plasma lactate at baseline showed no pathologic dependence of V_{O_2} on D_{O_2} in these studies.

To briefly summarize then, a growing number of studies of at least 170 patients have shown that V_{O_2} is not pathologically dependent on D_{O_2} when V_{O_2} and D_{O_2} are determined by mathematically independent techniques (Table 1.2.2).

We extended these studies by designing a study to focus on the potential importance of mathematical coupling of shared measurement error by applying the techniques of Stratton *et al.* (1987) to the mathematically coupled V_{O_2} and D_{O_2} data in patients with ARDS (Phang *et al.*, 1994). The study was designed so that the techniques of Stratton *et al.* could be applied both to individual patients (which Stratton *et al.* could not do) and to the pooled patient data (as Stratton *et al.* had already done). Following baseline determinations of D_{O_2}, calculated V_{O_2} and independently measured V_{O_2} using the metabolic cart, dobutamine was infused in increasing doses of 5, 10, and 15 µg/kg/min. At each dose of dobutamine the D_{O_2}, calculated V_{O_2}, and metabolic-cart-measured V_{O_2} were determined simultaneously. Thus, the study was designed so that we had three or four D_{O_2} versus V_{O_2} data points per patient over the full range of D_{O_2}.

As in previous studies, we found that the calculated V_{O_2} was dependent on the calculated D_{O_2}; however, the metabolic-cart-determined V_{O_2} was not dependent on D_{O_2} (Phang *et al.*, 1994). Using the technique of Stratton *et al.* we found that when the data on all patients was pooled, the calculated V_{O_2} versus D_{O_2} slope was 0.11 (statistically significant, $p < 0.001$). Secondly, we found that the slope of the measurement errors was positive and was greater than the observed slope. Because of this, the calculated V_{O_2} versus D_{O_2} slope was always significantly greater than the estimated true V_{O_2} versus D_{O_2} slope (observed slope 0.11, estimated true slope 0.06). Finally, the major result of the study was that the estimated true V_{O_2} versus D_{O_2} slope of *individual patients* was zero in all patients. Thus, the important and unique new finding of this study was that the mathematical coupling of shared measurement error could explain the dependence of the calculated V_{O_2} on D_{O_2} in individual patients.

A brief review of the studies of patients with ARDS and patients with sepsis in which oxygen delivery and oxygen consumption have been determined by mathematically independent techniques shows that V_{O_2} was not found to be dependent on D_{O_2} in the vast majority of these studies (Tables 1.2.1 and 1.2.2). Furthermore, in studies in which V_{O_2} was determined by both the Fick and the respiratory gas analysis techniques, pathologic dependence of V_{O_2} on D_{O_2} was associated with the Fick-determined V_{O_2} but not with respiratory-gas-determined V_{O_2}.

In summary, it is clear that the relationship between V_{O_2} and D_{O_2} should be studied by using mathematically independent techniques, as suggested by Stratton *et al.* (1987). The vast majority of studies that used this design, showed that V_{O_2} is not pathologically dependent on D_{O_2}.

One important criticism of this argument suggesting that mathematical coupling of shared measurement error explains the finding of a pathologic dependence of V_{O_2} on D_{O_2} is that the calculated V_{O_2} is found to be dependent on D_{O_2} in some subgroups of patients but not others. For example, several studies have shown that the calculated V_{O_2} is dependent on D_{O_2} in patients who had increased plasma lactate, but not in patients who had normal lactate levels. One interpretation of these results is that the risk of mathematical coupling of shared measurement errors is greater in subgroups of patients who have increased lactate, but this explanation has not been proven. An alternative interpretation is that patients who had increased lactate had true shock and, therefore, had physiologic dependence of V_{O_2} on D_{O_2}. A third explanation is that dependence of V_{O_2} on D_{O_2} could exist under specific conditions. This is one of the arguments against the proposal that the mathematical coupling of shared measurement errors is the sole explanation for a finding of a pathologic dependence of calculated V_{O_2} on calculated D_{O_2}.

It is relevant to note that errors arise in the measurement of V_{O_2} by the metabolic cart method. Furthermore, metabolic carts differ in their performance characteristics. In addition, clinical studies have been done using a variety of metabolic carts that have not been calibrated or validated. For these reasons we have focused on the validation of the measurement of V_{O_2} by the metabolic cart technique (Phang *et al.*, 1990; Ronco and Phang, 1991).

It is also important to note that the determination of V_{O_2} by the metabolic cart determines whole-body V_{O_2}. In contrast, the Fick-derived V_{O_2} excludes the lung V_{O_2}, because in this indirect technique the difference in arterial oxygen content and the mixed venous oxygen content is used to calculate V_{O_2}.

This exclusion of the lung V_{O_2} from the indirect Fick calculation is probably trivial in patients who have normal lungs, because lung V_{O_2} is normally very small. In contrast, critically ill patients may have an increased lung V_{O_2}, which would not be detected by the indirect Fick technique, and thus the assessment of the D_{O_2} versus V_{O_2} relationship may be affected. This suggestion is based on the elegant studies of Light (1988), who found that lung V_{O_2} is substantially increased in an animal model of pneumococcal pneumonia. He speculated that increased leukocyte numbers and leukocyte activity in the lung in pneumonia accounted for the significantly increased lung V_{O_2}. Therefore, it is plausible, but not yet proven, that humans who have pneumonia, ARDS, aspiration of gastric contents and other acute lung disease could have increased lung V_{O_2}. If this is true, then one would expect, and indeed one finds, higher global V_{O_2} values when using the metabolic cart method than when using the indirect Fick calculation (Hanique *et al.*, 1994).

ANALYSIS OF RANDOMIZED CONTROLLED TRIALS OF SUPRANORMAL OXYGEN DELIVERY IN THE CRITICALLY ILL

Several observations have led to the hypothesis that supranormal oxygen delivery decreases the mortality of critically ill patients. The first relevant observation is that survivors of critical illness have a higher cardiac index (>1.5 l/m/m^2), higher oxygen delivery ($D_{O_2} > 600$ ml/min/m^2) and higher oxygen consumption ($V_{O_2} > 170$ ml/min/m^2) than do non-survivors of critical illness (Shoemaker *et al.*, 1988b; Russell *et al.*, 1990). Secondly, the clinical studies described above that found a pathologic dependence of V_{O_2} on D_{O_2} suggested that the critical oxygen delivery in critically ill patients is higher than in normals. Thirdly, animal models of critical illness, such as bacteraemia and endotoxaemia, have also suggested that the critical oxygen delivery is increased in sepsis, a common admission diagnosis and complication of critical illness. These observations lead naturally to the hypothesis that increasing oxygen delivery to high levels (supranormal oxygen delivery) might improve multiple system organ failure and decrease the mortality of critically ill patients.

I use the term 'supranormal oxygen delivery' to define oxygen delivery applied to groups of patients in randomized controlled trials (RCTs) who are randomized to therapy to increase oxygen delivery to levels associated with survival of critical illness. It is relevant at this time to contrast the critical oxygen delivery defined in one study that identified the critical oxygen delivery of individual humans with the target oxygen delivery identified in randomized controlled trials of supranormal oxygen delivery. In this study the critical oxygen delivery of critically ill individual patients was 4.5 ml/min/kg (Ronco *et al.*, 1993a). In contrast, the target D_{O_2} in most of the RCTs of supranormal oxygen delivery was about 14 ml/min/kg, and thus the target oxygen delivery in these trials was much higher than the critical oxygen delivery identified in individual critically ill patients.

To date, there have been at least nine RCTs of supranormal oxygen delivery compared with usual oxygen delivery in a total of 852 critically ill patients (Table 1.2.3). The results of these trials are controversial because some trials found a decreased mortality in the supranormal oxygen delivery group (Shoemaker *et al.*, 1988a, b; Guiterrez *et al.*, 1992; Boyd *et al.*, 1993), some trials found no difference

Table 1.2.3 Randomized controlled trials of supranormal versus normal oxygen delivery in critically ill patients

| Study | Patient type | No. of patients | Mortality (%) | | p |
			Controls	Intervention	
Shoemaker *et al.* (1988a)	Surgical	88	28	4	<0.05
Boyd *et al.* (1993)	Surgical	107	22	6	<0.05
Tuchschmidt *et al.* (1992)	Septic shock	51	72	50	NS
Bone *et al.* (1989)	ARDS	100	48	60	NS
Fleming *et al.* (1992)	Trauma	67	44	24	NS
Yu *et al.* (1993)	Critical	67	34	34	NS
Gutierrez *et al.* (1992)	Critical, pH_i normal	141	53	28	<0.05
Gutierrez *et al.* (1992)	Critical, pH_i low	119	37	36	NS
Hayes *et al.* (1994)	Critical	109	34	54	<0.05
Gattinoni *et al.* (1995)	Critical	503	48.4	48.6	NS
Total		852			

ARDS, acute respiratory distress syndrome; NS, not significant.

in mortality (Bone *et al.*, 1989; Fleming *et al.*, 1992; Tuchschmidt *et al.*, 1992; Yu *et al.*, 1993; Gattinoni *et al.*, 1995) and one trial showed an increased mortality in the supranormal oxygen delivery group compared to the normal oxygen delivery group (Hayes *et al.*, 1994).

We have previously reviewed some of the methodological difficulties in the design, implementation, and analysis of these RCTs (Russell, 1993). For example, some of these RCTs do not give a clear definition of the clinical protocols and algorithms used to increase the oxygen delivery, some have deficiencies in the blinding of the randomization and of care-givers to ongoing results of the trial, some included prestudy sample size estimates, several negative RCTs lacked power testing, and some do not use a time-to-death life table analysis. Chalmers *et al.* (1981) have identified these important deficiencies in the quality of clinical trials, and identified a quantitative scoring instrument to make comparisons between trials. We have previously reported a wide range in the quantitative score of the quality of trials of supranormal oxygen delivery (Russell, 1993). The wide range of quality of these RCTs influences the interpretation of the results, because one may have less confidence in the results of RCTs that have a lower quality score.

I would like to propose that one additional technique for resolving the conflicting results of the RCTs of supranormal oxygen delivery is to use a physiologic rationale to understand the studies. Several of the studies were designed in a 'prophylactic' sense, by which I mean that the institution of supranormal oxygen delivery occurred prior to the development of tissue hypoxia. For example, studies of high-risk surgical patients (Shoemaker *et al.*, 1988a, b; Boyd *et al.*, 1993) and critically ill patients who had not yet shown tissue hypoxia, as reflected by low gastric mucosal pH (Gutierrez *et al.*, 1992), showed that supranormal oxygen delivery decreased mortality compared with the mortality in control groups. Therefore, these studies are consistent with the notion that supranormal oxygen delivery could be effective in preventing tissue hypoxia.

I would also like to suggest that many of the RCTs of supranormal oxygen delivery were designed to reverse tissue hypoxia and then prevent subsequent episodes of tissue hypoxia. For example, studies of general critically ill patients (Gattinoni *et al.*, 1995), patients with ARDS (Bone *et al.*, 1989), patients with septic shock (Tuchschmidt *et al.*, 1992) and a subgroup of patients with low gastric mucosal pH on admission to the ICU (Gutierrez *et al.*, 1992) showed the difference in mortality between the supranormal oxygen delivery group and the control group. One other study of patients who were general ICU patients found that patients in the supranormal oxygen delivery group had a higher mortality (54%) than patients in the control group (34%, $p < 0.05$) (Hayes *et al.*, 1994). Thus these studies are consistent with the notion that supranormal oxygen delivery is not effective in patients already suffering tissue hypoxia, and so is not effective in reversing tissue hypoxia. It is important to note that in the study by Hayes *et al.* (1994) increased mortality was associated with use of extremely large doses of catecholamines such as dobutamine, these being necessary to achieve the supranormal oxygen delivery targets. We consider this study especially important because it is the first one that evaluated patients who had not yet achieved supranormal oxygen delivery using volume expansion alone.

Therefore, one means of explaining the different results of the RCTs of supranormal oxygen delivery is that there could be different effects of supranormal oxygen delivery in different groups of patients. One hypothesis is that supranormal oxygen delivery could be effective in preventing, but not in reversing, tissue hypoxia. Another hypothesis is that supranormal oxygen delivery could be effective in high-risk surgical patients when applied pre-, intra- and postoperatively, but is not effective in general ICU patients.

A third approach to the attempt to resolve the controversial results of these RCTs is to undertake a meta-analysis. We have made a preliminary report of a meta-analysis of the RCTs of supranormal oxygen delivery in critical illness (Chittock *et al.*, 1996) in which we evaluated subgroups of trials that included the high-risk surgical patients separately from general ICU patients. We found that supranormal oxygen delivery was effective in reducing mortality in trials that included high-risk surgical patients (Shoemaker *et al.*, 1988a, b; Boyd *et al.*, 1993) and patients who had normal gastric mucosal pH on ICU admission (Gutierrez *et al.*, 1992). In contrast, the meta-analysis showed that there was no effect on mortality in trials that used the reversal of tissue hypoxia strategy (Bone *et al.*, 1989; Fleming *et al.*, 1992; Gutierrez *et al.*, 1992; Tuchschmidt *et al.*, 1992; Hayes *et al.*, 1994; Gattinoni *et al.*, 1995).

Another recent meta-analysis of the RCTs of supranormal oxygen delivery also suggested that supranormal oxygen delivery does not change the mortality in critically ill patients (Heyland *et al.*, 1996).

A CLINICAL APPROACH TO THE MANAGEMENT OF CLINICAL PERFUSION BY MANAGING OXYGEN DELIVERY AND OXYGEN CONSUMPTION IN CRITICAL ILLNESS

We continue to suggest that careful clinical assessment of the adequacy of oxygen delivery is fundamental to the management of perfusion in the critically ill. Clinicians must examine patients carefully to ensure normal mentation, warm skin with a normal capillary refill time, absence of extreme hypotension or tachycardia, presence of adequate urinary output, absence of peripheral cyanosis and presence of adequate arterial saturation using pulse oximetry assessment. We suggest that if clinical assessment indicates inadequate perfusion then oxygen delivery should be increased (by at least 25%) and clinical assessment repeated after this acute increase in oxygen delivery. To control for independent changes in oxygen demand, other treatment that could change oxygen delivery or oxygen demand should be maintained constant.

The direct measurement of V_{O_2} using a metabolic cart is not necessary for clinical management. Plasma lactate levels may be useful, but must be interpreted cautiously using a differential diagnosis approach because in the critically ill there can be hypoxic and non-hypoxic mechanisms of lactic acidosis. Gastric tonometry is suggested as a new, relatively non-invasive technology for assessing gastrointestinal perfusion. The measurement of intramucosal pH by tonometry is based on the principle that fluid in the stomach can be used to assess the carbon dioxide tension of the surrounding gastric tissues. Although one clinical trial has suggested an improved outcome in patients managed using gastric tonometry (Gutierrez *et al.*, 1992), we suggest that several methodological aspects need further evaluation before the technique is used routinely for clinical purposes (Russell, in press).

Oxygen consumption is the product of oxygen delivery and the oxygen extraction ratio ($V_{O_2} = D_{O_2} \times O_2ER$). As a result, V_{O_2}, D_{O_2}, and the O_2ER can be modified to prevent or reverse tissue hypoxia. To reiterate, tissue hypoxia may be prevented by balancing oxygen supply and oxygen demands.

Oxygen delivery may be increased by increasing cardiac output, haemoglobin and/or arterial oxygen saturation. Cardiac output may be increased using volume infusion, using inotropic agents (such as dobutamine, dopamine or dopexamine) or by using vasodilators (PGE_1 or PGI_2) in patients who are not profoundly hypotensive. Although there is some suggestion that vasodilators improve the abnormal critical oxygen extraction ratio found in animal models of sepsis, it is not clear whether such agents improve tissue oxygen extraction capability in critically ill humans.

The haemogloblin concentration may be increased by rapid red blood cell transfusion. In several of our studies, oxygen delivery could be increased by approximately 25–50% after RBC transfusion (Fenwick *et al.*, 1990; Russell *et al.*, 1990; Ronco *et al.*, 1991). However, there is evidence to suggest that red blood cell transfusion could paradoxically worsen tissue hypoxia in the critically ill. For example, red blood cell transfusion did not increase measured oxygen consumption in critically ill patients despite an important increase in oxygen delivery (Ronco *et al.*, 1991; Marik and Sibbald, 1993). Furthermore, red blood cell transfusion increased global oxygen delivery but did not increase the measured oxygen consumption, even in patients who had increased concentrations of plasma lactate (Ronco *et al.*, 1991; Marik and Sibbald, 1993). Also, studies in patients with sepsis indicated that red blood cell transfusion worsens gastric mucosal pH_i, as assessed by gastric tonometry (Silverman and Tuma, 1992; Marik and Sibbald, 1993). In addition, retrospective studies have shown an association between red blood cell transfusion and organ system failure after major abdominal surgery (Maetani *et al.*, 1986). Finally, a recent small randomized controlled trial of two different red blood cell transfusion strategies in the critically ill suggested that there was no difference in morbidity or mortality when patients were maintained either at a haemoglobin level of 70–90 g/l or 100–120 g/l. However, this preliminary pilot study did not have the power to be confident in the negative result. A larger multicentre trial of these two different transfusion strategies is currently underway in Canada (Hebert, personal communication).

The third component of oxygen delivery, the arterial oxygen saturation, may be increased (if low) by strategies such as increasing the oxygen fraction, by modifying the PEEP and by increasing the cardiac output if the mixed venous oxygen saturation is low.

The other general strategy for improving tissue oxygenation and clinical perfusion is to decrease the oxygen demand such that it is matched by the oxygen supply. Mechanical ventilation should be considered early in the course of patients with shock due to the increased work of breathing and as a result of the increased oxygen consumption by respiratory muscles in shock, and in acute respiratory failure. Acute respiratory distress increases respiratory muscle blood flow from about 2–3% of the cardiac output to as much as 30–40% of the cardiac output (Viires *et al.*, 1982). As a result, intubation and ventilation decrease the oxygen demand of the respiratory muscles and permit redistribution of perfusion and oxygen delivery to other vital organs (Viires *et al.*, 1982; Mantous *et al.*, 1995a). As already discussed, other measures such as sedation, cooling of the febrile patient and general ICU interventions directly influence oxygen demand.

SUMMARY

We have used the paradigm of the oxygen delivery–consumption relationship model to use a physiologic approach to the management of perfusion in the critically ill. Several of the key concepts that guide assessment and therapy are as follows. Below the critical oxygen delivery, oxygen consumption is physiologically dependent on oxygen delivery and, as a result, patients in shock do indeed have a physiologic dependence of V_{O_2} on D_{O_2}. The first priority in the assessment and management of perfusion is the prevention and reversal of tissue hypoxia by balancing the oxygen demand and supply. We suggest that a pathologic dependence of V_{O_2} on D_{O_2} has not yet been convincingly demonstrated in critically ill patients. Furthermore, we suggest that the contradictory results of the RCTs of supranormal oxygen delivery compared with normal oxygen delivery do not support routine use of supranormal oxygen delivery in the critically ill. Although some studies suggest a benefit of supranormal oxygen delivery in high-risk surgical patients, we suggest that this requires confirmation in further randomized controlled trials. Finally, we continue to suggest that intensivists must make a careful clinical assessment of perfusion by assessing oxygen delivery, oxygen consumption and oxygen demand. Unfortunately, the global assessment of D_{O_2} and V_{O_2} appears inadequate as a tool for detecting occult tissue hypoxia. We believe that careful clinical research focused on regional assessment of perfusion and oxygenation, such as the use of gastric tonometry for measuring gastric mucosal p_{CO_2}, could prove beneficial as a safe, convenient tool for detecting occult tissue hypoxia and occult inadequate perfusion in the critically ill (Russell, in press).

REFERENCES

Annat, G., Viale, J.P., Percival, C., Froment, M., Motin, J. (1986) Oxygen delivery and uptake in the adult respiratory distress syndrome. *Am Rev Respir Dis* **133**: 999–1001.

Astiz, M.E., Rackow, E.C., Falk, J.L., Kaufman, B.S., Weil, M.H. (1987) Oxygen delivery and consumption in patients with hyperdynamic septic shock. *Crit Care Med* **15**: 26–28.

Bihari, D., Smithies, M., Gimson, A., Tinker, J. (1987) The effects of vasodilation with prostacyclin on oxygen delivery and uptake in critically ill patients. *New Engl J Med* **317**: 397–403.

Bone, R.C., Slotman, G., Maunder, R., Silverman, H., Hyers, T.M., Kerstein, M.D., Ursprung, J.J., Prostaglandin E1 Study Group (1989) Randomized double-blind, multicenter study of prostaglandin E1 in patients with the adult respiratory distress syndrome. *Chest* **96**: 114–119.

Boyd, O., Grounds, M., Bennett, E.D. (1992) The dependency of oxygen consumption on oxygen delivery in critically ill postoperative patients is mimicked by variations in sedation. *Chest* **101**: 1619–1624.

Boyd, O., Grounds, R.M., Bennett, E.D. (1993) A randomized clinical trial of the effect of deliberate perioperative increase of oxygen delivery on mortality in high-risk surgical patients. *JAMA* **270**: 2699–2707.

Bredle, D.L., Reinhart, K. (1994) Critical oxygen delivery in patients with sepsis. *JAMA* **271**: 1158–1159 [Letter].

Cain, S.M. (1977) Oxygen delivery and uptake in dogs during anemic and hypoxic hypoxia. *J Appl Physiol* **42**: 228–234.

Carlile, P.V., Gray, B.A. (1989) Effect of opposite changes in cardiac output and arterial p_{O_2} on the relationship between mixed venous p_{O_2} and oxygen transport. *Am Rev Respir Dis* **140**: 891–898.

Chalmers, T.C., Smith, H., Blackburn, B., Silverman, B., Schroeder, B., Reitman, D., Ambroz, A. (1981) A method for assessing the quality of a randomized control trial. *Controlled Clinical Trials* **2**: 31–49.

Chittock, D., Baigorri, F., Russell, J.A. (1996) Randomized controlled trials (RCTs) of increased oxygen delivery (Do_2) in critical illness: a metaanalysis. *Am J Respir Crit Care Med* **153**: A466.

Danek, S.J., Lynch, J.P., Weg, J.G., Dantzker, D.R. (1980) The dependence of oxygen uptake on oxygen delivery in the adult respiratory distress syndrome. *Am Rev Respir Dis* **122**: 387–395.

Fenwick, J.C., Dodek, P.M., Ronco, J.J., Phang, P.T., Wiggs, B.R., Russell, J.A. (1990) Increased concentrations of plasma lactate predict pathologic dependence of oxygen consumption on oxygen delivery in patients with adult respiratory distress syndrome. *J Crit Care* **5**: 81–86.

Fleming, A., Bishop, M., Shoemaker, W., Appel, P., Sufficool, W., Kuvhenguwha, A., Kennedy, F., Wo, C. (1992) Prospective trial of supranormal values as goals of resuscitation in severe trauma. *Arch Surg* **127**: 1175–1181.

Gattinoni, L., Brazzi, L., Pelosi, P., Latini, R., Tognoni, G., Pesenti, A., Fumagalli, R. (1995) A trial of goal-oriented hemodynamic therapy in critically ill patients. *N Engl J Med* **333**: 1025–1032.

Gutierrez, G., Palizas, F., Doglio, G., Wainsztein, N., Gallesio, A., Pacin, J., Dubin, A., Schiavi, E., Jorge, M., Pusajo, J. (1992) Gastric intramucosal pH as a therapeutic index of tissue oxygenation in critically ill patients. *Lancet* **339**: 195–199.

Hanique, G., Dugernier, T., Laterre, P.F., Roeseler, J., Dougnac, A., Reynaert, M.S. (1994) Significance of pathologic oxygen supply dependency in the critically ill: comparison between measured and calculated methods. *Intensive Care Med* **20**: 12–18.

Hayes, M.A., Timmins, A.C., Yau, E.H.S., Palazzo, M., Hinds, C.J., Watson, D. (1994) Elevation of systemic oxygen delivery in the treatment of critically ill patients. *N Engl J Med* **330**: 1717–1722.

Heyland, D., Cook, D., King, D. *et al.* (1996) Maximizing oxygen delivery in critically ill patients: a methodologic appraisal of the evidence. *Crit Care Med* **24**: 517–522.

Kaufman, B.S., Rackow, E.C., Galk, J.L. (1984) The relationship between oxygen delivery and consumption during fluid resuscitation of hypovolemic and septic shock. *Chest* **85**: 336–340.

Komatsu, T., Shibutani, K., Okamoto, K., Kumar, V., Kubal, K., Sanchala, V., Lees, D.E. (1987) Critical level of oxygen delivery after cardiopulmonary bypass. *Crit Care Med* **15**: 194–197.

Light, B. (1988) Intrapulmonary oxygen consumption in experimental pneumococcal pneumonia. *J Appl Physiol* **64**: 2490–2495.

Lutch, J.S., Murray, J.F. (1972) Continuous positive-pressure ventilation: effects on systemic oxygen transport and tissue oxygenation. *Ann Intern Med* **76**: 193–202.

Maetani, S., Nishikawa, T., Hirakawa, A., Tobe, T. (1986) Role of blood transfusion in organ system failure following major abdominal surgery. *Ann Surg* **203**: 275–281.

Manthous, C.A., Shumacker, P.T., Pohlman, A., Schmidt, G.A., Hall, J.B., Samsel, R.W., Wood, L.D.H. (1993) Absence of supply dependence of oxygen consumption in patients with septic shock. *J Crit Care* **8**: 203–211.

Manthous, C.A., Hall, J.B., Kushner, R., Schmidt, G.A., Russo, G., Wood, L.D.H. (1995a) The effect of mechanical ventilation on oxygen consumption in critically ill patients. *Am J Respir Crit Care Med* **151**: 210–214.

Manthous, C.A., Hall, J.B., Olson, D., Sing, M., Chatila, W., Pohlman, A., Kushner, R., Schmidt, G.A., Wood, L.D.H. (1995b) Effect of cooling on oxygen consumption in febrile critically ill patients. *Am J Respir Crit Care Med* **151**: 10–14.

Marik, P.E., Sibbald, W.J. (1993) Effect of stored-blood transfusion on oxygen delivery in patients with sepsis. *JAMA* **269**: 3024–3029.

Mira, J.P., Fabre, J.E., Baigorri, F., Coste, J.. Annat, G., Artigas, A., Nitemberg, G., Dhainaut, J.F. (1994) Lack of oxygen supply dependency in patients with severe sepsis. A study of oxygen delivery increased by military antishock trouser and dobutamine. *Chest* **106**: 1524–1531.

Mohsenifar, Z., Goldbach, P., Tashkin, D.P., Campisi, D.J. (1983) Relationship between oxygen consumption and oxygen delivery in adult respiratory distress syndrome. *Chest* **84**: 267–271.

Nelson, D.P., Beyer, C., Samsel, R.W., Wood, L.D.H., Schumacker, P.T. (1987) Pathological supply dependence of O_2 uptake during bacteremia in dogs. *J Appl Physiol* **63**: 1487–1492.

Nelson, D.P., Samsel, R.W., Wood, L.G.H., Schumacker, P.T. (1988) Pathological supply dependence of systemic and intestinal O_2 uptake during endotoxemia. *J Appl Physiol* **64**: 2410–2419.

Phang, P.T., Rich, T., Ronco, J.J. (1990) A validation and comparison study of two metabolic monitors. *J Parent Enterol Nutr* **14**: 259–261.

Phang, P.T., Cunningham, K.F., Ronco, J.J., Wiggs, B.R., Russell, J.A. (1994) Mathematical coupling explains dependence of oxygen consumption on oxygen delivery in ARDS. *Am J Respir Dis Crit Care Med* **50**: 318–323.

Powers, S.R., Mannal, R., Neclerio, M., English, M., Marr, C., Leather, R., Ueda, H., Williams, G., Custead, W., Dutton, R. (1973) Physiologic consequences of positive end-expiratory pressure (PEEP) ventilation. *Ann Surg* **178**: 265–272.

Ronco, J.J., Phang, P.T. (1991) Validation of an indirect calorimeter to measure oxygen consumption in the ranges seen in critically ill patients. *J Crit Care* **6**: 36–41.

Ronco, J.J., Phang, P.T., Walley, K.R., Wiggs, B., Fenwick, J.C., Russell, J.A. (1991) Oxygen consumption is independent of changes in oxygen delivery in severe adult respiratory distress syndrome. *Am Rev Respir Dis* **143**: 1267–1273.

Ronco, J.J., Fenwick, J.C., Tweeddale, M.G., Wiggs, B.R., Phang, P.T., Cooper, D.J., Cunningham, K.F., Russell, J.A., Walley, K.R. (1993a) Identification of the critical oxygen delivery for anaerobic metabolism in critically ill septic and nonseptic humans. *JAMA* **270**: 1724–1730.

Ronco, J.J., Fenwick, J.C., Wiggs, B.R., Phang, P.T., Russell, J.A., Tweeddale, M.G. (1993b) Oxygen consumption is independent of increases in oxygen delivery by dobutamine in septic patients who have normal or increased plasma lactate. *Am Rev Respir Dis* **147**: 25–31.

Russell, J.A. (1993) Quantitative assessment of randomized controlled trials of increased oxygen delivery in critically ill adults. *Am Rev Respir Dis* **147**: A616.

Russell, J.A. (in press) Gastric tonometry: does it work? *Inten Care Med.*

Russell, J.A., Phang, P.T. (1994) The oxygen delivery consumption controversy. Approaches to management of the critically ill. *Am J Respir Crit Care Med* **149**: 533–537.

Russell, J.A., Ronco, J.J., Lockhat, D., Belzberg, A., Kiess, M., Dodek, P.M. (1990) Oxygen delivery and consumption and ventricular preload are greater in survivors than in nonsurvivors of the adult respiratory distress syndrome. *Am Rev Respir Dis* **141**: 659–665.

Shibutani, K., Komatsu, T., Kubal, K., Sanchala, V., Kumar, V., Bizzarri, D.V. (1983) Critical level of oxygen delivery in anesthetized man. *Crit Care Med* **11**: 640–643.

Shoemaker, W.C., Appel, P.L., Kram, H.B., Waxman, K., Lee, T.S. (1988a) Prospective trial of supranormal value of survivors as therapeutic goals in high-risk surgical patients. *Chest* **94**: 1176–1186.

Shoemaker, W.C., Appel, P.L., Kram, H.B. (1988b) Tissue oxygen debt as a determinant of lethal and nonlethal postoperative organ failure. *Crit Care Med* **16**: 1117–1120.

Silverman, H.J., Tuma, P. (1992) Gastric tonometry in patients with sepsis. Effects of dobutamine infusions and packed red blood cell transfusions. *Chest* **102**: 184–188.

Stratton, H.H., Feustel, P.J., Newell, J.C. (1987) Regression of calculated variables in the presence of shared measurement error. *J Appl Physiol* **62**: 2083–2093.

Tuchschmidt, J., Fried, J., Astiz, M., Rackow, E. (1992) Elevation of cardiac output and oxygen delivery improves outcome in septic shock. *Chest* **102**: 216–220.

Vermeij, C.G., Feenstra, B.W.A., Bruining, H.A. (1990) Oxygen delivery and oxygen uptake in postoperative and septic patients. *Chest* **98**: 415–420.

Vermeij, C.G., Feenstra, B.W.A., Adrichem, W.J., Bruining, H.A. (1991) Independent oxygen uptake and oxygen delivery in septic and postoperative patients. *Chest* **99**: 1438–1443.

Viires, N., Sillye, G., Aubier, M., Rassidakis, A., Roussos, C. (1982) Regional blood flow distribution in dog during induced hypotension and low cardiac output. Spontaneous breathing versus artificial ventilation. *J Clin Invest* **72**: 935–947.

Vincent, J.L., Roman, A., DeBacker, D., Kahn, R.J. (1990) Oxygen uptake/supply dependency. Effects of short-term dobutamine infusion. *Am Rev Respir Dis* **142**: 2–7.

Walley, K.R. (1996) Heterogeneity of oxygen delivery impairs oxygen extraction by peripheral tissues: theory. *J Appl Physiol* **81**: 885–894.

Weissman, C., Kemper, M. (1991) The oxygen uptake-oxygen delivery relationship during ICU interventions. *Chest* **99**: 430–435.

Weissman, C., Kemper, B.A., Elwyn, D.H., Askanazi, J., Hyman, A.I., Kinney, J.M. (1986) The energy expenditure of the mechanically ventilated critically ill patients. *Chest* **89**: 254–259.

Yu, M., Levy, M.M., Smith, P., Takiguchi, S.A., Miyasaki, A., Myers, S.A. (1993) Effect of maximizing oxygen delivery on morbidity and mortality rates in critically ill patients: a prospective, randomized, controlled study. *Crit Care Med* **21**: 830–838.

2

Inhaled Nitric Oxide in ARDS

Richard Straube, Janice L. Zimmerman, R. Phillip Dellinger

INTRODUCTION

The biological relevance of nitric oxide (NO) was first acknowledged in 1987 with its identification as an important endothelium derived relaxing factor (Palmer *et al.*, 1987). This simple gaseous molecule is now known or suspected to play a role in diverse and complex biological systems. Although previously thought of primarily as an environmental pollutant, the American Association for the Advancement of Science voted it the 'Molecule of the Year' for 1992 based on expanding knowledge of its biological role (Culotta and Koshland, 1992). Considerable research is ongoing into homeostatic and pathogenic properties of NO. It has been recognized that NO has potent bronchodilator and pulmonary vasodilator and weak bronchodilator actions. Therefore, administration of NO gas as an inhalational agent has been proposed for treatment of a number of cardiopulmonary diseases.

This review summarizes the pharmacologic properties of inhaled NO, its clinical applications in acute respiratory distress syndrome (ARDS), hypoxic respiratory failure of the neonate, other cardiopulmonary conditions, and delivery systems. Most clinical information results from uncontrolled studies involving small numbers of patients, a variety of delivery systems, and little outcome data. Only recently have well-designed trials been initiated to address the many questions regarding inhaled NO. Early enthusiasm for inhaled NO as a treatment modality has been tempered by the need to define carefully any detrimental as well as beneficial effects of inhaled NO in various disease states.

PHARMACOLOGY OF INHALED NITRIC OXIDE

Furchgott and Zawadski (1980) reported that the acetylcholine-induced relaxation of isolated arteries is dependent on the presence of an intact endothelial cell layer. The factor released from endothelium that caused smooth muscle relaxation was subsequently named endothelium-derived relaxing factor (EDRF). Nitric oxide is now known to produce the biological actions of EDRF.

The dilatory effect of NO is short lived with a half-life of 3–5 seconds. Endogenous NO is released from the endothelium and diffuses to subjacent smooth muscle cells. It has been shown to exert its dilatory effect by activating soluble guanylate cyclase intracellularly by binding to the heme moiety of the enzyme. This in turn causes cyclic guanosine monophosphate (cGMP) to rise, leading to smooth muscle relaxation.

Frostell *et al.* (1991) reported that in awake lambs inhalation of a gas mixture containing 40–80 ppm NO could reverse the acute pulmonary vasoconstriction induced by severe hypoxia. This dose-dependent pulmonary vasodilator effect of inhaled NO has now been demonstrated in a wide variety of states of pulmonary vasoconstriction. Since NO is rapidly inactivated by combination with hemoglobin, the vasodilating effect of inhaled NO is selectively exerted on the pulmonary vasculature. Both systemic arterial pressure and systemic vascular resistance appear to be unaffected clinically at dose ranges currently being utilized in human studies. Nitric oxide has great affinity for hemoglobin. The combination of NO with reduced hemoglobin takes place much faster than the reaction with oxygen, and is indeed the fastest direct action so far measured of an oxygen-carrying pigment with any ligand. The association rate constant with Fe^{2+} hemoglobin to form Fe^{3+} (methemoglobin) is about 300 times greater than for oxygen.

The diffusing capacity for inhaled NO is 4–5 times greater than for carbon monoxide. The anatomical proximity of the airspaces to muscular arterioles allows the diffusion of NO to reach the abluminal surface of those vessels. Because inhaled NO is preferentially delivered to better ventilated lung segments, its vasodilatory effect improves ventilation/perfusion (V_A/Q) matching in the presence of acute lung injury. Isolated perfused rabbit lungs have been used to study the localization of the site of vasodilation of inhaled NO in states of elevated pulmonary vascular resistance. When thromboxane was used to increase pulmonary artery pressures in this perfused model, the highest dose of inhaled NO (80 ppm) decreased mean pulmonary artery pressure by 3.5 mmHg, with equivalent proportional reductions at all segmental vascular resistance.

Inhaling high concentrations of NO have been reported to cause severe pulmonary edema and life-threatening methemoglobinemia. Because early studies were not designed to isolate the effects of NO from the effects of the reaction products of NO and O_2 (NO_x), it is unclear how much of the pulmonary toxic effects seen after NO exposure are the result of NO and how much are the result of NO_2 (see below). There is, however, little evidence of toxicity when the concentration of NO is 40 ppm or less. Animals have breathed inhaled NO in concentrations of 10–40 ppm for 6 days to 6 months with no evidence of toxicity (Oda *et al.*, 1976; Hugod, 1979). The Occupational Safety and Health Administration has published standards that limit 8 hour maximum working exposure levels for NO to 25 ppm.

The metabolites (nitrates and nitrites) of NO are cleared by the kidneys within 5–6 hours and methemoglobin levels rarely rise above 1–2% during administration of 40 ppm or less of inhaled NO. Dupuy *et al.* (1992) studied the introduction of inhaled NO in mechanically ventilated guinea-pigs at a dose of 100 ppm for 1 hour and did not induce substantial methemoglobinemia (concentrations remained less than 2%). Adatia *et al.* (1994) demonstrated transient methemoglobinemia of 9% in 1 of 5 patients after 10 hours of 10 ppm NO treatment. In a study by Date *et al.* (1996) of inhaled NO delivered to 32 patients with severe graft dysfunction after lung transplantation at doses of 20–60 ppm for an average of 84 hours (range 15–217 hours), transient methemoglobin levels of greater than 6% developed in only two patients, with no apparent complications. It is unlikely that clinically significant methemoglobinemia will be induced by inhaled NO concentrations of ≤ 40 ppm.

When NO is exposed to oxygen, nitric dioxide (NO_2) is formed. Nitric dioxide is potentially much more toxic than inhaled NO. Nitric dioxide, a strong oxidizing gas, initiates lipid peroxidation, which may result in cell injury or cell death. Pulmonary edema can be observed during exposure to nitric dioxide in concentrations above 50 ppm (Clutton-Brock, 1967). The magnitude of this reaction increases as the concentration of O_2 rises, as the square of the concentration of NO rises, and with time. Delivery devices should minimize NO and O_2 contact times. Within tissues, NO has a such greater affinity for hemoglobin than for oxygen that auto-oxidation is minimized.

Controversy exists with regard to the possible clinical significance of interactions of NO with reactive oxygen species. Inhaled NO combines with the superoxide anion to produce peroxynitrite, which through spontaneous homolysis forms a hydroxyl radical. Some studies would indicate NO to be protective against cytotoxic effects of reactive oxygen species (Wink *et al.*, 1994), whereas others raise concerns of potential toxicity via this route (Haddad *et al.*, 1994).

The potential ability of exogenous NO to suppress the ability to produce or respond to endogenous NO complicates the evaluation of the presence or absence of tachyphylaxis. In addition, the waxing and waning of the underlying cardiopulmonary disease process further complicates this evaluation. Nevertheless, during long-term inhalation of NO for 3–53 days, daily withdrawal of the inhaled NO was associated with deterioration in oxygenation and pulmonary artery pressures, and these improved once the inhaled NO was reinstated (Rossaint *et al.*, 1993).

Inhaled NO is converted to nitrate and nitrites in the blood which are excreted in the urine. Westfelt *et al.* (1995) studied 15 healthy subjects who inhaled 25 ppm of NO for 1 hour. Plasma and urine nitrate levels were followed for 2 and 48 hours, respectively. The conversion of inhaled NO to nitrate was demonstrated to be a major metabolic pathway accounting for more than 70% of the inactivation of NO. Valvini and Young (1995) demonstrated a 13-fold increase in combined nitrates and nitrites in a patient treated with 40–90 ppm of inhaled NO for acute respiratory failure due to leptospirosis.

Nitric oxide is supplied as a mixture of NO and N_2. In the absence of O_2 this mixture is stable indefinitely at room temperature and 1 atmosphere pressure. At increased pressure, however, the formation of N_2O and NO_2 may occur. This needs to be consider when NO is stored in pressurized cylinders.

Inhaled Nitric Oxide and Platelet Function

Nitric oxide plays a vital role in homeostasis by preventing adhesion of platelets to the vascular wall. Unstable NO can react with thiol containing molecules to form *S*-nitrosothiols, which are potent inhibitors of platelet aggregation in vitro. Högman *et al.* (1994) noted a prolongation of bleeding time from 51 to 72 seconds in rabbits receiving 30 ppm inhaled NO for 15 minutes. There were no changes in hematocrit, whole blood or plasma viscosity, erythrocyte aggregation tendency, or erythrocyte deformability. Högman *et al.* also noted mild prolongation of bleeding time in normal volunteers receiving 30 ppm inhaled NO (Frostel and Zapol, 1995). The same volunteers had no abnormality of bleeding time when breathing 10 ppm NO. In a larger study by Alberts *et al.* (1995), again with normal volunteers, these results could not be corroborated when no bleeding time prolongation was noted with concentrations of 30 and 80 ppm inhaled NO given for up to 50 minutes. Samama *et al.* (1995a) measured a decrease in platelet aggregation in patients with ARDS receiving 1–100 ppm inhaled NO in the absence of any increase in bleeding time. They postulated that the beneficial effects of inhaled NO might be linked to an antiplatelet effect. Since one theory of pathophysiology in ARDS relates to increased platelet aggregation in the lung with associated mediator injury, the effect of inhaled NO on this disorder is of interest for more than its oxygenation and pulmonary vascular resistance effects.

ACUTE RESPIRATORY DISTRESS SYNDROME (ARDS)

Our understanding of the pathophysiology of ARDS has increased substantially since the first description of the syndrome in 1967 by Ashbaugh *et al.* Multiple insults are capable of producing this syndrome which is characterized clinically by acute onset, compromised oxygenation, and the presence of diffuse infiltrates on a chest radiograph. The early pathophysiology of ARDS is characterized by pulmonary artery (PA) hypertension, inflammation, and altered vascular permeability which contributes to noncardiogenic pulmonary edema. Despite current supportive therapy, the mortality from ARDS ranges from 30% to 60%.

Physiologic Response to Inhaled NO

Vasodilator therapy to decrease pulmonary artery pressure (PAP) has been hypothesized to promote resolution of ARDS by decreasing extravasation of fluid into alveolar spaces. Intravenous vasodilators such as nitroprusside and prostacyclin (PGI_2) have been used to decrease PAP. However, these vasodilators cause systemic and non-selective pulmonary vasodilatation. This may result in systemic hypotension and, by increasing blood flow to poorly ventilated lung segments, increase intrapulmonary shunting and compromise arterial oxygenation. The selective delivery of inhaled NO to the lung with its lack of systemic hemodynamic effects is an attractive alternative to systemic vasodilators. The ability of inhaled NO to reverse PA hypertension has been hypothesized both to decrease pulmonary edema and to improve right ventricular (RV) function by decreasing RV afterload. Inhaled NO might also be expected to reduce intrapulmonary shunting because gas is distributed only to well-ventilated alveoli and not to collapsed or fluid-filled alveoli. Inhaled NO would cause vasodilation of the pulmonary vasculature in well-ventilated regions and divert PA blood flow to these areas. An improvement in V_A/Q matching would result in increased arterial oxygenation.

Many clinical studies document the physiologic effects of inhaled NO (Gerlach *et al.*, 1993; Rossaint *et al.*, 1993, 1995; Abman *et al.*, 1994; Bigatello *et al.*, 1994; Puybasset *et al.*, 1994a, b, 1995; Young *et al.*, 1994; Day *et al.*, 1996; Krafft *et al.*, 1996; Lowson *et al.*, 1996). Rossaint *et al.* (1993) published one of the first studies evaluating inhaled NO in adults with ARDS and compared it to prostacyclin infusion. Pulmonary gas exchange and pulmonary blood flow were characterized using the multiple inert-gas-elimination technique. Two concentrations of inhaled NO were used (18 and 36 ppm). Short-term inhalation of 18 ppm NO in nine patients revealed a statistically significant decrease in PAP (from 37 ± 3 to 30 ± 2 mmHg) with an associated decrease in pulmonary vascular resistance (PVR). There were no further incremental effects noted with the higher 36 ppm dose. Systemic blood pressure, cardiac output, and systemic vascular resistance remained unchanged. Inhalation of NO resulted in an increase in the P_aO_2/F_iO_2 ratio (from 152 ± 15 to 199 ± 23 mmHg) with a decrease in intrapulmonary shunting (Q_S/Q_T)/from $36 \pm 5\%$ to $31 \pm 5\%$. The inert-gas studies showed that inhaled NO increased the fraction of blood flowing to lung areas with normal V_A/Q ratios.

Prostacyclin infusion resulted in a similar decrease in PAP and PVR. However, systemic blood pressure and systemic vascular resistance were decreased and there was an increase in cardiac output. Prostacyclin resulted in a decrease in P_aO_2/F_iO_2 and an increase in intrapulmonary shunting. The inert-gas studies showed a decreased fraction of blood flowing to lung areas with normal V_A/Q ratios.

Similar physiologic effects of inhaled NO have been observed in pediatric patients with ARDS (Abman *et al.*, 1994; Day *et al.*, 1996). Day *et al.* (1996) evaluated the acute effects of 11 and 60 ppm inhaled NO in 19 patients. The acute hemodynamic effects of 11 and 60 ppm inhaled NO were similar with significant decreases in the PVR index. Pulmonary artery pressures were not reported. Oxygenation improved with increases in the P_aO_2/F_iO_2 ratio.

Currently, ventilatory strategies that limit inspiratory plateau pressures have been advocated in ARDS to minimize lung injury. (Slutsky, 1993). Progressive hypercapnia may result from volume and/or pressure limitations. Acute hypercapnia can cause PA hypertension through an increase in cardiac output and PVR (Horwitz *et al.*, 1968). The effects of inhaled NO (2 ppm) in normocapnic and hypercapnic conditions were investigated in 11 patients with ARDS by Puybasset *et al.* (1994b). In hypercapnic conditions, inhaled NO decreased PVR to values similar to NO levels in normocapnic conditions. Although PAP decreased in hypercapnic conditions, it did not return to values measured under normocapnic conditions. Increased cardiac output during hypercapnic conditions with inhaled NO was hypothesized to account for the higher PAP. Nitric oxide increased P_aO_2 during hypercapnia, but failed to improve intrapulmonary shunt. Thus inhaled NO appears to maintain many of its physiologic effects in ARDS when ventilatory techniques result in hypercapnia.

Since inhaled NO is delivered only to ventilated lung units, the techniques that increase lung unit recruitment were hypothesized to play an important role in the response to NO. An animal study of acute lung injury showed that inhaled NO decreased PAP with and without the application of continuous positive airway pressure (CPAP). (Putensen *et al.*, 1994). However, inhaled NO without CPAP had no significant effect on increasing P_aO_2 or improving V_A/Q matching. Inhaled NO and CPAP resulted in improvement in P_aO_2 and a decrease in blood flow to shunt units with an increased flow to normal V_A/Q units. In an elegant clinical study, Puybasset *et al.* (1995) demonstrated in 21 patients with ARDS that inhaled NO decreased PVR, PAP, and intrapulmonary shunt, and significantly increased P_aO_2. The effects of inhaled NO were augmented by the addition of 10 cmH_2O peak end-expiratory pressure (PEEP). In patients in whom PEEP was associated with alveolar recruitment as demonstrated by high resolution and spiral thoracic computed tomography (CT) scan, the increase in P_aO_2 with inhaled NO was significantly greater than the increase in patients without positive airway pressure. The optimal effects of inhaled NO in ARDS appear to depend on the ability to induce alveolar recruitment.

Another potential benefit of inhaled NO in ARDS would be improvement of RV function through amelioration of PA. Although PA hypertension severe enough to result in RV failure seldom occurs in ARDS, reduction of RV afterload may be important in some patients. Fierobe *et al.* (1995) evaluated RV function in patients with severe ARDS who received inhaled NO. Coincident with a fall in pulmonary resistance, an increase in RV ejection fraction (32 $\pm$ 5% vs 36 $\pm$ 6%) and a trend toward decreased RV end-systolic and end-diastolic volumes occurred. Further studies to characterize changes in RV function with the use of inhaled NO are needed.

Although the ability of inhaled NO to decrease PAP and to increase oxygenation have received the most attention, additional effects may be potentially beneficial in ARDS. Neutrophils play an important role in the pathophysiology of lung injury during ARDS. Recently, NO has been shown to prevent or reduce neutrophil adhesion to endothelial cells and oxygen free radical formation in an ischemia/reperfusion model (Kurose *et al.*, 1994). Chollet-Martin *et al.* (1996) evaluated the impact of inhaled NO on H_2O_2 production and adhesion molecule (CD11b/CD18) expression by lung neutrophils along with levels of cytokines (tumor necrosis factor (TNF), interleukin-6 and -8 (IL-6, IL-8)) in bronchoalveolar lavage (BAL) fluid from ARDS patients. This group was compared with a group of ARDS patients not receiving inhaled NO. Neutrophils from patients receiving inhaled NO showed a reduction in spontaneous H_2O_2 production and CD11b/CD18 expression. In addition, high levels of IL-8 and IL-6 in BAL decreased after NO inhalation compared to untreated patients. Although further study is necessary, these results suggest that longer term effects of inhaled NO may decrease lung inflammation in ARDS.

Dose Response of Inhaled NO

Several clinical studies have evaluated the dose–response characteristics of inhaled NO as well as acute physiologic responses. (Gerlach *et al.*, 1993; Bigatello *et al.*, 1994; Puybasset *et al.*, 1994; Young *et al.*, 1994; Day *et al.*, 1996; Lowson *et al.*, 1996). Gerlach *et al.* (1993) evaluated the time course and dose response of 0.01, 0.1, 1.0, 10, and 100 ppm inhaled NO in 12 patients with severe ARDS. The increase in P_aO_2 compared to baseline was significant at inhaled NO concentrations of $\geq$0.1 ppm. The 100 ppm concentration resulted in a worsening of oxygenation compared to the 10 ppm concentration. Significant decreases in PAP compared to baseline were noted with NO doses of $\geq$1 ppm. In contrast to the oxygenation effects, PAP had a continuous dose-dependent downward tendency over all doses tested. The time course for the effects of inhaled NO on oxygenation and PAP were also slightly different. An increase in P_aO_2 was noted within 1–2 minutes of gas initiation, whereas PAP did not decrease until 3 minutes of inhalation. Bigatello *et al.* (1994) reported a similar dose-related decrease of PAP with increasing concentrations of inhaled NO (5–40 ppm). The maximum reduction in PAP was achieved at NO concentrations of $\leq$20 ppm in 7 of 11 patients. They did not demonstrate a similar dose-response for the improvement in oxygenation. Higher concentrations of inhaled NO (20 ppm) increased the P_aO_2 less than did lower concentrations of 2–4 ppm in long-term treatment.

Puybasset *et al.* (1994a) evaluated lower doses of inhaled NO (100–5000 ppb) in patients with severe ARDS. They found that NO concentrations in the range 100–2000 ppb resulted in dose-dependent decreases in PAP and increases in P_aO_2. Lowson *et al.* (1996) described a dose-dependent effect for improvement in P_aO_2 with doses of 0.1, 1.0, and 10 ppm inhaled NO, but found no dose-related effects on the mean PAP. The maximum decrease in mean PAP occurred at an inhaled NO dose of 0.1 ppm, while maximum improvement in oxygenation occurred at 10 ppm.

The marked difference in dose–response characteristics for both oxygenation and lowering of PAP among studies may be related to differences in patient populations or techniques of measurement or delivery of inhaled NO. These factors make definitive conclusions as to precise dosaging difficult at this time. Several general conclusions, however, seem to be emerging. Currently, clinical studies would support the use of lower doses of inhaled NO (≤ 10 ppm). However, there may be individual patient variation in dose response based on severity of disease, etiology of ARDS, or ventilatory techniques used. It is unlikely that the optimum dose for improving oxygenation is identical to the dose necessary to produce the maximum decrease in PAP, or that either parameter predicts maximal clinical benefit (Zimmerman *et al.*, 1996).

Frequency of Acute Physiologic Response to Inhaled NO

As the number of clinical studies has expanded, it has become evident that not all patients with ARDS have an acute physiologic improvement after treatment with inhaled NO. Different investigators have defined acute physiologic improvements using different parameters with variable thresholds for classifying a response. Analysis of individual patient responses in the study by Rossaint *et al.* (1993) indicate that not all patients had a significant improvement in oxygenation or decrease in PAP. Rarely, a detrimental response to inhaled NO has been noted (Lowson *et al.*, 1996). Several clinical studies have attempted to describe the response rate and determine possible predictors of response. In the study by Puybasset *et al.* (1995), 81% of patients had improvement in PAP, PVR, and oxygenation. In 10%, no improvement in any hemodynamic or oxygenation variable was noted. In another 10% of patients, gas exchange improved and PVR decreased, but PAP did not change. In a recent study by Rossaint *et al.* (1995), 83% of patients were considered responders based on improvement in oxygenation, 87% responders based on improvement in venous admixture, and 63% responders by a decrease in PAP. In a study of NO inhalation in patients with septic shock and ARDS, 40% were classified as responders based on a rise in arterial oxygen tension and/or a decrease in mean PAP (Krafft *et al.*, 1996).

Interpretation of these clinical studies is difficult due to differences in patient populations, dose of inhaled NO, and definitions of response. Some studies have included primarily trauma patients, and others have included patients with late ARDS on extracorporeal membrane oxygenation (ECMO). The impact of various interventions such as ECMO, vasopressors, etc., on the response to inhaled NO is unknown. However, it might be reasonable to assume that the effects of NO may be differential based on the stage of disease. Likewise, definitions of responders have included an absolute increase in P_aO_2/F_iO_2 ratio, a percentage increase in P_aO_2, an absolute decrease in PAP, a percentage decrease in PAP, or a percentage decrease in intrapulmonary shunt fraction. None of these clinical trials have been blinded or involved concomitant control patients. A recent double-blind, placebo-controlled trial of inhaled NO in ARDS revealed a response rate (defined as a 20% increase in P_aO_2) of 60% in treated patients and a 24% response rate in placebo patients (Zimmerman *et al.*, 1996).

Several studies have attempted to identify factors that will predict response of individual patients (Bigatello *et al.*, 1994; Puybasset *et al.*, 1995; Rossaint *et al.*, 1995; Lowson *et al.*, 1996). Puybasset *et al.* (1995) found that the NO-induced decrease in PVR and PAP was proportional to the baseline level of PVR and PAP. A weak association was also noted between the increase in P_aO_2 and baseline PVR. Lowson *et al.* (1996) also found that the inhaled-NO-induced decrease in PVR and increase in P_aO_2 were significantly correlated with the baseline PVR. Other investigators have not found a correlation of improved oxygenation with the PVR or correlation of decrease in PAP with baseline PAP (Rossaint *et al.*, 1995). Standardization of definitions and larger clinical trials are necessary to further address response to inhaled NO in ARDS patients.

Toxicity of Inhaled NO in ARDS

Most ARDS studies utilizing NO concentrations ≤ 36 ppm report methemoglobin levels of $\leq 1.4\%$ (Rossaint *et al.*, 1993, 1995; Puybasset *et al.*, 1994a; Day *et al.*, 1996) Day *et al.* (1996) reported a significantly different maximum methemoglobin level at 10 ppm ($1.6 \pm 0.1\%$) compared to 40 ppm ($3.0 \pm 0.3\%$). Fewer studies report NO_2 levels. Puybasset *et al.* (1994a) reported a linear increase in NO_2 concentrations with NO concentrations of 100–2000 ppb. At the highest concentration, 5000 ppb, the NO_2 concentration was 103 ± 11 ppb, which is considered safe. However, potentially dangerous levels of 6 ppm NO_2 were detected in patients receiving inhaled NO at 128 ppm (Levy *et al.*, 1995).

The effects of inhaled NO on platelets was studied by Samama *et al.* (1995b) in six patients with ARDS. A non-dose-dependent but significant decrease in ex vivo platelet aggregation was noted with NO concentrations of 1, 3, 10, 30, and 100 ppm. This effect was not associated with prolongation of the bleeding time.

Clinical Benefits of Inhaled NO

Despite demonstration of the physiologic effects of inhaled NO in ARDS patients, clinical benefits have been more difficult to document. Theoretically, one could expect that improvement in oxygenation would lead to the ability to decrease the F_iO_2 and intensity of mechanical ventilation. Oxygen toxicity, barotrauma, and volutrauma would be minimized. Other potential clinical benefits might relate to decreases in lung edema as well as antiplatelet or anticytokine impact on the pulmonary circulation. The ultimate clinical benefit to be gained would be an improvement in survival. Other clinically relevant benefits of inhaled NO might include decreased time on mechanical ventilation with its attendant risks, decreased intensive care unit (ICU) stay, decreased hospital stay, or decreased cost. Thus far, no data have been reported from clinical trials that have prospectively addressed these issues. The complexity and heterogeneity of ARDS makes the design and implementation of such clinical trials problematic.

Several uncontrolled trials have reported outcomes with inhaled NO. Levy *et al.* added inhaled NO (5–10 ppm) to a regimen of therapeutic optimization in 20 ARDS patients (Levy *et al.*, 1995). Reversal of ARDS occurred in 16 patients, with 14 patients being discharged. Rossaint *et al.* (1995) evaluated the effects of NO inhalation in 30 patients with ARDS and compared their survival with similar patients without NO treatment in a retrospective manner. There was no difference in survival (69% vs 69%). An improved mortality was noted in patients with ARDS and septic shock who responded to NO (40%) versus nonresponders (67%) (Krafft *et al.*, 1996). The number of patients included in these studies is small and comparability of groups is not addressed. The pediatric study by Day *et al.* (1996) had no control group but found no difference in survival between patients treated with 10 and 40 ppm inhaled NO.

The Future of Inhaled NO and ARDS

Although inhaled NO has potentially beneficial physiologic effects in ARDS, rigorous clinical trials are required to answer many unanswered questions. The following are areas that need to be addressed:

- What is the optimum and safe dose of inhaled NO based on the desired effects?
- Is it possible to use clinical variables to predict which patients will respond to inhaled NO?
- What is the appropriate timing of intervention based on the stage of the disease process?
- What is the impact of other interventions such as ventilator management, use of vasopressors, etc., on the effects of inhaled NO?

- Does inhaled NO have a beneficial anti-inflammatory effect on the lung in ARDS?
- Are there clinically relevant benefits of the use of inhaled NO in ARDS?

HYPOXIC RESPIRATORY FAILURE OF THE NEONATE

During fetal life, the majority of blood bypasses the lungs and is shunted through the foramen ovale or the patent ductus arteriosus into the systemic circulatory system. At birth, the high pulmonary vascular resistance drops precipitously by up to 50% of the prenatal levels which, in turn, leads to a dramatic increase in pulmonary blood flow and a minimization of the extrapulmonary shunting (Walther *et al.*, 1993). A number of mechanisms have been identified which account for this rapid transition from fetal to postnatal life. Recently, it has been shown that increased endogenous production of NO is an important component in dropping the PA pressure during this transition period (Kinsella *et al.*, 1994; Abman *et al.*, 1995).

The failure of this normal sequence of events to occur leads to a clinical situation with continued intense pulmonary vasoconstriction, right-to-left extrapulmonary shunting and severe hypoxemia. If the infant has a structurally normal heart, the syndrome has been termed 'persistent pulmonary hypertension of the newborn' (PPHN) or 'persistent fetal circulation'. Although frequently idiopathic, PPHN is often associated with one of a variety of underlying diseases including meconium aspiration, pneumonia, perinatal asphyxia, sepsis, lung hypoplasia (including congenital diaphragmatic hernia), surfactant deficiency, and perinatal hypoxemia. Thus, many babies with PPHN will have both extrapulmonary shunting due to intense PA hypertension and intrapulmonary shunt resulting from V_A/Q mismatch.

Unfortunately, there is no generally accepted definition or therapy for PPHN (Weigel and Hageman, 1990). These patients are usually mildly preterm to post-term infants and usually become symptomatic within the first 24 hours of life (Davidson, 1993). Modalities used to treat this condition include: conventional mechanical ventilation, high frequency ventilation, alkalosis, muscle relaxants/paralytics, surfactant, and vasopressors (Weigel and Hageman, 1990; Kinsella *et al.*, 1994). Vasodilators (including tolazoline, nitroprusside, nitroglycerin, isoproterenol, and prostaglandins) are used to lower the PA pressure, but are limited by systemic hypotension. Currently, extracorporeal membrane oxygenation (ECMO) is considered to be the standard therapeutic modality for severe hypoxemia in full-term infants. It has reduced mortality in severe PPHN from 50–60% to 3–20%. Unfortunately, it is expensive, requires ligation of the common carotid artery and the internal jugular vein (although venous–venous ECMO is becoming increasingly common), and leads to significant morbidity in 15–30% of recipients. It also leads to intracranial infarcts or bleeding, major bleeding, seizures, metabolic abnormalities, infection, chronic lung disease, neurodevelopmental disorders, and hearing loss (Shanley *et al.*, 1994; Abman and Kinsella, 1995).

A selective pulmonary vasodilator is needed to overcome the intense PA hypertension associated with PPHN. Inhaled NO has been proposed as a potential therapy. Early studies demonstrated that hypoxic pulmonary vasoconstriction in adult sheep could be reversed with inhaled NO without causing changes in systemic blood pressures (Frostell *et al.*, 1991). These findings have been extended to neonatal animal models of hypoxia (F_iO_2 0.10–0.14) in either lambs (Roberts *et al.*, 1993) or piglets (Nelin *et al.*, 1994). In these models, hypoxia dramatically increased the PA pressures, increased PVR, and decreased pulmonary blood flow. These changes are completely reversed after several minutes of inhaled NO therapy. The levels of cGMP in the lungs of lambs with hypoxia doubled when treated with room air and tripled with treatment with 20 ppm of inhaled NO, suggesting that the reduction in PA pressures with both therapies acted through the NO/cGMP pathway (Roberts *et al.*, 1993). Similarly the increased PVR and PA hypertension induced by U46619 or U46619 plus hypoxia was reversed with inhaled NO in neonatal lambs (De Marco *et al.*, 1994).

Another model of PPHN was produced in neonatal lambs by closing the ductus arteriosus several days before delivery (Zayek *et al.*, 1993a, b). Again therapy with inhaled NO was associated with decreases in PVR and PA pressures and increased pulmonary blood flow in a dose-dependent fashion (Zayek *et al.*, 1993b). In this model, survival of lambs treated with 80 ppm was 83% compared to 0% in the control group (Zayek *et al.*, 1993a).

These encouraging results have led to the use of inhaled NO in neonates suffering from hypoxemia resulting from a variety of causes. Like the adult trials, however, few double-blind, placebo-controlled clinical trials examining clinically meaningful end-points have been reported. Thus, many questions remain concerning the appropriate patient population, dose, and duration for this therapy in neonates.

The original case series demonstrated that oxygenation could be improved with inhaled NO at initial doses of 6–80 ppm in neonates with severe PPHN (Kinsella *et al.*, 1992; Roberts *et al.*, 1992), but the effect was not sustained when inhaled NO was discontinued after

30 minutes (Roberts *et al.*, 1992). In patients treated with 6 ppm for 24 hours, there was a sustained improvement in oxygenation and echocardiographic evidence of improved pulmonary hypertension (Kinsella *et al.*, 1992). In this study, 13 of 15 patients meeting ECMO criteria were treated without ECMO. These findings were reproduced in a European study, and ECMO treatment was avoided in 2 of the 7 cases meeting ECMO criteria (Lönnqvist *et al.*, 1994). In another study of inhaled NO (5–80 ppm) in infants referred for ECMO, 13 of the 23 infants had clinically significant improvement in their oxygenation. There was no significant difference in the acute oxygenation response at the doses (5–80 ppm) studied (Finer *et al.*, 1994). In this study, patients with echocardiographic evidence of pulmonary hypertension were most likely to respond acutely to inhaled NO therapy. Of the 23 patients, 12 were treated without ECMO. Because there was no control group in any of these studies and the patients were treated in a non-blinded fashion, it is impossible to draw any conclusions about the utility of the inhaled NO in reducing the need for ECMO.

The first placebo-controlled trial examining clinical end-points in hypoxemic neonates comes from the joint National Institute of Childhood Health and Development and Canadian Neonatal Network's Neonatal Inhaled Nitric Oxide Study (NINOS) (presented at the American Pediatric Society and the Society for Pediatric Research, May 1996). This was a placebo-controlled, double-blind trial of the effects of inhaled NO on the rate of infants who either died or went on to require ECMO. Patients initially received 20 ppm inhaled NO or 'low flow' O_2. If the patient demonstrated suboptimal response to the initial gas, the flow rate was increased to deliver either 80 ppm inhaled NO or high-flow O_2. The two groups were well matched and critically ill with an oxygen index ((mean airway pressure $\times$ F_iO_2)/P_aO_2) of approximately 45 (the criterion for ECMO being 45 in this trial). The acute change in P_aO_2 was 7.8 and 43.6 T ($p < 0.001$) and the change in oxygen index was 2.2 and -15.5 ($p < 0.001$) in the control and inhaled-NO groups, respectively. The rate of infants who died or received ECMO was 73% in the control group compared to 51% in the inhaled-NO group ($p = 0.003$). Although mortality was decreased from 20% in the control group to 16% in the treatment group, this failed to reach statistical significance ($p = 0.54$). However, the decrease in the rate of ECMO from 62% to 42% was significant ($p = 0.009$).

Thus, it appears that inhaled NO can improve oxygenation and reduce the need for ECMO in severely hypoxemic neonates. Several questions remain to be answered, however. Most of the studies have suggested that doses above 20 ppm are rarely needed but no dose–response data are available to help establish the best dose of the drug. To date, all the data available suggest that inhaled NO is well tolerated with few side-effects. No data on the long-term outcomes of these infants are available. Because the developing organ systems of the neonate may be more affected by minor toxicities than is the case in adults, there is an increased concern regarding the potential long-term effects of nitrosylation of proteins, antiaggregation of platelets, and suppression of respiratory bursts in neutrophils associated with this therapy. Although these concerns remain purely theoretical, inhaled NO should be targeted at those severely ill neonates in whom the risk of the acute disaster clearly outweighs any subtle long-term risks.

INHALED NITRIC OXIDE: OTHER POTENTIAL USES

Asthma

Inhaled NO has been demonstrated to relax canine conducting airways by indirect as well as direct mechanisms. Brown *et al.* (1994) used high-resolution CT to measure changes in innervated canine airways greater than 1 mm in diameter. Inhaled NO completely reversed histamine-induced airway constriction in a dose-related fashion. With histamine-induced airway constriction of $60 \pm 3\%$ of baseline, the airway area increased to $85 \pm 5\%$, $102 \pm 5\%$, and $111 \pm 10\%$ with 100, 200, and 400 ppm inhaled NO, respectively. In contrast to histamine, inhaled NO only partially reversed methacholine-induced constriction. With methacholine-induced airway constriction of $63 \pm 3\%$ of baseline, the airway area increased to $67 \pm 3\%$, $75 \pm 3\%$, and $75 \pm 2\%$ after 100, 200, and 400 ppm inhaled NO, respectively. These high doses of inhaled NO would not be feasible in humans; however, lower levels of inhaled NO have been demonstrated to be a potent bronchodilator in guinea-pig studies. Dupuy *et al.* (1992) studied anesthetized and mechanically ventilated guinea-pigs. Intravenous methacholine was used to increase pulmonary resistance from 0.143 ± 0.008 to 0.474 ± 0.041 $cmH_2O/ml \cdot s$. Inhalation of 5–300 ppm inhaled NO produced a dose-related rapid, consistent, and reversible reduction in resistance. Onset of bronchodilation was rapid, beginning within 30 seconds of commencing inhalation. A 50% reduction in resistance was achieved with 15 ± 2.1 ppm. The addition of inhaled terbutaline was additive to the bronchodilating effects of inhaled NO.

Pfeffer *et al.* (1996) studied the effect of inhaled NO in pediatric asthma. They concluded that inhaled NO at 40 ppm had no apparent bronchodilatory effect in pediatric subjects with mild asthma.

Chronic Obstructive Pulmonary Disease

Moinard *et al.* (1994) examined the circulatory effects of inhalation of 15 ppm inhaled NO in 14 hypoxemic patients with chronic obstructive pulmonary disease (COPD). Four patients breathed 100% O_2 before inhaled NO. Ten minutes following NO inhalation there was a significant fall in mean pulmonary artery pressure and pulmonary vascular resistance of $19 \pm 10\%$ and $29 \pm 15\%$, respectively. The higher the baseline pulmonary artery hypertension, the greater the reduction in mean pulmonary artery pressure. No systemic circulatory effects were observed. The overall V_A/Q ratio was not altered, although there was a significantly higher percentage of ventilation in poorly and unperfused areas.

Lung Transplant

Early severe graft dysfunction, as manifested by hypoxemia and elevated PAP, occurs in approximately 15% of lung-transplant recipients. Inhaled NO has also been demonstrated to improve oxygenation and decrease PAP without systemic circulatory effects in patients with severe human lung allograft dysfunction. Date *et al.* (1996) compared treatment with and without inhaled NO in a retrospective study using historical controls. They analyzed postoperative hemodynamic data, gas exchange data, and clinical outcome in 32 lung-transplant recipients who developed immediate, severe graft dysfunction. Seventeen patients had received treatment without inhaled NO prior to its availability, while the subsequent 15 patients were treated with inhaled NO. Nitric oxide was delivered at 20–60 ppm for 15–217 hours (average 84 hours). Inhaled NO consistently lowered mean PAP (30 ± 2 to 26 ± 2 mmHg) and improved the P_aO_2/F_iO_2 ratio (88 ± 10 to 153 ± 30 T). These changes occurred within 1 hour and there were no effects on cardiac index or systemic arterial pressure. Using historical controls, the duration of mechanical ventilation was reduced from 17 ± 5 days in the control group compared to 12 ± 3 days in the group receiving inhaled NO. The number of airway complications was four in the historical controls and none in the inhaled NO treatment group. Mortality was 4/17 in the historical controls and 1/15 in the inhaled NO treatment group.

Adatia *et al.* (1994) also studied the use of 10 ppm inhaled NO in the treatment of severe postoperative graft dysfunction after lung transplantation. In five patients they demonstrated a clinically significant lowering of mean PAP from 38.4 ± 1.6 to 29.4 ± 3.1 mmHg, with a reduction of intrapulmonary shunt fraction from $28.6 \pm 8.3\%$ to $21.0 \pm 5.7\%$. There was a $28.4\% \pm 7.2\%$ reduction in transpulmonary pressure gradients. There were no major side-effects.

Inhaled NO has also been studied in lung ischemia/reperfusion injury in an isolated rat lung model (Eppinger *et al.*, 1995). Inhaled NO delivered at the start of reperfusion reversed postischemic pulmonary hypoperfusion, decreased lung neutrophil content, and decreased vascular permeability at 4 hours. Surprisingly, the vascular permeability injury was worse at 30 minutes. Superoxide dismutase given prior to reperfusion or delaying the inhaled NO until 10 minutes after reperfusion both prevented the early worsened injury. It was postulated that inhaled NO may increase toxicity early in reperfusion through its interaction with superoxide. Later, at 4 hours, it could be protective due to its pulmonary vasodilating properties and ability to reduce neutrophil-mediated injury. The interaction of inhaled NO and oxygen free radicals and its overall clinical impact is controversial (see Pharmacology of Inhaled Nitric Oxide, above). McDonald *et al.* (1995) have demonstrated successful treatment in humans of life-threatening acute reperfusion injury after lung transplantation using inhaled NO.

After Cardiac Surgery

Nitric oxide has been used as an effective pulmonary vasodilator after a wide variety of cardiac surgeries. It is thought to be particularly useful in selectively lowering RV afterload in patients with postoperative RV dysfunction. Fullerton *et al.* (1996) presented information from 20 patients studied in the operating room after weaning from cardiopulmonary bypass. They compared baseline hemodynamics with administration of 20 and 40 ppm inhaled NO. PVR was lowered from 343 ± 30 to 232 ± 25 dynes·s/cm^5 with 20 ppm NO, with no further lowering noted with 40 ppm NO. Mean PAP was lowered from 29 ± 1 to 22 ± 1 mmHg with 20 ppm and to 21 ± 1 mmHg with 40 ppm. Both PVR and PAP returned to baseline after withdrawal of inhaled NO. No changes were noted in either systemic vascular resistance or mean aortic pressure. Goldman *et al.* (1995) compared inhaled NO to prostacyclin for severe pulmonary hypertension after cardiac surgery. The mean pulmonary to systemic arterial pressure ratio was significantly lower during NO than with prostacyclin administration, as prostacyclin lowered systemic blood pressure. Inhaled NO is therefore a more effective and selective vasodilator than prostacyclin in severe postoperative pulmonary hypertension.

High-altitude Pulmonary Edema

The inhalation of NO has been shown to temporarily improve arterial oxygenation in high altitude pulmonary edema (HAPE). It was suggested that the beneficial effect might be related to a favorable action on the distribution of blood flow in the lungs. The data suggested that a defect in NO synthesis might contribute to the risk of HAPE. Scherrer *et al.* (1996) studied 36 mountaineers, 18 of whom were prone to HAPE and 18 of whom were resistant. The study was done in a high-altitude laboratory. In patients prone to HAPE, inhalation of NO at 40 ppm for 15 minutes produced a decrease in mean PAP that was three times larger than that in subjects classified as being resistant to HAPE. Inhaled NO elevated P_aO_2 significantly in the 10 subjects prone to HAPE who had radiographic evidence of pulmonary edema. Paradoxically, it worsened oxygenation in subjects resistant to HAPE.

Pulmonary Thromboembolism

Pinelli *et al.* (1996) reported the use of inhaled NO as an adjunct to pulmonary thromboendarterectomy. Following pulmonary thromboendarterectomy a patient developed acute and persistent pulmonary hypertension, gas exchange impairment, and right heart dysfunction which was improved with administration of inhaled NO

Estagnasié *et al.* (1994) have demonstrated the ability of inhaled NO ability to reverse flow through a patent foramen ovale occurring after pulmonary embolism.

Cardiac Transplantation Evaluation

A severe, fixed elevation in PVR is a contraindication for heart transplant. Currently, nitroprusside is used to evaluate the reversibility of PA hypertension. The nonselective vasodilation of nitroprusside and its dose-limiting systemic hypotension may limit its utility for this purpose. Semigran *et al.* (1994) demonstrated that inhaled NO as a selective pulmonary vasodilator may identify patients with reversible pulmonary vasoconstriction in whom agents such as nitroprusside fail to confirm its presence.

Primary Pulmonary Hypertension

Inhaled NO has been used as a screening vasodilator agent to screen for beneficial response of primary pulmonary hypertension in order to identify patients who are candidates for chronic vasodilator therapy.

In one study, when compared with prostacyclin, 10 ppm inhaled NO identified reversibility and did not induce any adverse systemic effect. Inhaled NO appeared to be an effective, safe, and reliable substitute for prostacyclin in screening for acute pulmonary vasodilator responsiveness for potential therapy for patients with a primary pulmonary hypertension (Sitbon *et al.*, 1995).

Pulmonary Artery Hypertension after Mitral Valve Replacement

Patients with mitral valve disease can develop severe life-threatening pulmonary artery hypertension after mitral valve replacement. Girard *et al.* (1992) administered inhaled NO postoperatively to six patients with mild pulmonary artery hypertension following mitral valve replacement. A dose of 36–38 ppm was inhaled for 10 minutes, with an approximately 10% reduction in mean PAP and a 22% reduction in PVR. There were no changes in systemic arterial or pulmonary artery occlusive pressure, and methemoglobin levels remained below 1%.

Delivery Devices for Inhaled NO

Commercial inhaled NO remains under development in the USA at this time. As previously discussed, NO readily combines with O_2 to form NO_2 which has been shown to be potentially toxic (Moncada *et al.*, 1991). This reaction is an important consideration in the design of delivery devices (Foubert *et al.*, 1992). The amount of NO_2 formed by the reaction of NO and O_2 depends on the contact time between the gases, the concentration of O_2, and the square of the NO concentration. Because the concentration of delivered O_2 is dictated by the patient's severity of disease and the NO concentration by a therapeutic threshold, the only way to minimize the amount of NO_2 delivered to the patient is by limiting the contact time between the two gases. In addition, soda lime canisters are inserted in-line in the inspiratory limb of the ventilator system to scavenge NO_2 prior to delivery of the patient breath (Pickett *et al.*, 1994). The current Occupational Safety and Health Administration (OSHA) recommendation for NO_2 exposure is 1 ppm.

Some patients may develop acute worsening in oxygenation and sudden rises in PAP if the concentration of inhaled NO is abruptly lowered. It is therefore important to have delivery devices that reliably deliver a set concentration of inhaled NO and allow small incremental changes to be made in the concentration delivered.

Injection of a NO/N_2 mixture into the inspiration limb of a ventilator circuit will cause a dilution of the delivered oxygen concentration delivered to the patient. The extent of the dilution depends on the final NO concentration desired and the concentration of the stock NO gas. Therefore, either the F_iO_2 delivered to the patient should be monitored or the dilutional effects of the N_2/NO compensated for by the device and/or the ventilator. Thus, an effective inhaled NO delivery device will deliver a constant dose of inhaled NO (preferably regardless of the mode of ventilation), limit the formation of NO_2 by minimizing the contact time of NO with O_2 as much as possible, and monitor the amount of NO, NO_2, and O_2 that the patient is receiving.

Several inhaled NO delivery systems have been described. The initial device was a Douglas bag in which NO and O_2 were mixed and allowed to interact for the duration of the therapy (Pepke-Zaba *et al.*, 1991). This system is no longer considered acceptable because of the indubitable build up of NO_2. More acceptable systems that address these safety concerns have been described (Stenqvist *et al.*, 1993; Tiballs *et al.*, 1993; Watkins *et al.*, 1993; Miller *et al.*, 1994; Wessel *et al.*, 1994; Young, 1994; Zapol *et al.*, 1994).

Although, the National Heart, Lung and Blood Institute (NHLBI) workshop recommended that NO and NO_2 concentrations be monitored during inhaled NO therapy (Zapol *et al.*, 1994), this monitoring has proven less straightforward than originally anticipated. Chemiluminescence devices developed for industrial use are highly accurate in many settings, but require large sample volumes (of the order of 700 ml/min (Wessel *et al.*, 1994)), have quenching problems at high oxygen concentration (Adatia and Wessel, 1994), are very large and expensive (Adatia and Wessel, 1994), have problems with water condensation (Wessel *et al.*, 1994), and in clinical settings can give unreliable NO_2 readings (Miller, 1994). Electrochemical monitors are less expensive, but are more sensitive to baseline drift and measurements may be affected by changes in airway pressure and gas flow (Adatia and Wessel, 1994). Neither system is optimal, and use of both types of monitor has been suggested (Frostell and Zapol, 1995).

The monitors for NO and NO_2 should measure the concentrations of these gases as they enter the patient as accurately as possible. The sample port for gases should be located on the inspiratory limb of the ventilator circuit as close to the patient as possible without risking contamination of the sample with expiratory gases. Ideally, the alveolar concentration of the gases would be most clinically relevant, but this is currently unobtainable. Sampling at the tip of the endotracheal tube allows measurement somewhat closer to the alveoli, and produces uninterpretable readings due to the inspiratory/expiratory gas mixing. Measurement of NO and NO_2 in the expiratory limb does not take into consideration the alteration in gas content that may occur in the distal airways and alveoli.

Finally, the manner in which the delivery device adds NO into the inspiratory limb of the ventilation circuit can affect the actual dose delivered. Systems that inject a constant flow of NO will deliver a constant concentration of NO to the patient only when the flow of gas from the ventilator is constant. If the flow of ventilator gas is intermittent and predictable (gated) or continually varying and unpredictable (such as with pressure support), a constant NO injection will deliver NO concentrations which vary over each breath cycle. Systems that sense the ventilator gas flow rate and inject NO proportionally to that flow provide for a constant NO concentration to be delivered, provided the response times of the sensors and flow valves are sufficiently fast. These design characteristics are likely to provide consistent NO delivery when used at the same flow rates and ventilation mode. It is difficult, however, to equate reported injected concentrations of NO among clinical studies when the gas is delivered via different delivery devices.

Until acceptable inhaled NO delivery devices are readily commercially available with all appropriate fail-safe systems and integrated monitoring, the safe delivery of inhaled NO remains a challenge for clinicians. Careful assessment of any delivery device is critical to assure that this potentially effective therapy can be administered efficiently and safely to critically ill patients.

ACKNOWLEDGEMENT

The authors are grateful for the organizational assistance and manuscript preparation provided by Toni Piper.

REFERENCES

Abman, S.H., Kinsella, J.P. (1995) Inhaled nitric oxide therapy of pulmonary hypertension and respiratory failure in preterm and term neonates. *Adv Pharmacol* **34**: 457–474.

Abman, S.H., Griebel, J.L., Parker, D.K., *et al.* (1994) Acute effects of inhaled nitric oxide in children with severe hypoxemic respiratory failure. *J Pediatr* **124**: 881–888.

Adatia, I., Wessel, D.L. (1994) Therapeutic use of inhaled nitric oxide. *Curr Opinion Pediatr* **6:** 583–590.

Adatia, I., Lillehei, C., Arnold, J.H., Thompson, J.E., Palazzo, R., Fackler, J.C., Wessel, D.L. (1994) Inhaled nitric oxide in the treatment of postoperative graft dysfunction after lung transplantation. *Ann Thorac Surg* **57**: 1311–1318.

Albert, J., Wallen, H., Brojiersen, A., Frostell, C., Hjemdahl, P. (1995) Effects of inhaled NO on platelet function in vivo in healthy volunteers. *FASEB J* **9**: A30 [abstract].

Ashbaugh, D.G., Bigelow, D.B., Petty, T.L., *et al.* (1967) Acute respiratory distress in adults. *Lancet* **ii**: 319–323.

Bigatello, L.M., Hurford, W.E., Kacmarek, R.M., *et al.* (1994) Prolonged inhalation of low concentrations of nitric oxide in patients with severe adult respiratory distress syndrome. *Anesthesiology* **80**: 761–770.

Brown, R.H., Zerhouni, E.A., Hirshman, C.A. (1994) Reversal of bronchoconstriction by inhaled nitric oxide. Histamine versus methacholine. *Am J Respir Crit Care Med* **150**: 233–237.

Chollet-Martin, S., Gatacel, C., Kermarrec, N., *et al.* (1996) Alveolar neutrophil functions and cytokine levels in patients with the adult respiratory distress syndrome during nitric oxide inhalation. *Am J Respir Crit Care Med* **153**: 985–990.

Clutton-Brock, J. (1967) Two cases of poisoning by contamination of nitrous oxide with higher oxides of nitrogen during anesthesia. *Br J Anaesth* **39**: 388–392.

Culotta, E., Koshland, D.E. (1992) NO news is good news. *Science* **258**: 1862–1865.

Date, H., Triantafillou, A.N., Trulock, E.P., Pohl, M.S., Cooper, J.D., Patterson, G.A. (1996) Inhaled nitric oxide reduces human lung allograft dysfunction. *J Thorac Cardiovasc Surg* **111**: 913–919.

Davidson, D. (1993) NO bandwagon yet. *Am Rev Respir Dis* **147:** 1078–1079 [editorial].

Day, R.W., Guarin, M., Lynch, J.M., *et al.* (1996) Inhaled nitric oxide in children with severe lung disease. Results of acute and prolonged therapy with two concentrations. *Crit Care Med* **24**: 215–21.

DeMarco, V., Skimming, J., Ellis, T.M., Cassin, S. (1994) Nitric oxide inhalation: effects on the ovine neonatal pulmonary and systemic circulations. *Chest* **105** (Suppl.): 91S–92S.

Dupuy, P.M., Shore, S.A., Drazen, J.M., Frostell, C., Hill, W.A., Zapol, W.M. (1992) Bronchodilator action of inhaled nitric oxide in guinea pigs. *J Clin Invest* **90**: 421–442.

Eppinger, M.J., Ward, P.A., Jones, M.L., Bolling, S.F., Deeb, G.M. (1995) Disparate effects of nitric oxide on lung ischemia-reperfusion injury. *Ann Thoracic Surg* **60**: 1169–1175.

Estagnaisé, P., Le Bourdellès, G., Mier, L., Coste, F., Dreyfuss, D. (1994) Use of inhaled nitric oxide to reverse flow through a patent foramen ovale during pulmonary embolism. *Ann Intern Med* **120**: 757–759.

Fierobe, L., Brunet, F., Dhainaut, J-F., *et al.* (1995) Effect of inhaled nitric oxide on right ventricular function in adult respiratory distress syndrome. *Am J Respir Crit Care Med* **151**: 1414–1419.

Finer, N.N., Etches, P.C., Kamstra, B., Tierney, A.J., Peliowski, A., Ryan, C.A.

(1994) Inhaled nitric oxide in infants referred for extracorporeal membrane oxygenation; Dose response. *J Pediatr* **124**: 302–308.

Foubert, L., Fleming, B., Latimer, R., Jonas, M., Oduro, A., Borland, C., Higenbottam, T. (1992) Safety guidelines for use of nitric oxide *Lancet* **339**: 1615–1616 [letter].

Frostell, C.G., Zapol, W.M. (1995) Inhaled nitric oxide, clinical rationale and applications. *Adv Pharmacol* **34**: 439–456.

Frostell, C., Fratacci, M.D., Wain, J.C., Jones, R., Zapol, W.M. (1991) Inhaled nitric oxide: a selective pulmonary vasodilator reversing hypoxic pulmonary vasoconstriction. *Circulation* **83**: 2038–2047.

Fullerton, D.A., Jones, S.D., Jaggers, J., Piedalue, F., Grover, F.L., McIntyre, R.C. (1996) Effective control of pulmonary vascular resistance with inhaled nitric oxide after cardiac operation. *J Thorac Cardiovasc Surg* **111**: 753–762.

Furchgott, R.F., Zawadzki, J.V. (1980) The obligatory role of endothelial cells in the relaxation of arterial smooth muscle by acetylcholine. *Nature* **288**: 373–376.

Gerlach, H., Rossaint, R., Rappert, D., Falke, K.J. (1993) Time-course and dose-response of nitric oxide inhalation for systemic oxygenation and pulmonary hypertension in patients with adult respiratory distress syndrome. *Eur J Clin Invest* **23**: 499–502.

Girard, C., Lehot, J.J., Pannetier, J.C., Filley, S., French, P., Estanove, S. (1992) Inhaled nitric oxide after mitral valve replacement in patients with chronic pulmonary artery hypertension. *Anesthesiology* **77**: 880–883.

Goldman, A.P., Delius, R.E., Deanfield, J.E., Macrae, D.J. (1995) Nitric oxide is superior to prostacyclin for pulmonary hypertension after cardiac operations. *Ann Thorac Surg* **60**: 300–305.

Haddad, I.Y., Crow, J.P., Hu, P., Ye, Y., Beckman, J., Matalon, S. (1994) Concurrent generation of nitric oxide and superoxide damages surfactant protein A. *Am J Physiol* **267** (3 Pt 1): L242–L249.

Högman, M., Frostell, C., Arnberg, H., Sandhagen, B., Hedenstierna, G. (1994) Prolonged bleeding time during nitric oxide inhalation in the rabbit. *Acta Physiol Scand* **151**: 125–129.

Horwitz, L.D., Bishop, V.S., Stone, H.L. (1968) Effects of hypercapnia on the cardiovascular system of conscious dogs. *J Appl Physiol* **25**: 346–348.

Hugod, C. (1979) Effective exposure to 43 ppm nitric oxide and 3.6 ppm nitrogen dioxide on rabbit lung: a light in electron microscopic study. *Intl Arch Occup Environ Health* **42**: 159–167.

Kinsella, J.P., Neish, S.R., Shafer, E., Abman, S.H. (1992) Low-dose inhalational nitric oxide in primary pulmonary hypertension of the newborn. *Lancet* **340**: 819–820.

Kinsella, J.P., Ivy, D., Abman, S.H. (1994) Ontogeny of NO activity and response to inhaled NO in the developing ovine pulmonary circulation. *Heart Circ Physiol* **36**: H1955–H1961.

Krafft, P., Fridrich, P., Fitzgerald, R.D., *et al.* (1996) Effectiveness of nitric oxide inhalation in septic ARDS. *Chest* **109**: 486–493.

Kurose, I., Wolf, R., Grisham, M.B., Granger, D.N. (1994) Modulation of ischemia/reperfusion-induced microvascular dysfunction by nitric oxide. *Circ Res* **74**: 376–382.

Levy, B., Bollaert, P.E., Bauer, P., *et al.* (1995) Therapeutic optimization including inhaled nitric oxide in adult respiratory distress syndrome in a polyvalent intensive care unit. *J Trauma* **38**: 370–374.

Lönqvist, P.A., Winberg, P., Lundell, B., Selldén, H., Olsson, G.L. (1994) Inhaled nitric oxide in neonates and children with pulmonary hypertension. *Acta Paediatr* **83**: 1132–1136.

Lowson, S.M., Rich, G.F., McArdle, P.A., *et al.* (1996) The response to varying concentrations of inhaled nitric oxide in patients with acute respiratory distress syndrome. *Anesth Analg* **82**: 574–581.

Macdonald, P., Mundy, J., Rogers, P., Harrison, G., Branch, J., Glanville, A., Keogh, A., Spratt, P. (1995) Successful treatment of life-threatening acute reperfusion injury after lung transplantation with inhaled nitric oxide. *J Thorac Cardiovasc Surg* **110**: 861–863.

Miller, C.C. (1994) Chemiluminescence analysis and nitrogen dioxide measurement. *Lancet* **343**: 300–301.

Miller, O.I., Celermajer, D.S., Deanfield, J.E., Macrae, D.J. (1994) Guidelines for the safe administration of inhaled nitric oxide. *Arch Dis Child* **70**: F47–F49.

Moinard, J., Manier, G., Pillet, O., Castaing, Y. (1994) Effect of inhaled nitric oxide on hemodynamics and VA/Q inequalities in patients with chronic obstructive pulmonary disease. *Am J Respir Crit Care Med* **149**: 1482–1487.

Moncada, S., Palmer, R.M.J., Higgs, E.A. (1991) Nitric oxide: physiology, pathophysiology, and pharmacology. *Pharmacol Rev* **43**: 109–142.

Nelin, L.D., Moshin, J., Thomas, C.J., Sasidharan, P., Dawson, C.A. (1994) The effect of inhaled nitric oxide on the pulmonary circulation of the neonatal pig. *Pediatr Res* **35**: 20–24.

Oda, H., Nogami, H., Kushumoto, S., *et al.* (1976) Long-term exposure to nitric oxide in mice. *J Jpn Soc Air Pollut* **11**: 150–160.

Palmer, R.M.J., Ferrige, A.G., Moncada, S.A. (1987) Nitric oxide release accounts for the biological activity of endothelium-derived relaxing factor. *Nature* **327**: 524–526.

Pepke-Zaba, J., Higgenbottam, T.W., Dinh-Xuan, A.T., Stone, D., Wallwork, J. (1991) Inhaled nitric oxide as a cause of selective pulmonary vasodilation in pulmonary hypertension. *Lancet* **338**: 1173–1174.

Pfeffer, K.D., Ellison, G., Robertson, D., Day, R.W. (1996) The effect of inhaled nitric oxide in pediatric asthma. *Am J Respir Crit Care Med* **153**: 747–751.

Pickett, J.A., Moors, A.H., Latimer, R.D., Mahmood, N., Ghosh, A., Oduro, A. (1994) The role of soda lime during administration of inhaled nitric oxide. *Br J Anaesth* **72**: 683–685.

Pinelli, G., Mertes, P.M., Carteaux, J.P., Hubert, T., Dopff, C., Burtin, P., Villemot, J.P. (1996) Inhaled nitric oxide as an adjunct to pulmonary thromboendarterectomy. *Ann Thorac Surg* **61**: 227–229.

Putensen, C., Räsänen, J., Lopéz, F.A., Downs, J.B. (1994) Continuous positive airway pressure modulates effect of inhaled nitric oxide on the ventilation-perfusion distributions in canine lung injury. *Chest* **106**: 1563–1569.

Puybasset, L., Rouby, J.J., Mourgeon, E. *et al.* (1994a) Inhaled nitric oxide in acute respiratory failure: dose–response curves. *Intensive Care Med* **20**: 319–327.

Puybasset, L., Stewart, T., Rouby, J-S. *et al.* (1994b) Inhaled nitric oxide reverses the increase in pulmonary vascular resistance induced by permissive hypercapnia in patients with acute respiratory distress syndrome. *Anesthesiology* **80**: 1254–1267.

Puybasset, L., Rouby, J-J., Mourgeon, E., *et al.* (1995) Factors influencing cardiopulmonary effects of inhaled nitric oxide in acute respiratory failure. *Am J Respir Crit Care Med* **152**: 318–328.

Roberts Jr, J.D., Polander, D.M., Lang, P., Zapol, W.M. (1992) Inhaled nitric oxide in primary pulmonary hypertension of the newborn. *Lancet* **340**: 818–819.

Roberts Jr, J.D., Chen, T.Y., Kawai, N., Wain, J., Dupuy, P., Shimouchi, A., Bloch, K., Polaner, D., Zapol, W.M. (1993) Inhaled NO reverses pulmonary vasoconstriction in the hypoxic and acidotic newborn lamb. *Circ Res* **72**: 246–254.

Rossaint, R., Falke, K.F., Lopez, F., *et al.* (1993) Inhaled nitric oxide for the adult respiratory distress syndrome. *N Engl J Med* **328**: 399–405.

Rossaint, R., Gerlach, H., Schmidt-Ruhnke, H., *et al.* (1995) Efficacy of inhaled nitric oxide in patients with severe ARDS. *Chest* **107**: 1107–1115.

Samama, C.M., Diaby, M., Fellahi, J-L., Mdhafar, A., Eyraud, D., Arock, M., Guillosson, J-J., Coriat, P., Rouby, J-J. (1995a) Inhibition of platelet aggregation by inhaled nitric oxide in patients with acute respiratory distress syndrome. *Anesthesiology* **83**: 56–65.

Samama, C.M., Diaby, M., Fellachi, J-L., *et al.* (1995b) Inhibition of platelet aggregation by inhaled nitric oxide in patients with acute respiratory distress syndrome. *Anesthesiology* **83**: 56–65.

Scherrer, U., Vollenweider, L., Delabays, A., Savcic, M., Eichenberger, U., Kleger, G-R., Fikrle, A., Ballmer, P.E., Nicod, P., Bartsch, P. (1996) Inhaled nitric oxide for high-altitude pulmonary edema. *N Engl J Med* **334**: 624–629.

Semigran, M.J., Cockrill, B.A., Kacmarek, R., Thompson, B.T., Zapol, W.M. (1994) Hemodynamic effects of inhaled nitric oxide in heart failure. *J Am Coll Cardiol* **24**: 982–988.

Shanley, C.J., Hirschl, R.B., Shumacher, R.E., Overbeck, M.C., Delosh, T.N., Chapman, R.A., Coran, A.G., Barlett, R.H. (1994) Extracorporeal life support for neonatal respiratory failure. A 20-year experience. *Ann Surg* **220**: 269–280.

Sitbon, O., Brenot, F., Denjean, A., Bergeron, A., Parent, F., Azarian, R., Herve, P., Raffestin, B., Simonneau, G. (1995) Inhaled nitric oxide as a screening vasodilator agent in primary pulmonary hypertension. A dose-response study and comparison with prostacyclin. *Am J Respir Crit Care Med* **151**: 384–399.

Slutsky, A.S. (1993) ACCP consensus conference – mechanical ventilation. *Chest* **104**: 1833–1859.

Stenqvist, O., Kjelltoft, B., Lundin, S. (1993) Evaluation of a new system for ventilatory administration of nitric oxide. *Acta Anaesthesiol Scand* **37**: 687–691.

Tiballs, J., Hochmann, M., Carter, B., Osborne, A. (1993) An appraisal of techniques for administration of gaseous nitric oxide. *Anaesth Intensive Care* **21**: 844–847.

Valvini, E.M., Young, J.D. (1995) Serum nitrogen oxides during nitric oxide inhalation. *Br J Anaesth* **74**: 338–339.

Walther, F.J., Benders, M.J., Leighton, J.O. (1993) Early changes in the neonatal circulatory transition. *J Pediatr* **123**: 625–632.

Watkins, D.N., Jenkins, I.R., Rankin, J.M., Clarke, G.M. (1993) Inhaled nitric oxide in severe acute respiratory failure. Its use in intensive care and description of a delivery system. *Anaesth Intensive Care* **21**: 861–875.

Weigel, T.J., Hageman, J.R. (1990) National survey of diagnosis and management of persistent pulmonary hypertension of the newborn. *J Perinatol* **10**: 369–375.

Wessel, D.L., Adatia, I., Thompson, J.E., Hickey, P.R. (1994) Delivery and monitoring of inhaled nitric oxide in patients with pulmonary hypertension. *Crit Care Med* **22**: 930–938.

Westfelt, U.N., Benthin, G., Lundin, S., Stenqvist, O., Wennmalm, A. (1995) Conversion of inhaled nitric oxide to nitrate in man. *Br J Pharmacol* **114**: 1621–1624.

Wink, D.A., Hanbauer, I., Laval, F. (1994) Nitric oxide protects against the cytotoxic effects of reactive oxygen species. *Ann NY Acad Sci* **738**: 265–278.

Young, J.D. (1994) A universal nitric oxide delivery system. *Br J Anaesth* **73**: 700–702.

Young, J.D., Brampton, W.J., Knighton, J.D., Finfer, S.R. (1994) Inhaled nitric oxide in acute respiratory failure in adults. *Br J Anaesth* **73**: 499–502.

Zapol, W.M., Rimar, S., Gillis, N., Marletta, M., Bosken, C.H. (1994) NHLBI workshop summary: nitric oxide and the lung. *Am J Respir Crit Care Med* **149**: 1375–1380.

Zayek, M., Wild, L., Roberts, J.D. Jr, Morin III, F.C. (1993a) Effect of nitric oxide on the survival rate and incidence of lung injury in newborn lambs with persistent pulmonary hypertension. *J Pediatr* **123**: 947–952.

Zayek, M., Cleveland, D., Morin III, F.C. (1993b) Treatment of persistent pulmonary hypertension in the newborn lamb by inhaled nitric oxide. *J Pediatr* **122**: 743–750.

Zimmerman, J.L., Taylor, R.W., Dellinger, R.P., *et al.* (1996) Acute response to inhaled nitric oxide (NO) in acute respiratory distress syndrome (ARDS). *Chest* **110** (Suppl.): 58S.

3

The Choice of Inotropic Drugs in Patients with Sepsis

Andreas Meier-Hellmann, Konrad Reinhart

INTRODUCTION

An appropriate choice of catecholamines in the treatment of patients with sepsis requires, first, a clear understanding of the various pharmacological effects of catecholamines and, secondly, a concept of which physiological targets should be reached in septic patients. The first of these is much more easily achieved than the second. There is widespread knowledge of the effects of catecholamines on the different catecholamine receptors (Table 3.1) which, when coupled with knowledge of the location of catecholamine receptors in the various regions, should allow us to predict fairly clearly the advantages and disadvantages of the various catecholamines on the global and regional perfusion (Table 3.2). Unfortunately, the physiological endpoints for the treatment of patients with sepsis are not so clear. The long-standing practice of many intensivists to try to reach maximal or supranormal haemodynamic goals with catecholamine treatment (Kaufman *et al.*, 1984; Schumacker and Cain, 1987; Sibbald *et al.*, 1989; Tuchschmidt *et al.*, 1989) is being increasingly questioned as studies

Table 3.1 Effects of the different catecholamines on the different receptors

Catecholamine	Receptor					
	α_1	α_2	β_1	β_2	DA_1	DA_2
Dobutamine	++	0	+++	++	0	0
Epinephrine	+++	+++	++	+++	0	0
Norepinephrine	+++	+++	++	+	0	0
Dopamine:						
0–3 µg/kg/min	0	+	0	0	+++	++
2–10 µg/kg/min	+	+	++	+	++	++
>10 µg/kg/min	++	++	++	+	+	+
Dopexamine	0	0	+	+++	++	+

Table 3.2   Effects of the different catecholamines on regional blood flow

Catecholamine	Kidney	Brain	Heart	Splanchnic	Muscle	Skin
Dobutamine	+	+	+	+	++	+
Epinephrine	−/+	+	+	−/+	+/0	−
Norepinephrine	−/+	+	+	−/+	−/0	0
Dopamine:						
0–3 µg/kg/min	+++	+	0	+++	0	0
2–10 µg/kg/min	++/+	+	+	++/+	0	0
>10 µg/kg/min	−/+	+	+	−/+	−	−
Dopexamine	+++	+	+	+++	+	+

demonstrate that large increases in cardiac index or oxygen delivery (D_{O_2}) are not beneficial for all patients and may even be harmful in some (Hayes *et al.*, 1994; Gattinoni *et al.*, 1995). On the other hand, tissue hypoxia, especially in the splanchnic area, is still considered to be an important co-factor in the pathogenesis of multiple organ failure (MOF) (Deitch *et al.*, 1987; Marshall *et al.*, 1988; Meakins and Marshall, 1989; Fiddian-Green, 1991). Thus, the specific effects of inotropic drugs on splanchnic perfusion is of particular interest. Nelson *et al.* (1988) demonstrated that the critical D_{O_2} of the small intestine in septic sheep was higher than whole-body D_{O_2}. Therefore, the achievement of critical whole-body D_{O_2} does not exclude oxygen supply dependency in specific tissues (Nelson *et al.*, 1988). Previous studies have not conclusively demonstrated a reduction of splanchnic perfusion in sepsis, perhaps because different models and methods were used to measure splanchnic perfusion (Dahn *et al.*, 1989). In laboratory experiments of sepsis (Lang *et al.*, 1984; Wang *et al.*, 1991), it has been reported that redistribution of blood flow and relative improvement in hepatic and small intestine perfusion occur. In healthy individuals, an infusion of endotoxin doubled splanchnic blood flow (Fong *et al.*, 1990). In septic patients, Dahn *et al.* (1987) demonstrated that splanchnic perfusion increased to the same extent as the cardiac output (CO), although the splanchnic oxygen consumption (V_{O_2}hep) increased to a far greater extent than whole-body oxygen consumption (V_{O_2}). We found that 60% of the cardiac output in septic patients was distributed through the splanchnic region, in comparison to 18–30% in healthy individuals. (Leevy *et al.*, 1961; Johnson and McNamara, 1981). Considering this marked change in splanchnic blood flow, it is not surprising that the effects of catecholamines are different in septic and non-septic patients. However, little is known with certainty about the influence of various catecholamines on regional blood flow and oxygenation under the specific conditions of sepsis (Brown *et al.*, 1996).

Therefore, the current clinical practices outlined below, which are typical of those used in many institutions, are based on very limited scientific and clinical data:

- The use of β-mimetics to counteract the negative inotropic effects of sepsis on the heart and to increase D_{O_2} to very high levels.
- Avoidance, or infusion at as low doses as possible, of vasopressors due to the risk of deterioration in splanchnic and renal perfusion.
- The use of dopaminergic agents to increase perfusion in the renal and splanchnic regions.

It has not yet been proven how useful these three guiding recommendations are in the treatment of patients with sepsis. There is evidence that the effects of catecholamines on global and regional perfusion (see Tables 3.1 and 3.2), which were typically investigated in patients without sepsis, may be different in sepsis or septic shock (Bersten *et al.*, 1992). Therefore, a re-evaluation of the various catecholamine effects under the special conditions of sepsis is needed.

CATECHOLAMINES GENERALLY USED

Dobutamine

Many authors suggest that dobutamine, due to its predominant β_1-receptor-mediated effects, is the catecholamine of choice for increasing myocardial contractility and achieving supranormal CO and D_{O_2} levels (Dhainaut *et al.*, 1990; Reinhart *et al.*, 1990; Shoemaker *et al.*, 1989, 1993). Animal investigations (Vincent *et al.*, 1987) and clinical studies (Gilbert *et al.*, 1986; Vincent *et al.*, 1990) have shown that an increase in D_{O_2} following dobutamine infusion leads to an increased V_{O_2}. Furthermore, it is hypothesized that the β_2-mediated effects counteract peripheral vasoconstriction and hence improve tissue oxygenation (Shoemaker *et al.*, 1989).

The concept that increasing D_{O_2} by the use of β-mimetic catecholamines can be beneficial in septic patients is supported by data from Gutierrez *et al.* (1994), who found an increase in gastric mucosal pH (pH_i) in septic patients after treatment with dobutamine despite an unchanged V_{O_2}. Under the conditions of an adequate volume replacement, dobutamine increases cardiac output and D_{O_2} to a greater extent than does dopamine (Vincent *et al.*, 1987). Vincent *et al.* (1990) demonstrated that an infusion of dobutamine at 5 µg/kg/min in adequately volume-resuscitated septic patients increased the D_{O_2} by 29% and the V_{O_2} by 18%. Furthermore, they speculated that dobutamine decreased the maldistribution of tissue perfusion. Hannemann *et al.* (1995) demonstrated in septic patients that a combination of dobutamine with norepinephrine, in comparison to dopamine alone, infused to achieve a similar mean arterial pressure, is associated with a lower heart rate, lower filling pressures, and lower intrapulmonary shunting. A higher D_{O_2} with dopamine alone was not associated with a higher oxygen consumption; therefore, the authors concluded that, by comparison, dopamine did not improve tissue oxygenation but induced a greater myocardial stress and impaired pulmonary gas exchange.

To our knowledge, it is not yet clear whether dobutamine selectively influences splanchnic or renal perfusion. Improvement in splanchnic perfusion and oxygenation is supported by the results of Silverman and Tuma (1992), who found that infusion of dobutamine at 5 µg/kg/min increased a pathologically reduced pH_i. In contrast, blood transfusion alone did not influence pH_i but increased D_{O_2} to a similar extent. In septic pigs, Schneider *et al.* (1987) found that adequate volume substitution alone restored a decreased cardiac output and led to redistribution of blood flow in favour of the splanchnic region. An additional infusion of dobutamine did not influence the distribution of blood flow to the kidneys and the splanchnic region. In patients with congestive heart failure, Leier (1988) found that those who received dobutamine at 7.5 µg/kg/min experienced an increase in CO, and to a lesser extent renal perfusion, but a decrease in splanchnic perfusion. Mousdale *et al.* (1988) were able to measure only minor increases in renal blood flow under dobutamine and dopexamine, while various doses of dopamine induced remarkable increases in the renal flow.

Hayes *et al.* (1994) demonstrated that there was no difference in global V_{O_2} between a group of 50 patients treated with dobutamine up to 200 µg/kg/min to achieve three goals (cardiac index >4.5 l/min/m^2, D_{O_2} >600 ml/min/m^2, V_{O_2} >170 ml/min/m^2) established on the basis of previously published recommendations (Shoemaker *et al.*, 1988a, b; Bland *et al.*, 1995) and 50 patients who were treated only with an adequate-volume therapy. Contrary to what might have been expected, the survival in the patients with the dobutamine treatment was lower than in the control group. The authors speculated that the aggressive dobutamine treatment in an attempt to increase V_{O_2} may have been detrimental in some patients.

In conclusion, when dobutamine is used to increase D_{O_2} there is some evidence of an improvement in tissue oxygenation. Nevertheless, there is no clear recommendation as to what extent the D_{O_2} should be increased, and it is doubtful that there is an optimum D_{O_2} level appropriate for all septic patients. Therefore, the increase of D_{O_2} by the use of dobutamine should be monitored carefully using methods that indicate changes in tissue oxygenation, such as the measurement of lactate, or the measurement of regional CO_2 production (pH_i), or changes in Vo_2. Whether dobutamine selectively influences regional blood flow remains unknown. Management of septic shock with dobutamine alone is often not sufficient to restore adequate blood pressure; in most patients it must be combined with a vasopressor. Whether the combination of dobutamine and norepinephrine is superior to the treatment with dopamine alone has not yet been conclusively demonstrated, but there is evidence that the use of dobutamine is at least as effective as dopamine.

Norepinephrine

Norepinephrine has only moderate β_1- and β_2-mimetic effects. In experimental models it increased splanchnic vascular resistance and decreased splanchnic blood flow (Granger *et al.*, 1980). In fact, norepinephrine is used in animal studies to induce renal failure (Mills *et al.*, 1960). Consequently, norepinephrine is often only used as a last resort if haemodynamic stabilization is not achieved with other catecholamines (Shoemaker *et al.*, 1991).

Melchior *et al.* (1987) found that an infusion of 0.5 or 1.0 µg/kg/min norepinephrine did not change whole-body Vo_2, despite an increased cardiac index (CI) and mean arterial pressure (MAP). They concluded that the beneficial β-mimetic effects of norepinephrine outweigh the possible deleterious effects mediated by α-receptors. In septic dogs, Bakker and Vincent (1993) demonstrated an increase in right and left ventricular stroke work index with an infusion of norepinephrine ranging from 0.1 to 0.2 µg/kg/min and an increase in Do_2 and Vo_2 with an infusion of norepinephrine from 0.5 to 1.0 µg/kg/min. Schneider *et al.* (1987) recommended norepinephrine over dobutamine for the treatment of right heart failure in septic shock, since an increase in diastolic blood pressure improves myocardial perfusion. Schreuder *et al.* (1989) reported that a norepinephrine infusion in patients in septic shock increased Vo_2 but did not change Do_2. However, it remains unknown how much of the increase in Vo_2 is due to an improvement in perfusion pressure, which increased simultaneously from 57 to 75 mmHg. This finding underlines the importance of an adequate perfusion pressure and shows that treatment with norepinephrine is indicated if an adequate perfusion pressure cannot be maintained with volume substitution and dobutamine or dopamine. In six patients with septic shock in whom haemodynamic stabilization by dopamine or dobutamine infusion was not achieved, Do_2 and Vo_2 values were inconsistent when they were treated with norepinephrine

(Meadows *et al.*, 1988). In our own investigations (Specht *et al.*, 1993), the change in catecholamine treatment from dobutamine to norepinephrine in patients with septic shock led to a decrease in Do_2 but Vo_2 remained unchanged, suggesting an unchanged tissue oxygenation. However, redistribution of blood flow with norepinephrine treatment alone, undetected by the measurement of the global oxygen transport-related variables, cannot be excluded.

Several authors have demonstrated an increase in urine output in patients with septic shock treated with norepinephrine (Desjars *et al.*, 1987; Hesselvik and Brodin, 1989; Martin *et al.*, 1990); however, it should be emphasized that these patients had markedly decreased blood pressures. In the study by Desjars *et al.* (1987), the infusion of 0.5–1.0 µg/kg/min norepinephrine increased the MAP from 48 to 62 mmHg. Hesselvik and Brodin (1989) reported an increase in MAP from 50 to 69 mmHg after the infusion of 0.5 µg/kg/min norepinephrine. The principal mechanism of improved renal function in these studies is the increase in perfusion pressure to an adequate level. Redl-Wenzl *et al.* (1993) reported an increase in creatinine clearance after treatment with norepinephrine in 56 patients with septic shock. However, in this study the patients also had an inadequate perfusion pressure of 56 mmHg before treatment with norepinephrine. There is a lack of knowledge about whether treatment with norepinephrine has beneficial effects on renal function in the presence of an adequate perfusion pressure. Fukuoka *et al.* (1989) reported in septic patients with lactate levels in a normal range that a norepinephrine infusion increased urine output and did not change creatinine clearance, whereas in patients with elevated lactate levels norepinephrine had no effect on urine output but decreased creatinine clearance.

The findings concerning the effects of norepinephrine on splanchnic perfusion are inconsistent. Bersten *et al.* (1992) compared the effects of different catecholamines on regional blood flow in septic and non-septic sheep as measured by the microsphere technique. In the non-septic animals there was a redistribution of blood flow to the heart and away from brain, kidneys, liver and pancreas with norepinephrine, dobutamine, dopamine, dopexamine or salbutamol treatment. Thus, a deleterious effect of norepinephrine on splanchnic perfusion is demonstrated in these animals. In contrast, in septic animals no such redistribution of regional blood flow was found. The authors explained these findings by a decreased sensitivity of α-adrenergic receptors and a direct sepsis-associated vasodilatation (Baker and Wilmoth, 1984; Seaman and Greenway, 1984; Kato *et al.*, 1988; Gray *et al.*, 1990; Hollenberg *et al.*, 1992).

Schneider *et al.* (1987) infused pigs with *Escherichia coli* and stabilized the animals initially only by volume substitution. Further treatment with dobutamine or norepinephrine did not influence the distribution of the given volume, measured with radiolabelled erythrocytes. There was a decreased pooling of blood in the legs after norepinephrine infusion. Breslow *et al.* (1987) infused pigs with *E. coli* and kept the pulmonary capillary wedge pressure within the normal range by infusing isotonic solutions. Under these conditions norepinephrine, dopamine and phenylepinephrine given in doses to achieve a MAP of 75 mmHg were without selective effects on regional blood flow. A beneficial effect of norepinephrine on splanchnic oxygenation in septic patients was shown in a study by Marik and Mohedin (1994), who compared norepinephrine and dopamine given as vasopressors. Patients who were treated with norepinephrine had an increased pH_i, whereas dopamine led to a decrease in pH_i.

We measured the splanchnic blood flow in 10 patients with septic shock by the green dye dilution technique. After changing the catecholamine treatment from a combination of dobutamine with norepinephrine to norepinephrine alone we observed a parallel decrease in splanchnic perfusion and cardiac output. The relationship between splanchnic perfusion and cardiac output remained unchanged. Furthermore, the splanchnic VO_2 remained unchanged (Table 3.3). These findings are in contrast to the widespread opinion

Table 3.3 Effects of changing catecholamine treatment from a combination of dobutamine with norepinephrine to norepinephrine alone in 10 patients with septic shock

	Dobutamine + norepinephrine	Norepinephrine	p
DO_2 (ml/min/m^2)	796 ± 151	598 ± 113	*
VO_2 (ml/min/m^2)	159 ± 27	152 ± 26	NS
CI (l/min/m^2)	6.0 ± 1.2	4.3 ± 0.8	*
DO_2hep (ml/min/m^2)	210 ± 108	171 ± 88	*
VO_2hep (ml/min/m^2)	77 ± 41	72 ± 21	NS
HBF (l/min/m^2)	1.6 ± 0.8	1.1 ± 0.6	*
DO_2/DO_2hep	4.3 ± 1.4	4.1 ± 1.7	NS
VO_2/VO_2hep	4.9 ± 2.5	4.8 ± 1.3	NS
CI/HBF	4.3 ± 1.4	4.1 ± 1.7	NS
S_vO_2 (%)	76 ± 4	71 ± 6	*
$S_{hv}O_2$ (%)	58 ± 13	49 ± 15	*

DO_2, Oxygen delivery; VO_2, oxygen consumption; CI, cardiac index; DO_2hep, splanchnic oxygen delivery; VO_2hep, splanchnic oxygen consumption; HBF, hepatic blood flow; S_vO_2, mixed venous oxygen saturation; $S_{hv}O_2$, hepatic venous oxygen saturation.
* Statistically significant ($p < 0.5$); NS, not significant.

generated from studies in non-septic animals (Granger *et al.*, 1980; Reilly *et al.*, 1981; Giraud and MacCannell, 1984) that norepinephrine selectively decreases splanchnic perfusion, whereas a study in septic animals (Bersten *et al.*, 1992) also reported an unchanged splanchnic perfusion with norepinephrine. Nevertheless, due to the decrease in splanchnic D_{O_2}, hepatic venous oxygen extraction increased in our study. Therefore, in situations where there is a further decrease in splanchnic D_{O_2}, there is an increased risk that splanchnic V_{O_2} may become supply dependent with norepinephrine treatment alone.

In conclusion, treatment with vasopressors is often indispensable in the therapeutic management of septic shock. Provided that the D_{O_2} is in a supranormal range, treatment with norepinephrine alone is probably without negative tissue-oxygenation effects. Both animal and human studies have shown that the negative effect of norepinephrine on splanchnic perfusion is only seen in non-septic conditions.

Epinephrine

The rationale for using epinephrine in the treatment of septic shock is its β-receptor-mediated increase in cardiac output and α-receptor-mediated increase in perfusion pressure (Bollaert *et al.*, 1990; Lipman *et al.*, 1991; Mackenzie *et al.*, 1991). Low doses of epinephrine have predominantly β-mimetic effects, and only at higher doses do the α-mimetic effects become predominant (Innes & Nickerson, 1975). Bollaert *et al.* (1990) investigated the effects of epinephrine in doses of 0.5–1.0 µg/kg/min in 13 patients with septic shock who could not be stabilized by 15 µg/kg/min dopamine. Epinephrine increased MAP, systemic vascular resistance and cardiac output in these patients. Furthermore, the D_{O_2} and V_{O_2} increased. Elevated arterial lactate levels were interpreted as a direct metabolic effect of the epinephrine. Moran *et al.* (1993) reported an increase in D_{O_2} from 481 to 531 ml/min/m^2 and an increase in V_{O_2} from 165 to 193 ml/min/m^2 with epinephrine infusion in doses up to 18 µg/min in patients with septic shock. In animal studies, epinephrine has produced both a dose-dependent reduction (Haddy *et al.*, 1962, 1967; Pawlik *et al.*, 1975) and an increase in splanchnic perfusion (Greenway and Lawson, 1966). Little is known about the effects of epinephrine on splanchnic and renal perfusion shock states.

In our own investigations in septic patients, changing the catecholamine treatment from a combination of dobutamine and norepinephrine to epinephrine alone, titrated to achieve the same MAP, decreased the $S_{hv}O_2$ but did not change the S_vO_2, indicating a redistribution of blood flow at the expense of the splanchnic region (Meier-Hellmann *et al.*,

1994). Dahn *et al.* (1988) reported a parallel decrease in $S_{hv}O_2$ and S_vO_2 during hypoxia. In contrast, in 33 patients undergoing liver surgery the $S_{hv}O_2$ decreased and the S_vO_2 did not change after skin incision (Kainuma *et al.*, 1991). The authors explained this discrepancy as being a selective decrease in splanchnic perfusion mediated by endogenous catecholamines liberated following the incision. The selective decrease in $S_{hv}O_2$ seems to be a marker for deterioration in splanchnic oxygenation. We measured splanchnic perfusion, DO_2 and VO_2 in eight patients with septic shock treated with a combination of dobutamine and norepinephrine (Meier-Hellmann *et al.*, in press). After a change in treatment to epinephrine alone, titrated to achieve the same MAP as before, the DO_2 and VO_2 were unchanged, but splanchnic perfusion decreased in the presence of an unchanged cardiac output (Table 3.4). The decrease in splanchnic DO_2 led to a decrease in splanchnic VO_2. These changes in splanchnic oxygenation were not detected by whole-body DO_2 or VO_2, which both remained unchanged. This indicates the limitations of global measurements of DO_2 and VO_2 as markers of changes in tissue oxygenation. Deterioration of tissue oxygenation was also supported by an increase in lactate levels and a decrease in pH_i with the epinephrine. Similar findings were reported by Levy *et al.* (1995) who, in comparing a combination of dobutamine and norepinephrine to a treatment with epinephrine alone, also found an increase in lactate and a decrease in pH_i with epinephrine.

Table 3.4   Effects of changing catecholamine treatment from a combination of dobutamine with norepinephrine to epinephrine alone in 8 patients with septic shock

	Dobutamine + norepinephrine	Epinephrine	p
DO_2 (ml/min/m^2)	819 ± 120	822 ± 249	NS
VO_2 (ml/min/m^2)	145 ± 27	152 ± 45	NS
CI (l/min/m^2)	5.9 ± 0.9	5.9 ± 1.7	NS
DO_2hep (ml/min/m^2)	380 ± 170	222 ± 92	*
VO_2hep (ml/min/m^2)	107 ± 59	78 ± 39	*
HBF (l/min/m^2)	2.8 ± 1.4	1.6 ± 0.6	*
Fractional HBF (%)	47 ± 19	29 ± 14	*
Lactate:			
Arterial (mmol/l)	1.6 ± 0.8	2.9 ± 1.5	*
Mixed venous (mmol/l)	1.6 ± 0.8	3.0 ± 1.6	*
Hepatic venous (mmol/l)	1.3 ± 0.8	2.4 ± 1.5	*
Gastric mucosal pH	7.27 ± 0.08	7.19 ± 0.05	*

DO_2, oxygen delivery; VO_2, oxygen consumption; CI, cardiac index; DO_2hep, splanchnic oxygen delivery; VO_2hep, splanchnic oxygen consumption; HBF, hepatic blood flow.
* Statistically significant ($p < 0.5$); NS, not significant.

In conclusion, these findings point to a very limited role for epinephrine in septic patients, and in our opinion norepinephrine should be the vasopressor of first choice.

Dopamine

Dopamine has effects on α- and β-adrenergic as well as dopaminergic receptors, which are found in renal, mesenteric and hepatic vessels (Goldberg, 1972), and can be divided into presynaptic (DA_1) and post-synaptic (DA_2) receptors. Stimulation of DA_1 receptors causes renal and splanchnic vasodilatation. Stimulation of DA_2 receptors blocks norepinephrine output from sympathetic nerves (Goldberg, 1972). The effects of dopamine are dose dependent. In doses up to $3\,\mu g/kg/min$, dopamine selectively stimulates the dopaminergic receptors. In doses up to $5\,\mu g/kg/min$ there is stimulation of β-receptors, and in doses greater than $5\,\mu g/kg/min$ the α-receptors are also stimulated.

Vincent and Preiser (1993) advocated dopamine as the primary drug of choice in the management of decreased MAP in patients in septic shock. It is the opinion of other authors that the α-mimetic effects of dopamine are a disadvantage because a previously disturbed microcirculation could be further compromised (Vincent *et al.*, 1987; Shoemaker *et al.*, 1989). In 437 critical care patients, Shoemaker *et al.* (1991) were more frequently able to induce an increase in DO_2 and VO_2 with dobutamine than with dopamine. In brain-dead patients treatment with dopamine to elevate MAP to within a normal range caused a lower mitochondrial redox state in liver cells as compared to patients with a lower MAP who were not treated with dopamine (Nakatani *et al.*, 1991). This effect of dopamine can be interpreted as hypoxia-mediated organ failure.

Dopamine in low doses is often recommended as an additional drug for the improvement of renal function and splanchnic perfusion. In non-septic patients, Duke *et al.* (1994) showed that low-dose dopamine increased urine output without changing creatinine clearance, whereas low-dose dobutamine did not change urine output but increased creatinine clearance. In animals and healthy humans an increase in inulin clearance, renal plasma flow and sodium excretion has been shown after dopamine infusion (Goldberg, 1972). Mousdale *et al.* (1988) demonstrated that dopamine in doses of 2.5, 5.0 and $10.0\,\mu g/kg/min$ induced a significantly higher renal plasma flow than dobutamine in a similar dosage or dopexamine in doses of 1.0, 2.0 and $4.0\,\mu g/kg/min$ in healthy humans. Lherm *et al.* (1996) demonstrated in a group of septic patients that low-dose dopamine increased the urine output and the creatinine clearance in patients with severe sepsis, whereas there was no effect in patients with septic shock. Nevertheless, the beneficial effects in the patients with severe sepsis were only seen for 48 hours, and therefore the authors raised the possibility of down-regulation of the dopaminergic receptors. The effects of dopamine on renal function in patients with septic shock are not completely understood. It is not known whether dopamine affects the incidence of renal failure in septic shock patients.

Dopamine improved a decreased hepatic blood flow in dogs ventilated with positive end-expiratory pressure (Johnson *et al.*, 1991). In septic rats, dopamine induced a selective improvement in hepatic blood flow (Townsend *et al.*, 1987). It should be recognized that an increase in hepatic blood flow does not guarantee improved splanchnic oxygenation because a redistribution of blood flow in the splanchnic area may lead to a deterioration in tissue oxygenation. For example, Giraud and MacCannell (1984) infused dogs with dopamine and were able to measure an increase in blood flow in the superior mesenteric artery and in the muscularis of the gut, but they found decreased blood flow to the gut mucosa accompanied by a decrease in splanchnic V_{O_2}. Pawlik *et al.* (1976) demonstrated that intraarterial infusion of dopamine (1 μg/kg/min) in dogs caused splanchnic vasoconstriction with reduction of blood flow and splanchnic V_{O_2}. In the same investigation, epinephrine also led to a reduction in splanchnic blood flow but did not influence the splanchnic V_{O_2}. Therefore, the authors suggested that dopamine is a drug with deleterious side-effects on splanchnic oxygenation. In contrast to these findings, however, Kullmann *et al.* (1983) showed an increased blood flow to the intestinal organs and an improved perfusion of the mucosa and submucosa in rabbits as measured using a microsphere technique. In the above-mentioned study by Marik and Mohedin (1994), septic patients who were stabilized from septic shock with dopamine had a lower pH_i than did patients who received norepinephrine. Leier (1988) reported in congestive heart failure patients that 3 μg/kg/min dopamine significantly increased renal blood flow and did not change splanchnic blood flow. In nonseptic pigs, Roytblat *et al.* (1990) measured a dose-independent increase in splanchnic D_{O_2} and a dose-dependent increase in splanchnic V_{O_2} after dopamine infusion. Since higher doses of dopamine increased splanchnic V_{O_2} to a greater extent than splanchnic D_{O_2}, the authors concluded that dopamine did not improve splanchnic oxygenation and explained the increased splanchnic V_{O_2} as a calorigenic effect of dopamine (Jackson *et al.*, 1982; Ruttimann *et al.*, 1989; Regan *et al.*, 1990). In our studies, the addition of 2.8–3.0 μg/kg/min dopamine to norepinephrine increased $S_{hv}O_2$ more than S_vO_2, indicating redistribution of global blood flow in favour of splanchnic perfusion (Meier-Hellmann *et al.*, 1994). On one hand this finding correlates with the reported improvement of splanchnic blood flow under dopamine (Winsö *et al.*, 1985; Lundberg *et al.*, 1990; Johnson *et al.*, 1991). On the other hand, there is no guarantee that the increased $S_{hv}O_2$ is not the result of a decreased splanchnic V_{O_2}. In 11 patients with septic shock treated with norepinephrine we added dopamine in a dose of 2.8–3.0 µg/kg/min. In the patients who had a fractional splanchnic flow in a normal range, low-dose dopamine increased splanchnic perfusion, whereas in patients with an elevated fractional splanchnic flow before treatment we found no further increase, or even some decrease, in splanchnic flow (Meier-Hellmann *et al.*, 1997). This finding suggests that the effect of dopamine depends on the individual baseline splanchnic flow, which could vary from normal to markedly elevated in septic patients.

Furthermore, it is well known that prolonged dopamine infusion suppresses the circulating concentrations of pituitary-dependent hormones. This may be harmful to the already threatened metabolic and immunological homeostasis in critically ill patients. Dopamine infusion may induce hypoprolactinaemia, which can lead to impaired lymphocyte function and depressed lymphokine-dependent macrophage activation (Lucas *et al.*, 1990; Van den Berghe *et al.*, 1994b). Growth hormone and insulin-like growth factor-I concentrations are lower under dopamine infusion, which may be one reason for the difficulty of inducing anabolism by adequate feeding (Van den Berghe *et al.*, 1994b, c). It has been shown that dopamine reduces the serum concentrations of dehydroepiandrosterone sulphate, a steroid which plays an important role in the modulation of the immune response (Van den Berghe *et al.*, 1995). Dopamine infusion can induce or aggravate a low T_3 syndrome, and it is well known that T_3 has important effects on cardiac and haemodynamic function such as positive chronotropy and inotropy and reduced systemic vascular resistance (Van den Berghe *et al.*, 1994a).

In conclusion, it remains questionable whether management of septic shock with higher doses of dopamine alone, compared to the combination of dobutamine and norepinephrine, is advantageous. Whether low-dose dopamine can prevent renal failure has also not yet been proven. The improvement in some indicators of renal function would be an argument for the use of low-dose dopamine, although there are only a few studies to support this concept under the conditions of septic shock. Animal studies have reported deleterious effects of dopamine on splanchnic oxygenation. One study demonstrated an increased splanchnic V_{O_2} after dopamine infusion, but it remained unclear if the increased V_{O_2} was the result of improved oxygenation or simply the calorigenic effect of the catecholamine. Thus, to date the evidence favours the use of synthetic catecholamines over low-dose dopamine insofar as the effects on the pituitary-dependent hormones, which may adversely affect immunologic and haemodynamic function, are concerned.

Dopexamine

The relatively new catecholamine dopexamine has predominantly β_2- and dopaminergic-receptor activity. Many animal and human studies have described the usefulness of dopexamine in heart failure (Baumann *et al.*, 1988; De Marco *et al.*, 1988; Parratt *et al.*, 1988; Svenson *et al.* 1988). For example, Tan *et al.* (1987) have demonstrated a direct inotropic effect of dopexamine in patients with low-output cardiac failure.

To date, only a few studies have examined the effects of dopexamine in patients with septic shock. For example, Colardyn *et al.* (1989) reported an increase in cardiac index and heart rate and a decrease in systemic vascular resistance. Unfortunately, no data regarding DO_2 and VO_2 were mentioned. Among animal experiments, Cain and Curtis (1991) found no difference in mesenteric venous blood flow in a group of septic dogs treated with dopexamine and in a control group without catecholamine treatment. The gut of the dopexamine-treated animals produced less lactate and the authors concluded that dopexamine caused gut mucosa to be preferentially perfused. Biro *et al.* (1988) measured a relatively higher skeletal muscle and gastric blood flow in non-septic dogs with dopexamine in comparison to dobutamine. In dogs in haemorrhagic shock, Lokhandwala and Jandhyala (1992) demonstrated an increase in splanchnic perfusion of 40–50% from baseline after blood retransfusion, whereas splanchnic perfusion increased 80–90% from baseline if dopexamine was added to the transfusion.

Uusaro *et al.* (1995b) reported an increase in whole-body DO_2 and splanchnic DO_2 to a similar extent after dopexamine infusion in cardiac surgery patients. They did not find a specific effect on splanchnic blood flow after dopexamine infusion, as indicated by an unchanged fractional splanchnic blood flow. However, they did observe a decrease in pH_i, which could be a sign of severe splanchnic hypoxia induced by the cardiac surgery, but could be also an indicator of a redistribution of splanchnic blood flow and an underperfusion of gut mucosa, similar to the effect of low-dose dopamine. Smithies *et al.* (1994) reported an increase in pH_i in 10 septic patients treated with dopexamine to a maximum dose of 6.0 µg/kg/min. In patients meeting the criteria for the systemic inflammatory response syndrome, Maynard *et al.* (1995) demonstrated that 1 µg/kg/min dopexamine increased the pH_i, the indocyanin green (ICG) plasma disappearance rate and the monoethylglycinexylidide (MEGX) production rate, whereas 2.5 µg/kg/min dopamine had no effect on these parameters. A beneficial effect on outcome in 54 high-risk patients was reported by Boyd *et al.* (1993), who treated patients perioperatively with dopexamine to achieve a DO_2 of >600 ml/min/m^2. To clarify whether the reduced mortality in the study from Boyd *et al.* was truly an effect of the dopexamine treatment is the purpose of an ongoing multicentre trial.

In our own studies, the addition of 4.0 µg/kg/min dopexamine had no influence on the difference between S_vO_2 and $S_{hv}O_2$ (Meier-Hellmann *et al.*, 1994). This finding is consistent with the report by Leier (1988), who found that an increase in cardiac output in patients with heart failure accompanied an increase in splanchnic perfusion. Kuhly *et al.* (1995) demonstrated an increase in DO_2 and VO_2 in septic patients being treated with dopexamine, but they found no effect on the gastric or sigmoid pH_i.

Several studies have examined the effect of dopexamine on renal blood flow, although to date little is known about such effects in patients with septic shock. In both healthy subjects and patients with heart failure, dopexamine has been shown to increase urine output (Baumann *et al.*, 1990). In patients undergoing hepatic surgery, dopexamine caused no further increase in urine output in comparison to dopamine (Gray *et al.*, 1991). Stephan *et al.* (1990) demonstrated a more profound decrease in renal vascular resistance under dopamine than under dopexamine in cardiac surgery patients. The increase in renal blood flow was proportional to the increase in cardiac output. The authors therefore concluded that no selective dopaminergic effect of dopexamine was proven. Magrini *et al.* (1988) reported an increase in renal blood flow to a higher extent than an increased cardiac output in patients with hypertension receiving dopexamine. Mousdale *et al.* (1988) demonstrated that dopamine in doses of 2.5, 5.0 and 10.0 µg/kg/min increased renal plasma flow more than dopexamine in doses of 1.0, 2.0 and 4.0 µg/kg/min.

In conclusion, although some investigators recommend the use of dopexamine to improve splanchnic oxygenation and renal function, further studies are required to prove the usefulness of dopexamine in the treatment of septic shock patients and to compare the effects with those of low-dose dopamine.

Phosphodiesterase Inhibitors

Phosphodiesterase III decomposes cyclic adenosine-3′,5′ monophosphate (cAMP) in the myocardium. Inhibition of this enzyme (e.g. by enoximone or amrinone), results in an elevation of cAMP levels in cardiac cells. In cardiogenic shock patients, enoximone increases the left ventricular stroke work index and decreases the pulmonary capillary wedge pressure (Chaterjee, 1988). This is accompanied by a significant increase in Do_2 and Vo_2 (Vincent *et al.*, 1988a, b). A further increase in myocardial contractility can be achieved by combining phosphodiesterase inhibitors with a catecholamine such as dobutamine (Gage *et al.*, 1986). This potentially desired boost of cardiac function has also been observed in an endotoxaemic shock model where amrinone was combined with norepinephrine (De Boelpape *et al.*, 1989). Kox and Brydon (1991) have demonstrated increased Do_2 and Vo_2 in patients with septic shock being treated with enoximone, and they interpreted this as being due to improved tissue oxygenation.

Side-effects of phosphodiesterase inhibitors include an increase in pulmonary shunt volume accompanied by a drop in P_aO_2 (Vincent *et al.*, 1988a) and marked vasodilation. The latter can reduce venous return, making it necessary to restore cardiac filling pressures by fluid administration (Vincent *et al.*, 1988a, b). Furthermore, the long half-life of these substances makes the handling of these drugs difficult. Phosphodiesterase inhibitors have not been investigated in septic patients in a controlled manner. Therefore, these substances should only be used in this syndrome if cardiac failure occurs and does not respond to conventional catecholamine treatment.

Limitations

To give recommendations for the use of inotropic and vasopressor drugs in sepsis is difficult due not only to the lack of data on clinical outcome and organ dysfunction, but also to some limitations in the methods applied to assess regional perfusion and oxygenation. It is still unclear whether the pH_i really reflects the whole splanchnic area (Lang *et al.*, 1984; Uusaro *et al.*, 1995b). It is well known that sepsis markedly changes the relationship between blood flow from the portal system and the hepatic artery (Imamura and Clowes, 1975), and the measurement of splanchnic blood flow by a hepatic venous catheter technique cannot separate these two. An increase in splanchnic blood flow could be induced by increased blood flow in the hepatic artery with a simultaneous decrease in blood flow in the gut. The interpretation of the indocyanin green clearance or of lactate values is not easy and results are often unclear (Mizock and Falk, 1992; Uusaro *et al.*, 1995a).

The finding that the effects of low-dose dopamine on renal function may depend on the diagnosis of severe sepsis or septic shock, and that the effects on splanchnic blood flow may depend on whether the splanchnic blood flow was in a normal or in an elevated range before treatment, indicates that it is impossible to give universally valid recommendations for the use of catecholamines in septic patients. It seems logical that the use of catecholamines should be guided by the individual conditions in regional blood flow, but the estimation of regional blood flow under clinical conditions still has marked limitations.

Conclusion

In evaluating the guidelines listed at the outset for the use of catecholamines in septic patients against the different and sometimes controversial findings from the available studies, the first recommendation – to increase D_{O_2} by the use of β-mimetics – seems to be beneficial in some patients. It should be pointed out that there is no clear end-point for the increase of D_{O_2}, and therefore the D_{O_2} level should be guided by the measurement of parameters assessing global and regional oxygenation. At this point, the differences between dobutamine and dopamine do not appear large. Because dopamine led to a higher D_{O_2} but without increasing V_{O_2}, as well as a leading to higher heart rate and intrapulmonary shunting, the recommendation to use dobutamine as the catecholamine of first choice seems to be justified.

The second recommendation – to avoid vasopressors – is based on the experience with vasopressors in non-septic patients. For norepinephrine, no negative effects on regional perfusion have been demonstrated, provided the patient is adequately volume resuscitated and the D_{O_2} is normal or slightly elevated. Therefore, after volume resuscitation and treatment with dobutamine, norepinephrine should be used to achieve an adequate perfusion pressure. Unfortunately, similar to the increase in D_{O_2}, there are no clear end-points for volume loading and perfusion pressure. In various studies in critically ill and septic patients (Edwards *et al.*, 1989; Tuchschmidt *et al.*, 1992; Gattinoni *et al.*, 1995), the MAP target was between 74 and 88 mmHg and the PCWP target was between 12 and 16 mmHg. Whether these common end-points are really meaningful remains unclear, and thus the use of norepinephrine should also be guided by methods that detect tissue hypoxia. Because there is evidence that epinephrine could decrease splanchnic perfusion, it should not be used in septic patients.

We could find little evidence to support the third recommendation – the use dopaminergic drugs to increase renal or splanchnic perfusion. Neither low-dose dopamine nor dopexamine have been proven to prevent renal failure in septic patients. Furthermore, there is evidence that low-dose dopamine may reduce the mucosal perfusion in the gut in some patients, and thus its use is not recommended in septic patients. There is some suggestion that dopexamine can improve splanchnic perfusion as indicated by the measurement of pH_i, ICG plasma disappearance rate or MEGX production. But, since these effects remain somewhat controversial, there is no reason for a general recommendation for dopexamine in septic patients.

Thus, a reasonable approach in the use of catecholamines in septic patients includes, the following:

- To counteract the negative inotropic effects of sepsis and to increase DO_2, dobutamine may have slight advantages over dopamine.
- To achieve an adequate organ perfusion pressure use norepinephrine, or a combination of dobutamine with norepinephrine, which may have some advantages over high-dose dopamine. Epinephrine should be avoided because it seems to redistribute blood flow away from the splanchnic region.
- There are no convincing data to support the routine use of low-dose dopamine or dopexamine in patients with sepsis.

These recommendations are, of course, limited by the lack of definitive outcome studies and methods of measurement of regional perfusion/oxygenation. Until such limitations can be overcome, other alternative catecholamine regimens should not necessarily be dismissed as inferior.

COMMENTARY   Jeff Lipman, *Brisbane*

A positive inotropic agent is one that increases contractility. Contractility is an increase in force of contraction independent of preload and independent of afterload. The intravenous inotropic agents are dobutamine, epinephrine, norepinephrine, dopamine, dopexamine, isuprenaline, the phosphodiesterase inhibitors and the digitalis derivatives. All these agents also have peripheral vascular effects, i.e. they are not pure inotropic agents. Not infrequently, when choosing which inotropic agent to use the choice often incorporates these peripheral effects. For example, the neonatologists will use isuprenaline to increase cardiac output, as cardiac output is so heart-rate dependent in the neonate. However, 'marginal issues often make the most noise'. Seldom will experts differ on the drug of choice for a young, previously well, patient with rapid onset of community-acquired lobar pneumonia who has Gram-positive cocci on a sputum stain. When everyone has a different opinion on the 'drug of choice' for inotropic use in sepsis it suggests there is not one ideal agent and that there are many correct answers, or certainly many answers that are as imprecise as any other.

Tables 3.1 and 3.2 in Meier-Hellmann and Reinhart's article are the standard text outlines of the peripheral autonomic nervous system effects of the agents they describe. These effects are reproducible in animals and in human volunteers. One of the problems in sepsis is that these effects are not identically reproducible in septic patients. There is down-regulation of cardiac and vascular receptors, circulating negative inotropic factors, nitric oxide vascular effects and many other confounding effects, all complicating the cardiovascular and peripheral vascular effects of these drugs. The result of all this is that in the septic patient both the vascular and the cardiac effects of all these agents are highly unpredictable. To stress this, we and others have shown that the amount of drug needed to produce any desired end-point in sepsis varies from patient to patient, from day to day and that the vascular effect profile 'kicks in' at different doses in different patients. It is not possible to prescribe a dose *x* of inotropic agent for all patients for any desirable end-point (compare this to antibiotic use in sepsis).

Meier-Hellmann and Reinhart have produced an excellent review of the current literature covering inotropic agents in sepsis. I sometimes differ with their interpretation of the literature they quote, and therefore with some of their section conclusions, but that shouldn't detract from this admirable dissertation.

Our differences (and the ultimate problem) stems from the fact that there are no published outcome studies specifically comparing the different inotropic agents in sepsis. This necessitates the use of surrogate end-points in benefit analysis. Meier-Hellmann and Reinhart place enormous emphasis on decrements in stomach pH_i as an indication of splanchnic hypoperfusion to index danger and early warning of multi-organ dysfunction (Fiddian-Green, 1991). Many physicians may agree with this point of view, but in the last analysis this parameter can, at best, be regarded only as a surrogate end-point of outcome.

In the era of cost containment, I think a few words on costs would have been appreciated. Obviously the cost of a drug may vary from country to country, but epinephrine and norepinephrine are far cheaper than the other (synthetic) agents. A burning issue in my mind is what drug is the most cost-effective? I doubt whether we will ever have the answer to this.

BASIC RECIPE

Many intensive care units have a 'set of rules' for managing the haemo-dynamics of patients with severe sepsis. Ours is as follows:

- Attend to preload first, i.e. see that the patient is volume loaded.
- Maintain an adequate diastolic blood pressure.
- Maintain an adequate urine output (without a diuretic).
- Try to avoid too much tachycardia.
- Monitor serum lactate as a surrogate marker of morbidity, and if it rises increase (or alter) therapy; if it falls you are on the correct track.

One could easily dovetail the recommendations of the above article to this.

REFERENCES

Baker, C.H., Wilmoth, F.R. (1984) Microvascular responses to *E. coli* endotoxin with altered adrenergic activity. *Circ Shock* **12**: 165–176.

Bakker, J., Vincent, J.L. (1993) Effects of norepinephrine and dobutamine on oxygen transport and consumption in a dog model of endotoxic shock. *Crit Care Med* **21**: 425-432.

Baumann, G., Gutting, M., Pfafferott, C., *et al.* (1988) Comparison of acute haemodynamic effects of dopexamine hydrochloride, dobutamine and sodium nitroprusside in chronic heart failure. *Eur Heart J* **9**: 503–512.

Baumann, G., Felix, S.B., Filcek, S.A.L. (1990) Usefulness of dopexamine hydrochloride versus dobutamine in chronic congestive heart failure and effects on hemodynamics and urine output. *Am J Cardiol* **65**: 748–754.

Bersten, A.D., Hersch, M., Cheung, H., *et al.* (1992) The effect of various sympathomimetics on the regional circulations in hyperdynamic sepsis. *Surgery* **112**: 549–561.

Biro, G.P., Douglas, J.R., Keon, W.J., *et al.* (1988) Changes in regional blood flow distribution induced by infusions of dopexamine hydrochloride or dobutamine in anesthetized dogs. *Am J Cardiol* **62**: 30C–36C.

Bland, R.D., Shoemaker, W.C., Abraham, E., *et al.* (1995) Hemodynamic and oxygen transport patterns in surviving and nonsurviving postoperative patients. *Crit Care Med* **13**: 85–90.

Bollaert, P.E., Bauer, Ph., Audibert, G., *et al.* (1990) Effects of epinephrine on hemodynamics and oxygen metabolism in dopamine-resistant septic shock. *Chest* **98**: 949–953.

Boyd, O., Grounds, R.M., Bennett, E.D. (1993) A randomized clinical trial of the effect of deliberate perioperative increase of oxygen delivery on mortality in high-risk surgical patients. *JAMA* **270**: 2699–2707.

Breslow, M.J., Miller, C.F., Parker, S.D., *et al.* (1987) Effect of vasopressors on organ blood flow during endotoxin shock in pigs. *Am J Physiol* **252**: H291–H300.

Brown, R.S., Carey, J.S., Mohr, P.A., *et al.* (1966) Comparative evaluation of sympathomimetic amines in clinical shock. *Circulation* **34**: 260–271.

Cain, S.M., Curtis, S.E. (1991) Systemic and regional oxygen uptake and delivery and lactate flux in endotoxic dogs infused with dopexamine. *Crit Care Med* **19**: 1552–1560.

Chaterjee, K. (1988) Enoximone in heart failure: mechanisms of action. *Br J Clin Pract* **64**: 19–25.

Colardyn, F.C., Vandenbogaerde, J.F., Vogelaers, D.P., *et al.* (1989) Use of dopexamine hydrochloride in patients with septic shock. *Crit Care Med* **17**: 999–1003.

Dahn, M.S., Lange, P., Lobdell, K., *et al.* (1987) Splanchnic and total body oxygen consumption differences in septic and injured patients. *Surgery* **101**: 69–80.

Dahn, M.S., Lange, P., Jacobs, L.A. (1988) Central mixed and splanchnic venous oxygen saturation monitoring. *Intensive Care Med* **14**: 373–378.

Dahn, M.S., Lange, P., Lobdell, K., *et al.* (1989) Hepatic blood flow and splanchnic oxygen consumption measurements in clinical sepsis. *Surgery* **107**: 295–301.

De Boelpape, C., Vincent, J.L., Contempré, B. (1989) Combination of norepinephrine and amrinone in the treatment of endotoxin shock. *J Crit Care* **4**: 202–207.

Deitch, E.A., Berg, R., Specian, R. (1987) Endotoxin promotes the translocation of bacteria from the gut. *Arch Surg* **122**: 185–190.

De Marco, T., Kwasman, M., Lau, D., *et al.* (1988) Dopexamine hydrochloride in chronic congestive heart failure with improved cardiac performance without increased metabolic cost. *Am J Cardiol* **62**: 57C–62C.

Desjars, P., Pinaud, M., Potel, G., *et al.* (1987) A reappraisal of norepinephrine in human septic shock. *Crit Care Med* **15**: 134–137.

Dhainaut, J.F., Edwards, J.D., Grootendorst, A.F., *et al.* (1990) Practical aspects of oxygen transport: conclusions and recommendations of the Round Table Conference. *Intensive Care Med* **16**: 179–180.

Duke, G.J., Briedis, J.H., Weaver, R.A. (1994) Renal support in critically ill patients: low dose dopamine or low dose dobutamine. *Crit Care Med* **22**: 1919–1925.

Edwards, J.D., Brown, G.C., Nightingale, P., *et al.* (1989) Use of survivors' cardiorespiratory values as therapeutic goals in septic shock. *Crit Care Med* **17**: 1098–1103 .

Fiddian-Green, R.G. (1991) Role of gut in shock and resuscitation. In: Stoutenbeck, C.P., van Saene, H.K.F. (eds) *Infection and the Anesthetist*, Vol. 5 (1), pp. 75–99. London: Baillière Tindall/W.B. Saunders.

Fong, Y., Marano, M.A., Moldawer, L.L., *et al.* (1990) The acute splanchnic and peripheral tissue metabolic response to endotoxin in humans. *J Clin Invest* **85**: 1896–1904.

Fry, D.E., Pearlstein, L., Fulton, R.L. (1980) Multiple-system organ failure: the role of uncontrolled infection. *Arch Surg* **115**: 136–140.

Fukuoka, T., Nishimura, M., Imanaka, H., *et al.* (1989) Effects of norepinephrine on renal function in septic patients with normal and elevated lactate levels. *Crit Care Med* **17**: 1104–1107.

Gage, J., Rutman, H., Lucido, D., *et al.* (1986) Additive effects of dobutamine and amrinone on myocardial contractility and ventricular performance in patients with severe heart failure. *Circulation* **74**: 367–373.

Gattinoni, L., Brazzi, L., Pelosi, P., *et al.* (1995) A trial of goal-oriented hemodynamic therapy in critically ill patients. *N Engl J Med* **333**: 1025–1032.

Gilbert, E.M., Haupt, M.T., Mandanas, R.Y., *et al.* (1986) The effect of fluid loading, blood transfusion, and catecholamine infusion on oxygen delivery and consumption in patients with sepsis. *Am Rev Respir Dis* **134**: 873–878.

Giraud, G.D., MacCannell, K.L. (1984) Decreased nutrient blood flow during dopamine- and epinephrine-induced intestinal vasodilatation. *J Pharm Exp Ther* **230**: 214–220.

Goldberg, L.I. (1972) Cardiovascular and renal actions of dopamine. Potential clinical applications. *Pharmacol Rev* **24**: 1–29.

Granger, D.N., Richardson, P.D.I., Kvietys, P.R., *et al.* (1980) Intestinal blood flow. *Gastroenterology* **78**: 837–863.

Gray, G.A., Furman, B.L., Parratt, J.R. (1990) Endotoxin-induced impairment of vascular reactivity in the pithed rat: role of arachidonic acid metabolites. *Circ Shock* **31**: 395–406.

Gray, P.A., Bodenham, A.R., Park, G.R. (1991) A comparison of dopexamine and dopamine to prevent renal impairment in patients undergoing orthotopic liver transplantation. *Anaesthesia* **46**: 638–641.

Greenway, C.V., Lawson, A. (1966) The effects of adrenaline and noradrenaline on venous return and regional blood flow in the anesthetized cat with special reference to intestinal blood flow. *J Physiol (Lond)* **187**: 579–595

Gutierrez, G., Clark, C., Brown, S.D., *et al.* (1994) Effect of dobutamine on oxygen consumption and gastric mucosal pH in septic patients. *Am J Respir Crit Care Med* **150**: 324–329.

Haddy, F.J., Molnar, J.I., Borden, C.W., *et al.* (1962) Comparison of direct effects of angiotensin, and other vasoactive agents on small and large blood vessels in several vascular beds. *Circulation* **25**: 239–246.

Haddy, F.J., Chou, C.C., Scott, J.B., *et al.* (1967) Intestinal vascular responses to naturally occurring vasoactive substances. *Gastroenterology* **52**: 444–451.

Hannemann, L., Reinhart, K., Grenzer, O., *et al.* (1995) Comparison of dopamine to dobutamine and norepinephrine for oxygen delivery and uptake in septic shock. *Crit Care Med* **23**: 1962–1970.

Hayes, M.A., Timmins, A.C., Yau, E.H.S., *et al.* (1994) Elevation of systemic oxygen delivery in the treatment of critically ill patients. *N Engl J Med* **330**: 1717–1722.

Hesselvik, J.F., Brodin, B. (1989) Low dose norepinephrine in patients with septic shock and oliguria: Effects on afterload, urine flow, and oxygen transport. *Crit Care Med* **17**: 179–180.

Hollenberg, S.M., Cunnion, R.E., Parrillo, J.E. (1992) Effect of septic serum on vascular smooth muscle: In vitro studies using rat aortic rings. *Crit Care Med* **20**: 993–998.

Imamura, M., Clowes, G.H.A. (1975) Hepatic blood flow and oxygen consumption in starvation, sepsis and septic shock. *Surg Gynecol Obstet* **141**: 27–34.

Innes, I.R., Nickerson, M. (1975) Norepinephrine, epinephrine and the sympathomimetic amines. In: Goodman, L.D., Gilman, A. (eds) *The Pharmacological Basis of Therapeutics.* pp. 483–504, New York: MacMillan.

Jackson, L.K., Key, B.M., Cain, S.M. (1982) Total and hindlimb O_2 uptake and blood flow in hypoxic dogs given dopamine. *Crit Care Med* **10**: 327–331.

Johnson, D.J., Johannigman, J.A., Branson, R.D., *et al.* (1991) The effect of low dose dopamine on gut hemodynamics during PEEP ventilation for acute lung injury. *J Surg Research* **50**: 344–349.

Johnson, G.A., McNamara, J.J. (1981) Organ ischemia after hemorrhagic shock. *Surg Forum* **32**: 24–26.

Kainuma, M., Fujiwara, Y., Kimura, N., *et al.* (1991) Monitoring hepatic venous hemoglobin oxygen saturation in patients undergoing liver surgery. *Anesthesiology* **74**: 49–52.

Kato, T., Hayashi, K., Takamizawa, K. (1988) Response of femoral arteries to norepinephrine following endotoxicosis. *Circ Shock* **26**: 383–390.

Kaufman, B.S., Rackow, E.C., Falk, J.L. (1984) The relationship between oxygen delivery and consumption during fluid resuscitation of hypovolemic and septic shock. *Chest* **85**(3): 337–340.

Kox, W.J., Brydon, C. (1991) Improvement of tissue oxygenation with enoximone in septic shock. In: Vincent. J.L. (ed.) *Update in Intensive Care and Emergency Medicine*, Vol. 14, pp. 137–143. Berlin: Springer-Verlag.

Kuhly, P., Oschmann, G., Specht, M., *et al.* (1995) Dopexamine hydrochloride does not improve gastric and sigmoid mucosal acidosis in critically ill patients. *Crit Care Med* **23**: (Suppl.): A106.

Kullmann, R., Breull, W.R., Reinsberg, J., *et al.* (1983) Dopamine produces vasodilation in specific regions and layers of the rabbit gastrointestinal tract. *Life Sciences* **32**: 2115–2122.

Lang, C.H., Bagby, G.J., Ferguson, J.L., *et al.* (1984) Cardiac output and redistribution of organ blood flow in hypermetabolic sepsis. *Am J Physiol* **246R**: 331–337.

Leevy, C.M., George, W., Lesko, W., *et al.* (1961) Observations on hepatic oxygen metabolism in man. *JAMA* **178**: 565–567.

Leier, C.V. (1988) Regional blood flow responses to vasodilators and inotropes in congestive heart failure. *Am J Cardiol* **62**: 86E–93E.

Levy, B., Bollaert, P.E., Nace, L., *et al.* (1995) Norepinephrine-dobutamine is better for splanchnic circulation than epinephrine in dopamine resistant septic shock. *Intensive Care Med* **21**: (Suppl. 1): S4 .

Lherm, T., Troché, G., Rossignol, M., *et al.* (1996) Renal effects of low-dose dopamine in patients with sepsis syndrome or septic shock treated with catecholamines. *Intensive Care Med* **22**: 213–219.

Lipman, J., Roux, A., Kraus, P. (1991) Vasoconstrictor effects of adrenaline in human septic shock. *Anaesth Intensive Care* **19**: 61–65.

Lokhandwala, M.F., Jandhyala, B.S. (1992) Effects of dopaminergic agonists on organ blood flow and function. *Clin Intensive Care* **3** (1) (Suppl.): 12–16.

Lucas, A., Baker, B.A., Cole, T.J. (1990) Plasma prolactin and clinical outcome in preterm infants. *Arch Dis Child* **65**: 977–983.

Lundberg, J., Lundberg, D., Norgren, L., *et al.* (1990) Intestinal hemodynamics during laparotomy: effects of thoracic epidural anesthesia and dopamine in humans. *Anesth Analg* **71**: 9–15 .

Mackenzie, S.J., Kapadia, F., Nimmo, G.R., *et al.* (1991) Adrenaline in treatment of septic shock: effects on hemodynamics and oxygen transport. *Intensive Care Med* **17**: 36–39.

Magrini, F., Foulds, R.A., Roberts, N., *et al.* (1988) Renal hemodynamic effects of dopexamine hydrochloride. *Am J Cardiol* **62**: 53C–56C.

Marik, P.E., Mohedin, M. (1994) The contrasting effects of dopamine and norepinephrine on systemic and splanchnic oxygen utilization in hyperdynamic sepsis. *JAMA* **272**: 1354–1357.

Marshall, J.C., Christou, N.V., Horn, R., *et al.* (1988) The microbiology of multiple organ failure: the proximal GI tract as an occult reservoir of pathogens. *Arch Surg* **123**: 309–315.

Martin, C., Eon, B., Saux, P., *et al.* (1990) Renal effects of norepinephrine used to treat septic shock patients. *Crit Care Med* **18**: 282–285.

Maynard, N.D., Bihari, D.J., Dalton, R.N., *et al.,* (1995) Increasing splanchnic blood flow in the critically ill. *Chest* **108**: 1648–1654.

Meadows, D., Edwards, J.D., Wilkins, R.G., *et al.* (1988) Reversal of intractable septic shock with norepinephrine therapy. *Crit Care Med* **16**: 663–666.

Meakins, J.L., Marshall, J.C. (1989) The gut as the motor of multiple system organ failure. In: Marston, A., Bulkley, G.B., Fiddian Green, R.G. *et al.* (eds) *Splanchnic Ischemia and Multiple Organ Failure*, pp. 339–348. St Louis: C.V. Mosby.

Meier-Hellmann, A., Hannemann, L., Specht, M., *et al.* (1994) The relationship between mixed venous and hepatic venous O_2 saturation in patients with septic shock. *Adv Exp Med Biol* **345**: 701–707.

Meier-Hellmann, A., Reinhart, K., Bredle, D.L., *et al.* (1997): The effects of low-dose dopamine on splanchnic perfusion and oxygen uptake in patients with septic shock. *Intensive Care Med* **23**: 31–37.

Meier-Hellmann, A., Reinhart, K., Bredle, DL., *et al.* (in press): Epinephrine impairs splanchnic perfusion in septic shock. *Crit Care Med.*

Melchior, J.C., Pinaud, M., Blanloeil, Y., *et al.* (1987) Hemodynamic effects of continuous norepinephrine infusion in dog with and without hyperkinetic endotoxic shock. *Crit Care Med* **15**: 687–691.

Mills, L.C., Moyer, J.H., Handley, C.A. (1960) Effects of various sympathicomimetic drugs on renal hemodynamics in normotensive and hypotensive dogs. *Am J Physiol* **198**: 1279 .

Mizock, B.A., Falk, J.L. (1992) Lactic acidosis in critical illness. *Crit Care Med* **20**: 80–93.

Moran, J.L., O'Fathartaigh, M.S., Peisach, A.R., *et al.* (1993) Epinephrine as an inotropic agent in septic shock: a dose-profile analysis. *Crit Care Med* **21**: 70–77.

Mousdale, S., Clyburn, P.A., Mackie, A.M., *et al.* (1988) Comparison of the effects of dopamine, dobutamine, and dopexamine upon renal blood flow: a study in normal healthy volunteers. *Br J Clin Pharmacol* **25**: 555–560.

Nakatani, T., Isihkawa, Y., Kobayashi, K., *et al.* (1991) Hepatic mitochondrial redox state in hypotensive brain-dead patients and an effect of dopamine administration. *Intensive Care Med* **17**: 103–107.

Nelson, D.P., Samsel, RW., Wood, L.D., *et al.* (1988) Pathologic supply dependence of systemic and intestinal O_2 uptake during endotoxemia. *J Appl Physiol* **64**: 2410–2419.

Parratt, J.R., Wainwright, C.L., Fagbemi, O. (1988) Effect of dopexamine hydrochloride in the early stages of experimental myocardial infarction and comparison with dopamine and dobutamine. *Am J Cardiol* **62**: 18C–23C.

Pawlik, W., Shepherd, A.P., Jacobson, E.D. (1975) Effects of vasoactive agents on intestinal oxygen consumption and blood flow in dogs. *J Clin Invest* **56**: 484–490.

Pawlik, W., Shepherd, A.P., Mailman, D., *et al.* (1976) Effects of dopamine and epinephrine on intestinal blood flow and oxygen uptake. In Grote, J., Reneau, D., Thews, G. (eds) *Oxygen Transport to the Tissue*, Vol. II, pp. 511–516. New York: Plenum Press.

Redl-Wenzl, E.M., Armbruster, C., Edelmann, G., *et al.* (1993) The effects of norepinephrine on hemodynamics and renal function in severe septic shock states. *Intensive Care Med* **19**: 151–154.

Regan, C.J., Duckworth, R., Fairhurst, J.A., *et al.* (1990) Metabolic effects of low-dose dopamine infusion in normal volunters. *Clin Sci* **79**: 605–611.

Reilly, F.D., McCusky, R.S., Cilento, E. (1981) Hepatic microvascular regulatory mechanisms. I. Adrenergic mechanisms. *Microvasc Res* **21**: 103–116.

Reinhart, K., Hannemann, L., Kuss, B. (1990) Optimal levels of O_2 delivery in the critically ill. *Intensive Care Med* **16**: 149–154.

Roytblat, L., Gelman, S., Bradley, E.L., *et al.* (1990) Dopamine and hepatic oxygen supply–demand relationship. *Can J Physiol Pharmacol* **68**: 1165–1169.

Ruttimann, Y., Chioléro, R., Jéquier, E., *et al.* (1989) Effects of dopamine on total oxygen consumption and oxygen delivery in healthy men. *Am J Physiol* **257**: E541–546.

Schneider, A.J., Groeneveld, A.B.J., Teule, G.J.J., *et al.* (1987) Volume expansion, dobutamine and noradrenaline for treatment of right ventricular dysfunction in porcine septic shock: a combined invasive and radionuclide study. *Circ Shock* **23**: 93–106.

Schreuder, W.O., Schneider, A.J., Groeneveld, A.B.J., *et al.* (1989) Effect of dopamine vs norepinephrine on hemodynamics in septic shock. Emphasis on right ventricular performance. *Chest* **95**: 1282–1288.

Schumacker, P., Cain, S. (1987) The concept of a critical oxygen delivery. *Intensive Care Med* **13**: 223–229.

Seaman, K.L., Greenway, C.V. (1984) Loss of hepatic venous responsiveness after endotoxin in anesthetized cats. *Am J Physiol* **246**: H658–H663.

Shoemaker, W.C., Appel, P.L., Kram, H.B., *et al.* (1988a) Prospective trial of supranormal values of survivors as therapeutic goals in high risk surgical patients. *Chest* **94**: 1176–1186.

Shoemaker, W.C., Appel, P.L., Kram, H.B. (1988b) Tissue oxygen debt as a determinant of lethal and nonlethal postoperative organ failure. *Crit Care Med* **16**: 117–120.

Shoemaker, W.C., Appel, P.L., Kram, H.B., *et al.* (1989) Comparison of hemodynamic and oxygen transport effects of dopamine and dobutamine in critically ill surgical patients. *Chest* **96**: 120–126.

Shoemaker, W.C., Appel, P.L., Kram, H.B. (1991) Oxygen transport measurements to evaluate tissue perfusion and titrate therapy: dobutamine and dopamine effects. *Crit Care Med* **19**: 672–688.

Shoemaker, W.C., Appel, P.L., Kram, H.B., *et al.* (1993) Hemodynamic and oxygen transport monitoring to titrate therapy in septic shock. *New Horizons* **1**: 145–159.

Sibbald, W.J., Bersten, A., Rutledge, F.S. (1989) The role of tissue hypoxia in multiple organ failure. In: Reinhart K., Eyrich, K. (eds) *Clinical Aspects of Oxygen Transport and Tissue Oxygenation*, pp. 102–114. Berlin: Springer-Verlag.

Silverman, H.J., Tuma, P. (1992) Gastric tonometry in patients with sepsis. Effects of dobutamine infusions and packed red blood cell transfusions. *Chest* **102**: 184–188.

Smithies, M., Yee, T.H., Jackson, L., *et al.* (1994) Protecting the gut and the liver in the critically ill: effects of dopexamine. *Crit Care Med* **22**: 789–795.

Specht, M., Meier-Hellmann, A., Hannemann, L. *et al.* (1993) Effects of dobutamine vs norepinephrine therapy on oxygen supply and oxygen consumption in septic patients. *Crit Care Med* **21** (Suppl.): S276.

Stephan, H., Sonntag, H., Henning, H., *et al.* (1990) Cardiovascular and renal haemodynamic effects of dopexamine: comparison with dopamine. *Br J Anaesth* **65**: 380–387.

Svenson, G., Strandberg, L.E., Lindvall, B., *et al.* (1988) Haemodynamic response to dopexamine hydrochloride in postinfarction heart failure: lack of tolerance after continuous infusion. *Br Heart J* **60**: 489–496.

Tan, L.B., Littler, A., Murray, R.G. (1987) Beneficial haemodynamic effects of intravenous dopexamine in patients with low-output heart failure. *J Cardiovasc Pharmacol* **10**: 280–286.

Townsend, M.C., Schirmer, W.J., Schirmer, J.M., *et al.* (1987) Low-dose dopamine improves effective hepatic blood flow in murine peritonitis. *Circ Shock* **21**: 149–153.

Tuchschmidt, J., Fried, J., Swinney, R., *et al.* (1989) Early hemodynamic correlations of survival in patients with septic shock. *Crit Care Med* **17**: 719–723.

Tuchschmidt, J., Fried, J., Astiz, M., *et al.* (1992) Elevation of cardiac output and oxygen delivery improves outcome in septic shock. *Chest* **102**: 216–220.

Uusaro, A., Ruokonen, E., Takala, J. (1995a) Estimation of splanchnic blood flow by the Fick principle in man and problems in the use of indocyanine green. *Cardiovasc Res* **30**: 106–112.

Uusaro, A., Ruokonen, E., Takala, J. (1995b) Gastric mucosal pH does not reflect changes in splanchnic blood flow after cardiac surgery. *Br J Anaesth* **74**: 149–154.

Van den Berghe, G., de Zegher, F., Lauwers, P. (1994a) Dopamine and the sick euthyroid syndrome in critical illness. *Clin Endocrinol* **41**: 731–737.

Van den Berghe, G., de Zegher, F., Lauwers, P. (1994b) Dopamine suppresses pituitary function in infants and children. *Crit Care Med* **22**: 1747–1753.

Van den Berghe, G., de Zegher, F., Lauwers, P., *et al.* (1994c) Growth hormone secretion in critical illness: effect of dopamine. *J Clin Endocrinol Metab* **79**: 1141–1146

Van den Berghe, G., de Zegher, F., Schetz, M., *et al.* (1995) Dehydroepiandrosterone sulphate in critical illness: effect of dopamine. *Clin Endocrinol* **43**: 451–463.

Vincent, J.L., Preiser, J.C. (1993) Inotropic agents. *New Horizons* **1**: 137–144.

Vincent, J.L., Van der Linden, P., Domb, M., *et al.* (1987) Dopamine compared with dobutamine in experimental septic shock: Relevance to fluid administration. *Anesth Analg* **66**: 565–571.

Vincent, J.L., Carlier, E., Berré, J., *et al.* (1988a) Administration of enoximone in cardiogenic shock. *Am J Cardiol* **62**: 419–423.

Vincent, J.L., Domb, M., van der Linden, P., *et al.* (1988b) Amrinone administration in endotoxic shock. *Circ Shock* **26**: 75–83.

Vincent, J.L., Roman, A., Kahn, R.J. (1990) Dobutamine administration in septic shock: addition to a standard protocol. *Crit Care Med* **18**: 689–693.

Wang, P., Ba, Z.F., Chaudry, I.H. (1991) Hepatic extraction of indocyanine green is depressed early in sepsis despite increased hepatic blood flow and cardiac output. *Arch Surg* **126**: 219–224.

Winsö, O., Biber, B., Martner, J. (1985) Does dopamine suppress stress-induced intestinal and renal vasoconstriction? *Acta Anaesthesiol Scand* **29**: 508–514.

4

Adequacy of Renal Replacement in Intensive Care Medicine: A Case for Continuous Techniques

Rinaldo Bellomo, Claudio Ronco

INTRODUCTION

The importance of adequate dialysis in patients with end-stage renal failure is widely recognized. The technique has been analysed in many studies and reviewed in a number of papers and editorials (Gotch and Krueger, 1975; Lowrie *et al.*, 1981; Lowrie and Laird, 1983; Hakim, 1990; Vanholder and Ringoir, 1992; Owen *et al.*, 1993; Depner, 1994). In particular, despite a long-standing controversy about biochemical and clinical markers of physiologically adequate renal replacement therapy in such patients (Fuerst *et al.*, 1976; Teschan *et al.*, 1979; Lewis *et al.*, 1980; Luke, 1981; Bourne and Teschan, 1983; Gilli and De Bastiani, 1983; Laird *et al.*, 1983; Hoerl and Heidland, 1984; Schoots *et al.*, 1984; Marsh *et al.*, 1986; Lindsay and Henderson, 1988; Blake *et al.*, 1991; Hakim *et al.*, 1992a; Depner, 1993; Ritz *et al.*, 1994), it is widely accepted that the issue has important clinical repercussions and deserves much laboratory research and attention in clinical practice (Lowrie and Laird, 1983; Hakim, 1990; Vanholder and Ringoir, 1992; Depner, 1994). It is, therefore, somewhat curious that very little attention has been paid to the concept of 'adequacy of dialysis' in patients with acute renal failure. It is also disappointing that almost no attention has been paid to this issue where it is likely to matter most, i.e. in the intensive care unit (ICU).

In the following discussion, it will be argued that the concept of adequacy of dialysis for critically ill patients with acute renal failure is pivotal to the choice and application of renal replacement therapy. It will also be argued that 'adequacy of dialysis' in the critically ill is determined by a number of variables ranging from blood biochemistry to nutrition, from haemodynamics to biocompatibility, and that more laboratory and clinical research should be devoted to its definition and to the consequences of its use in clinical practice.

WHAT IS ADEQUACY?

There is no agreed definition of what the word 'adequate' means with respect to dialysis. In some ways the term has continually changed in meaning as our understanding of uraemia control has evolved. In end-stage renal failure, for instance, previously so-called adequate dialysis, continues to be demonstrated to be 'inadequate' on a regular basis (Owen *et al.*, 1993; Collins *et al.*, 1994; Hakim *et al.*, 1994a; Linsay *et al.*, 1994; Parker *et al.*, 1994).

In the management of the critically ill with acute renal failure, the issue of adequacy is not discussed. There are several reasons for this. The use of conventional forms of renal replacement with bioincompatible membranes has been so fraught with technical and pathophysiological problems (Kaplow and Foffinet, 1968; Johnson *et al.*, 1970; Bischel *et al.*, 1973, 1975; Von Hartizch *et al.*, 1974; Craddock *et al.*, 1977; Endou *et al.*, 1978; Kirkendol *et al.*, 1978; Korchik *et al.*, 1978; Carlton *et al.*, 1979; Kjellstrand *et al.*, 1980a; Swartz *et al.*, 1980; Patterson *et al.*, 1981; Hakim and Lowrie, 1982; Mault *et al.*, 1982; Chenoweth *et al.*, 1983; Romaldini *et al.*, 1984; Vas, 1985; Bouffard *et al.*, 1986a; Luger *et al.*, 1987; Gutierrez *et al.*, 1990a; Aunsholt and Larsen, 1992; Dieber *et al.*, 1993; Ronco and Burchardi, 1993; Smit and Gareth Jones, 1993; Manns *et al.,* 1994) that providing a treatment which controls hyperkalaemia, limits oedema and acidosis, and lowers the blood urea concentration to 'acceptable' levels (similar to that of end-stage renal failure patients) was considered 'adequate'. The heterogeneity of the patient population (Lien and Chan, 1985; Wheeler *et al.*, 1986; Lange *et al.*, 1987; Groeneveld *et al.*, 1991; Spiegel *et al.*, 1991; Chew *et al.*, 1993) makes it nearly impossible to evaluate the impact of different approaches to dialytic therapy in the absence of very large multicentre studies. The variability in illness severity, the many confounding factors inherent in intensive care therapy, and the small numbers obtained in single institutions further aggravate the problem of defining 'adequacy' in this setting.

While the problems described above have not disappeared, progress has been made in several directions. We now have several safe, effective and flexible forms of renal replacement therapy (Kramer *et al.*, 1977; Geronemus and Schneider, 1984; Wendon *et al.*, 1989; McDonald and Mehta, 1991; Bellomo *et al.*, 1992a; Hakim, 1993; Schiffe *et al.*, 1994). Illness severity scores have been developed and validated (Knaus *et al.*, 1985, 1991; Lemeshow *et al.*, 1993; Le Gall *et al.*, 1993). Such scores now make it possible to make more accurate comparisons of populations of critically ill patients from the same or different ICUs. Ventilator techniques, haemodynamic manipulations and approaches to the management of sepsis are increasingly performed according to consensus principles (European Society of Intensive Care Medicine Expert Panel, 1991; ACCP/SCCM Consensus Conference Committee, 1992; Bidani *et al.*, 1994; Slutsky, 1994a,b). The ability to organize multicentre studies is increasing because of recent advances in telecommunications. These changes open the door to the possibility of testing the concept of adequacy of dialysis for acute renal failure in the near future.

At present, however, any discussion of the concept of adequacy of dialysis in the critically ill with acute renal failure has to rely on indirect data and physiologic principles. Such principles, however, are still helpful in defining a priori the necessary properties of an adequate renal replacement therapy.

PHYSIOLOGICAL PRINCIPLES OF ADEQUACY

The first indirectly established principle in the management of critically ill patients is that the degree of physiological derangement in the first 24 hours after admission to the ICU (but also thereafter) 'drives' prognosis to hospital discharge. This principle has been widely tested and demonstrated in multiple studies of illness severity scoring systems which have evaluated it prospectively in thousands of ICU patients (Knaus *et al.*, 1985, 1991; Lemeshow *et al.*, 1993; Le Gall *et al.*, 1993). A corollary of this principle is that early correction or prevention of any physiological derangement is an important therapeutic goal in critical care medicine. Acute renal failure should be no exception. Adequate therapy, therefore, means a renal replacement therapy that is applied early to prevent hyperkalaemia, hyponatraemia, uraemia, acidosis and pulmonary and peripheral oedema. It also means a therapy that does not generate derangements of its own.

The second principle is that the adequacy of any artificial organ support in the ICU is measured by how closely such support mimicks the flexibility, versatility and efficacy of the organ system it seeks to substitute. This is true for mechanical ventilation, cardiac assistance devices and artificial oxygenators. It should also be true of any artificial kidney.

The third principle is that the use of any artificial organ support should not delay the recovery from injury of the native organ.

The fourth principle is that, particularly in the setting of multisystem organ failure, any organ replacement therapy should have absent or minimal proinflammatory effects.

Another observation is important in defining adequacy of dialysis in the ICU. In critically ill patients, the time frame of renal support delivery is different from that in the ambulatory setting. While, in the latter situation, it is important to deliver treatment over a relatively short period of time to enable the patient to achieve as normal a lifestyle as possible, in the ICU no such time constraints exist. The amount of time per day spent receiving renal replacement therapy matters little to a sedated and mechanically ventilated patient. What matters to the patient and the treating physician is that recovery should be speedy and the outcome favourable.

PATHOPHYSIOLOGICAL DERANGEMENTS AND RENAL REPLACEMENT

Several serious pathophysiological derangements occur as a consequence of acute renal failure in the ICU. First is the development of azotaemia. In critically ill patients, azotaemia develops rapidly. It is sustained by the need to administer full nutritional support and by a high degree of catabolism.

Physiological adequacy of renal replacement in this setting implies early and steady control of such azotaemia. It makes little physiological sense to wait for the blood urea nitrogen concentration to rise above some scientifically unvalidated and biologically magical number such as 100 or 120 mg/dl before initiating dialytic therapy. It makes no sense at all to wait for any of the clinical manifestations of uraemia to appear. No clinician would wait for established hypoxaemia to develop before initiating mechanical ventilation or for profound hypotension to cause end-organ dysfunction before initiating fluid and pressor resuscitation. The very reason for the existence of ICUs is the maintenance of homeostasis. There should be no reason to treat acute renal failure any differently where appropriate facilities are available.

A delay in the dialytic treatment of acute renal failure means that acid–base derangements inevitably develop. Adequacy of dialysis means the early treatment or the prevention of such derangements. If acetate is used as dialysate buffer during intermittent haemodialysis a number of therapy-induced acid–base derangements may be added to those already present in the critically ill patient (Gattinoni and Feriani, 1993). In the first 30 minutes of acetate dialysis, for instance, acetate metabolism may not be fast enough to balance bicarbonate losses. This may worsen metabolic acidosis (Kveim and Nesbakken, 1975). Acetate haemodialysis also significantly increases oxygen consumption while decreasing carbon dioxide production. This results in hypoventilation and hypoxaemia (Oh *et al.*, 1970; Bouffard *et al.*, 1986b). If bicarbonate is used as a buffer the correction of metabolic acidosis is more physiological and predictable. However, because of the intermittent nature of treatment, metabolic acidosis will redevelop in the interval between dialysis sessions and require renewed correction at the time of dialysis. The pathophysiological consequences of such swings in pH are presently unknown. Continuous haemofiltration, on the other hand, allows the titration of infused bicarbonate to achieve the desired target serum concentration and pH. Indeed, continuous haemofiltration has been shown to be effective in the correction of lactic acidosis (Barton *et al.*, 1991; Kirschbaum *et al.*, 1993). When replacement fluids contain lactate and the patient is lactate intolerant, however, hyperlacticaemia may develop (Davenport *et al.*, 1990). Although it remains controversial whether such hyperlacticaemia has a major proacidotic effect (Davenport *et al.*, 1990; Nimmo *et al.*, 1991, 1993), lactate is best avoided as a buffer in patients with severe liver disease.

In summary, adequate control of serum bicarbonate and pH can be achieved reliably and maintained near constant with haemofiltration but not with intermittent haemodialysis. The importance of this aspect of dialytic adequacy remains unknown.

The same principles of homeostasis apply to imbalances of serum potassium, sodium, magnesium, chloride, calcium and phosphate and to derangements of total body water and total body sodium.

The 'conventional' indications for initiating dialytic treatment, when applied to critically ill patients, are probably physiologically suboptimal and clinically unwise. From a strictly physiological point of view, it is also less than ideal to treat a state like acute renal failure intermittently. Safe and effective continuous renal replacement therapies are now available and are physiologically more desirable.

THE REAL KIDNEY AND DIALYSIS

The concept that any artificial form of renal support should closely mimick the features of the native organ is an important criterion for the assessment of adequacy. In the case of the kidney, replacement therapy should ideally provide steady control of uraemia, acid–base balance, serum electrolytes, total body water and total body salt content. It should also provide an adequate stimulus to erythropoiesis, participate in the control of mineral balance and bone physiology, assist in the control of vascular tone and contribute to the elimination of a variety of middle molecules, including cytokines (Pessina *et al.*,

1987; Klapproth *et al.*, 1989; Bocci, 1991). It should do all this to a degree similar to that of the human kidney and provide such therapy for 24 hours a day. No such replacement therapy currently exists, but any renal replacement that more closely approaches these goals can also be said to approximate more closely the concept of 'adequacy'.

Of the renal replacement techniques currently available (intermittent haemodialysis, peritoneal dialysis, continuous haemofiltration/haemodiafiltration) only continuous forms can fulfil the criterion of offering renal replacement for 24 hours a day. However, in a number of ICU patients receiving aggressive protein-rich nutritional support, peritoneal dialysis is unable to achieve the small molecular clearances and daily nitrogen extraction rates needed to contol uraemia optimally (Howdieshell *et al.*, 1992). Accordingly, the use of supplemental haemodialytic therapy may be required. Modern techniques of haemofiltration, such as continuous arteriovenous haemodiafiltration (CAVHD), continuous veno-venous haemofiltration (CVVH), and continuous veno-venous haemodiafiltration (CVVHD), on the other hand, have been shown to predictably and steadily control uraemia in all treated critically ill patients, irrespective of their nutritional therapy (Conand *et al.*, 1988; Pattison *et al.*, 1988; Stevens *et al.*, 1988; Bellomo *et al.*, 1990, 1992c; Reynolds *et al.*, 1991; Schaefer *et al.*, 1991; Voerman *et al.*, 1994). They also permit rapid and steady control of total body water and salt content according to clinical needs. Such ability to control the volume state may have powerful positive implications in the management of patients with pulmonary oedema and the acute respiratory distress syndrome. In both these conditions, the achievement of a negative fluid balance has been associated with improved outcome (Humphrey *et al.*, 1990).

Standard intermittent haemodialysis fails this test of adequacy because of its episodic nature. The need to remove volume over a short period of time in these patients, who require at least 2 l/day of intravenous fluids for nutritional and pharmacological purposes, is frequently associated with hypotension. Often, in order to avoid such hypotension, fluid removal is suboptimal, resulting in the persistence of oedema (Ronco *et al.*, 1990).

A superficial analysis of continuous versus intermittent therapies would reveal that the latter achieve a significantly greater K_t/V (K_t, urea clearance time by dialysis; V, volume of distribution of urea) and must, therefore, offer superior control of uraemia. In fact, however, prescription and delivery of intermittent dialysis often differ even in chronic renal failure patients (Gotch *et al.*, 1990; Sargent, 1990; Depner *et al.*, 1991a; Le Febre *et al.*, 1991; Kjellstrand *et al.*, 1991; Delmez *et al.*, 1992) for reasons that vary from changes in the true time spent receiving therapy to solute disequilibrium, and the use of the K_t/V in comparing continuous therapy with intermittent therapy is misleading (Ronco *et al.*, 1993, 1994a, b, c).

The rapid fall in blood urea nitrogen concentration during intermittent haemodialysis, the failure of extracirculatory body pools of urea to equilibrate rapidly (Depner *et al.*, 1991b; Schneditz *et al.*, 1992) and the regional blood flow dependence of such re-equilibration mean that, for an equal K_t/V, a continuous form of therapy would remove vastly more urea nitrogen from the total body pool and accomplish much greater blood purification (Clark *et al.*, 1994). The importance of tissue urea pool disequilibrium is likely to be even greater in diminishing the true delivery of dialysis in the setting of critical illness and continuous vasopressor infusion.

That standard dialysis falls short of the mark is clearly demonstrated by the work of Clark *et al.* (1994) who have recently shown that an intermittent haemodialysis frequency of at least 5 times a week would be required to match the degree of uraemia control achieved with CVVH at an ultrafiltration rate of 1 l/h. Their work is also supported by the findings obtained comparing the weekly K_t/V achieved with different techniques of continuous renal replacement therapy with that achieved with thrice-weekly standard haemodialysis as shown in Figure 4.1. Furthermore, if the peak concentration hypothesis (Keshaviah *et al.*, 1989) (the peak level of urea correlates best with toxicity) were true, once again, standard haemodialysis would be found wanting. We recently retrospectively analysed two cohorts of critically ill patients treated with either intermittent haemodialysis or CVVHD. The groups were comparable in terms of illness severity and demographic features and in terms of urea and creatinine levels prior to treatment. After the first 24 hours of treatment, however, CVVHD-treated patients had a significantly ($p < 0.0001$) lower plasma urea concentration. This difference persisted throughout therapy. The mean urea level in intermittent haemodialysis patients was 35 versus 23.4 mmol/l for CVVHD ($p < 0.0001$) (Figure 4.2). Clearly, when compared to CVVHD, intermittent haemodialysis is biochemically inadequate.

Even though continuous therapies are rarely at work for the full 24 hours a day as intended (the mean operational time per day has recently been reported at 21.8 hours) (Frankenfield *et al.*, 1989), they offer better small molecular clearances (CAVHD or CVVHD) than intermittent haemodialysis, with a weekly urea nitrogen extraction averaging 196 g (Frankenfield *et al.*, 1989). It would theoretically take approximately 7 hours of intermittent haemodialysis each day to achieve such levels of blood purification. Intermittent haemodialysis would then start to look remarkably similar to continuous therapy!

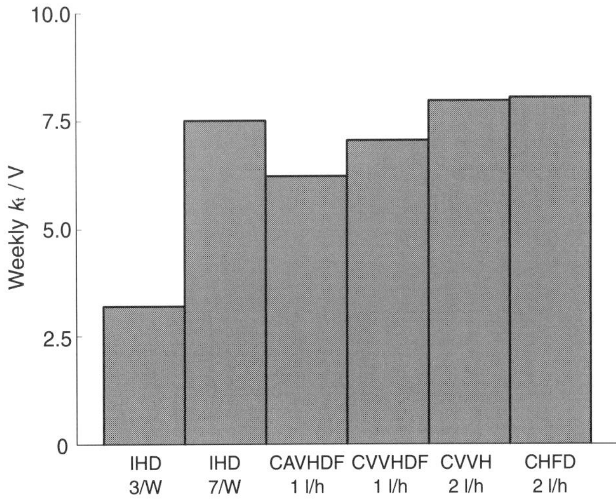

Figure 4.1.   Diagram illustrating the approximate weekly urea K_t/V obtained with different forms of renal replacement therapy. Intermittent haemodialysis applied three times a week (IHD 3/W) is clearly much less effective than continuous therapies such as continuous arteriovenous haemodiafiltration at 1 l/h of dialysate flow (CAVHDF 1 l/h), continuous veno-venous haemodiafiltration at 1 l/h of dialysate flow (CVVHDF 1 l/h), continuous veno-venous haemofiltration at 2 l/h of controlled ultrafiltration (CVVH 2 l/h) and continuous high-flux haemodialysis with controlled dialysate flow at 2 l/h (CHFD 2 l/h). Intermittent haemodialysis must be performed for 4 h/day (IHD 7/W) to achieve similar levels of weekly urea K_t/V.

In addition, recent work by Frankenfield *et al.* (1994) has clearly demonstrated that urea nitrogen extraction during continuous haemodiafiltration was quantitatively equal to that achieved by the native kidneys of a control group of critically ill septic patients without acute renal failure who were matched for illness severity. Such data strongly support the concept that continuous techniques more closely approach the performance of the native kidney. In addition, mean blood urea nitrogen concentrations could be maintained at approximately 70 mg/dl despite nutritional support with >2 g protein/kg/day. These findings are in keeping with those of others (Bellomo *et al.*, 1991, 1997) and underscore the nutritional implications of being able to provide adequate renal replacement.

In terms of control of serum electrolytes and acidosis, there are no prospective data demonstrating a difference in adequacy between intermittent haemodialyis, peritoneal dialysis and haemofiltration techniques. Retrospective data, however, suggest that, once again, continuous renal replacement therapies may be superior (Keshaviah *et al.*, 1989; Bellomo *et al.*, 1992b).

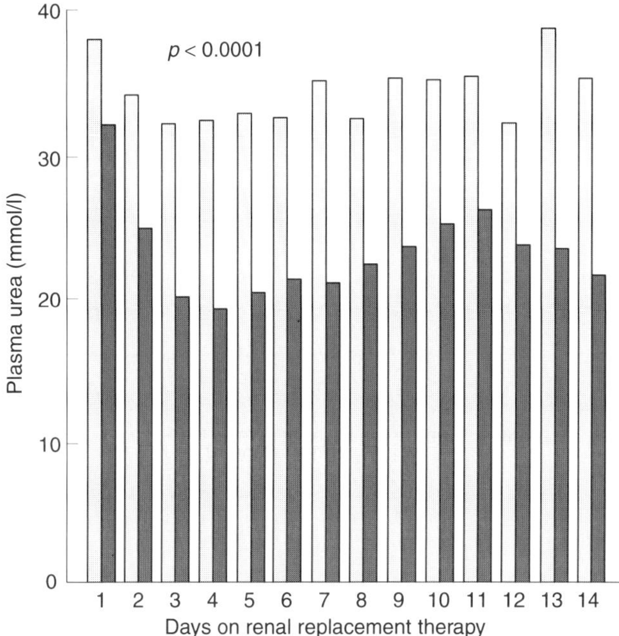

Figure 4.2. Graph illustrating the difference in uraemic control during continuous haemofiltration and intermittent haemodialysis in critically ill patients with acute renal failure. From the start of therapy, continuous haemofiltration (shaded columns) is associated with plasma urea levels of around 20 mmol/l. Intermittent haemodialysis (open columns) is associated with mean urea levels above 30 mmol/l. The difference is highly significant.

As argued previously, one of the corollaries of intensive-care management is the maintenance of homeostasis. This demands that preventive early intervention be applied in the form of mechanical ventilation, fluid and pressor resuscitation and renal replacement therapy if necessary. In the ICU, the time-honoured criteria for the initiation of renal replacement therapy are associated with a physiologically unacceptable degree of derangement from homeostasis. More appropriate criteria must be applied that are in keeping with the higher level of physiological care applied to the failure of other organ systems. We offer a set of criteria (Table 4.1) that we believe more closely approximate the needs of critically ill patients.

If adequate renal replacement means early intervention, then techniques associated with earlier application of replacement therapy are clearly preferable. Once again available data support the use of continuous therapy (Bellomo *et al.*, 1992b, 1993a). The reasons for earlier intervention with haemofiltration include the ease of implementation

Table 4.1 Proposed criteria for the initiation of renal replacement therapy in critically ill patients

- Oliguria (urinary output <5 ml/kg/day)
- Anuria (no urinary output for >12 hours)
- Serum creatinine concentration >600 µmol/l (>6.7 mg/dl)
- Plasma urea concentration >35 mmol/l (>100 mg/dl)
- Hyperkalaemia (serum potassium concentration >6.5 mmol/l)
- Pulmonary oedema not responsive to conventional therapy and diuretics
- Metabolic acidosis (pH < 7.2)
- Uraemic encephalopathy
- Uraemic pericarditis
- Uraemic neuropathy

Note: The presence of one of the above criteria is sufficient grounds for the initiation of renal replacement therapy in a critically ill patient. The presence of two of these criteria makes renal replacement urgent and mandatory.

within the ICU, the rapid preparation of the extracorporeal circuit, the lack of a need for surgical intervention and the ability to start therapy at any time of the day or night without concerns about personnel availability.

The haemodynamic consequences of renal replacement therapy constitute an important aspect of clinical 'adequacy'. The evidence that standard haemodialysis is associated with the induction of hypotension in 10–50% of haemodynamically stable end-stage renal failure patients is overwhelming (Endou *et al.*, 1978; Korchik *et al.*, 1978; Ogden, 1978; Leski *et al.*, 1979; Nies *et al.*, 1979; Kjellstrand *et al.*, 1980b; Rosa *et al.*, 1980; Ronco and Burchardi, 1993; Hakim *et al.*, 1994b). This hypotensive effect of haemodialysis as seen in the critically ill was the prime stimulus to the development of continuous therapies. Such therapies have been shown to lead to outstanding haemodynamic stability (Lauer *et al.*, 1983; Coraim *et al.*, 1986; Alarabi *et al.*, 1991; Canand *et al.*, 1991; Keller *et al.*, 1991; Laggner *et al.*, 1991; Bandouin *et al.*, 1993; Vandenbogaede *et al.*, 1988), an important measure of dialytic adequacy in the ICU. It has been argued (Henrich, 1993) that the use of several techniques (bicarbonate dialysis, high sodium dialysate, cold dialysate and the like) to compensate for the hypotensive effects of standard haemodialysis, will result in the maintenance of haemodynamic stability (Henrich *et al.*, 1982; Velez *et al.*, 1984; Sherman *et al.*, 1985; Agarwal *et al.*, 1992). This may be true in chronic patients, but remains to be proved in critically ill patients with acute renal failure. Current evidence continues to suggest that continuous therapies are superior.

Another important aspect of adequacy relates to the effect of therapy on renal recovery. There are no data available to compare prospectively the effects of standard haemodialysis and continuous therapies on the rate of renal recovery, although retrospective data suggest a trend in favour of continuous therapies (Bellomo *et al.*, 1993a). Recent work (Manns *et al.*, 1994) (Figure 4.3) indicates that renal injury occurs during and after intermittent haemodialysis and could result in deterioration of residual renal function.

This adverse effect may be independent of any decrease in blood pressure and simply relate to the use of bioincompatible membranes such as cuprophane (Schulman *et al.*, 1991; Hakim *et al.*, 1992b; Hakim, 1993). A recent clinical study by Schiffl *et al.* (1994) demonstrated that critically ill patients with acute renal failure treated with intermittent cuprophane haemodialysis had intense activation of the complement system and lipo-oxygenase pathway, alterations in neutrophil function, a higher incidence of sepsis, a need for prolonged haemodialysis, delayed resolution and recovery from renal failure and decreased survival when compared to a matched control group treated with poly-acrylonitrile membranes. Hakim *et al.* (1994b) confirmed the extreme importance of membrane biocompatibility in determining the outcome of patients with acute renal failure. Their randomized controlled trial comparing cuprophane dialysis with dialysis with a biocompatible polymethylmethacrylate membrane showed that patients treated with a biocompatible membrane had a 62% rate of renal recovery versus 37% for cuprophane-treated patients ($p < 0.04$ after adjustment for illness severity), required fewer dialysis treatments and showed a

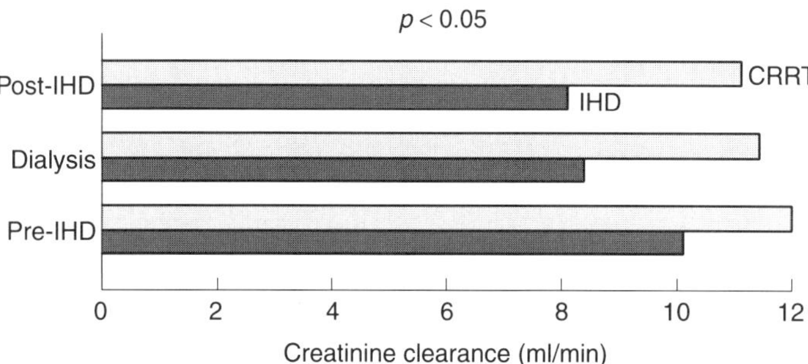

Figure 4.3.   Graph displaying the effects of intermittent haemodialysis (IHD) and continuous renal replacement therapy (CRRT) on residual creatinine clearance in patients with acute renal failure. IHD results in a significant decrease in creatinine clearance, while CRRT does not ($p < 0.05$). (From data reported in Manns *et al.* (1994).)

strong trend towards increased overall survival. One of the mechanisms by which continuous therapies appear to be superior to standard haemodialysis may, therefore, simply be that the former use biocompatible membranes.

The issue of biocompatibility stretches beyond that of immunological dysfunction into the area of nutrition. Simple exposure (not dialysis) to cellulosic membranes may result in net protein catabolism (Gutierrez *et al.*, 1990) which continues for up to 9 hours following exposure to the bioincompatible membrane. No such effect is seen with biocompatible membranes. The significance of such adverse biochemical effects, seen in conjunction with the activation of a myriad of inflammatory cascades (Hakim, 1993), should be dismissed as clinically unimportant.

The dismal nitrogen balances achieved with standard approaches (low-protein diet and conventional haemodialysis) to the nutritional mangement of these patients (Bouffard *et al.*, 1987) are unacceptable in view of current thinking in the area of nutrition for the critically ill (Elwyn, 1980; Cerra, 1987; Berger and Adams, 1989; Daly *et al.*, 1990; Deitch *et al.*, 1992; Jeejeebhoy, 1992) and acute renal failure (Toback *et al.*, 1983; Garza-Quintero *et al.*, 1987). With the use of continuous therapies and the increased administration of protein nitrogen, patients with critical illness can progressively move toward the nutritionally important goal of a near-neutral nitrogen balance (Kierdorf *et al.*, 1986; Kierdorf, 1991; Bellomo *et al.*, 1991, 1997) as shown in Figure 4.3. Adequate protein supplementation does not only have positive repercussions on the maintenance of respiratory muscle mass and function (Pingleton and Harmon, 1987; Weissman and Heyman, 1987), but is also likely to have a favourable effect on renal recovery (Toback, 1977; Toback *et al.*, 1983), another important aspect of clinical adequacy.

Particular environments where unique issues of clinical dialytic adequacy apply are the neurosurgical and liver ICUs. Critically ill neurosurgical patients and patients with combined liver and renal failure have a high incidence of cerebral oedema. Such patients require a dialytic therapy that can both deal with their extreme nutritional needs and not induce swings in intracranial pressure. There is strong evidence that intermittent haemodialysis induces measurable increases in intracerebral water (Kishimoto *et al.*, 1980; La Greca *et al.*, 1980, 1982; Winney *et al.*, 1986; Davenport *et al.*, 1993a). Such changes are likely to aggravate any previous cerebral oedema and may pose a serious threat to the life of such patients. However, even other intermittent techniques, such as intermittent haemofiltration, which have been shown to be better than intermittent haemodialysis (Kishimoto *et al.*, 1980) in this area of cerebral physiology, have been clearly shown to be inferior to continuous therapies in high-risk patients (Davenport *et al.*, 1989a–c, 1993a, b). These data make continuous haemofiltration techniques the renal replacement therapy of choice under these circumstances. In addition, continuous haemofiltration therapies have never been reported to induce the disequilibrium syndrome (Arieff, 1994) and may have further beneficial effects in liver failure patients by removing noxious middle molecules from the circulation (Matsubara *et al.*, 1990). These data show that, once again, intermittent therapies do not meet the criteria of clinical adequacy in this subgroup of patients, while continuous haemofiltration techniques do.

There is strong consensus that many important adverse aspects of sepsis are mediated by circulating molecules including interleukins, tumour necrosis factor, leukotrienes, thromboxane and platelet activating factor (Ayres, 1985; Balk and Bone, 1989; Kirschbaum *et al.*, 1993). As a consequence of such consensus, the development of antagonists to these 'soluble mediators of sepsis' has become an accepted therapeutic goal (Fisher *et al.*, 1993; Marshall, 1994) in critically ill septic patients. In the case of patients with acute renal failure, it is important to note that the kidney is involved in the excretion of a number of these molecules (Pessina *et al.*, 1987; Klapproth *et al.*, 1989; Bocci, 1991; Graziani *et al.*, 1993). Therefore, it is possible that kidney failure would result in a greater cumulative inflammatory load with its predictable adverse consequences. An adequate form of renal replacement would seek to replicate this potentially useful immunomodulatory renal activity.

This is, in part, achieved during continuous haemodiafiltration (Bellomo *et al.*, 1993b; Braun *et al.*, 1993; Hoffman *et al.*, 1994). The opposite is true of intermittent haemodialysis (Arnout *et al.*, 1985; Hakim and Schafer, 1985; Luger *et al.*, 1987, Dinarello, 1990; Himmelfarb *et al.*, 1991; Strasser and Schiffl, 1991). This opposing effect on inflammatory mediators is likely to explain the emerging difference in outcome between patients treated with biocompatible and bioincompatible membranes. The significance of the 'blood purification' effect achieved during continuous haemofiltration/haemodiafiltration may well go beyond the mere avoidance of inflammatory stimulation. Growing evidence indicates that continuous therapies may have a place as adjunctive therapy in sepsis and that their 'blood purification' effect is clinically important (Ossenkoppele *et al.*, 1985; Gotloib *et al.*, 1986; Barzilay *et al.*, 1989; Gomez *et al.*, 1990; Coraim *et al.*, 1991; Steiner *et al.*, 1991; Grootendorst *et al.*, 1992, 1993; Lee *et al.*, 1993). The biological impact of these techniques and the importance of using the correct membrane type and size has recently been highlighted by work performed in septic acute renal failure patients revealing the major impact of continuous haemofiltration on circulating levels of complement factor D (Gasche *et al.*, 1996). In addition, recent work by van Bommel *et al.* (1995) has clearly demonstrated the complex and dynamic nature of the interactions between the dialysing membrane, the ultrafiltration process, and several mediators of sepsis. Such a process involves membrane adsorption of mediators, saturation-dependent sieving of such mediators, release of mediators after membrane saturation and possible mediator generation. In addition, different membranes appear to behave differently with regard to adsorption and sieving. Much is yet to be learned in this area.

OBSTACLES TO THE USE OF CONTINUOUS THERAPIES

There appear to be two major obstacles to the more widespread application of continuous renal replacement therapies. The first is one of technical competence on the part of nursing and medical staff, and the second is the fear of increased cost.

The answer to the former is obvious: training. Saying that members of an ICU with its support nephrology staff feel technically uncomfortable with continuous therapies is like saying that an intensivist is uncomfortable with the insertion of a pulmonary artery catheter or that a nephrologist is uncomfortable with performing a renal biopsy. In both cases, time should be set aside to become competent in the use of the technique.

The problem of cost is controversial and subtle. In Australia and Europe, if disposables only are taken into account, the weekly cost of continuous veno-venous haemofiltration with a polyacrylonitrile membrane of an expected mean filter life of 48 hours, would be approximately US $700. The equivalent cost in disposables of four sessions of intermittent haemodialysis would be about US $100–150. The difference would add less than US $100/day to the cost of patient care, close to the cost of 1 day of treatment with some third-generation cephalosporin or a newer multicidal penicillin (other therapies not tested in prospective controlled randomized trials the ICU). With the average daily cost of an ICU bed at US $2000–3000, the additional financial burden of continuous therapies is minimal.

Other facts, however, merit discussion. In many ICUs (including the authors'), continuous renal replacement is carried out without additional nursing costs. On the other hand, intermittent haemodialysis requires approximately 25 h/week of additional nursing time, at an estimated cost of close to US $500. This alone makes the cost of intermittent haemodialysis essentially the same as that of CVVH in Australia and in many parts of Europe and probably in some USA centres. Furthermore, the capital expenditure for a haemodialysis machine is substantially greater than that needed for a peristaltic pump system.

Clearly, there are local factors that play a role in these approximate cost assessments but, no matter what they are, the introduction of continuous renal replacement therapy does *not* represent a major financial burden in the care of a critically ill patient with acute renal failure. There is little doubt that, if continuous therapies had historically preceded the development of standard techniques, the latter would rarely, if ever, be considered for use in the ICU.

THE FUTURE OF RENAL REPLACEMENT THERAPY IN THE ICU

Given the absence of prospective controlled randomized studies and accepted definitions of dialytic adequacy in acute renal failure in the ICU, one option is to continue to apply the therapies of the 1970s (standard cellulose-based intermittent haemodialysis) until such trials are performed and definitions become established. This option, although wrapped in the cloth of scientific righteousness, ignores the fact that if critical care physicians and nephrologists steadfastedly refused to implement therapies that have not been tested and proven to increase survival under prospective, controlled and randomized conditions, every ICU in the world would have to be dismantled and haemodialysis for acute renal failure ceased. More to the point, such widely embraced technologies as volume-cycled ventilators, the pulmonary artery catheter and the pulse oximeter have never been shown, in controlled trials, to affect patient outcome favourably. It is therefore much more likely that a less scientifically 'pure' but more pragmatic option will emerge, i.e. a progressive shift toward continuous therapies.

The trend in this direction is essentially complete in Australia and relatively strong in Europe where continuous haemofiltration techniques are now the common forms of renal replacement therapy in the ICU. The USA has lagged behind such trends for a number of complex medical and non-medical reasons. Other trends are also emerging. They include an earlier start of renal replacement therapy, a tighter control of blood urea concentration and the provision of more aggressive, nitrogen rich, nutritional support.

Despite all the above changes, it seems unwise to move to continuous therapies by attrition and to other newer therapeutic options without some documentation of their impact. We need to test the wisdom of tentative definitions of dialytic adequacy and that of new criteria for the initiation of dialysis (see Table 4.1). We have a unique opportunity to tackle these issues in a more systematic way than has been possible for chronic haemodialysis, and should not miss it.

REFERENCES

ACCP/SCCM Consensus Conference Committee (1992) Definitions for sepsis and organ failure and guidelines for the use of innovative therapies in sepsis. *Chest* **101**: 1644–1655.

Agarwal, R., Jost, C., Khair-el-din, T., Victor, R., Grayburn, P., Henrich, W.L. (1992) 35°C dialysis increases peripheral resistance and improves hemodynamic stability in patients. *J Am Soc Nephrol* **3**: 351.

Alarabi, A.A., Wilstrom, B., Danielson, B.G. (1991) Continuous arteriovenous hemodialysis and hemofiltration in acute renal failure: comparison of uremic control. *Contrib Nephrol* **93**: 61–64.

Arieff, A.I. (1994) Dialysis disequilibrium syndrome: current concepts on pathogenesis and prevention. *Kidney Int* **45**: 629–635.

Arnout, M.A., Hakim, R.M., Todd, R.F., Dana, N., Colten, H.R. (1985) Increased expression of an adhesion promoting glycoprotein in the granulocytopenia of hemodialysis. *N Engl J Med* **312**: 457–462.

Aunsholt, N.A., Aa, Larsen, C. (1992) The arterial oxygen extraction tension and oxygen compensation factor during acetate and bicarbonate dialysis. *Blood Purif* **10**: 317–325.

Ayres, S.M. (1985) SCCM's New Horizons Conference on sepsis and septic shock. *Crit Care Med* **13**: 864–866.

Balk, R.A., Bone, R.C. (1989) The septic syndrome: definitions and clinical implication. *Crit Care Clin* **5**: 1–8.

Bandouin, S.V., Wiggins, J., Keogh, B.F., Morgan, C.J., Evans, T. (1993) Continuous veno-venous haemofiltration following cardio-pulmonary bypass. *Intensive Care Med* **19**: 290–293.

Barton, I.K., Streather, C.P., Hilton, P.J., Bradley, R.D. (1991) Successful treatment of severe lactic acidosis by haemofiltration using a bicarbonate-based replacement fluid. *Nephrol Dial Transplant* **6**: 368–370.

Barzilay, E., Kessler, D., Berlot, G., Gullo, A., Geber, D., Ben Zeev, I. (1989) Use of extracorporeal supportive techniques as additional treatment for septic-induced multiple organ failure patients. *Crit Care Med* **17**: 634–637.

Bellomo, R., Ernest, D., Love, J., Parkin, G., Boyce, N. (1990) Continuous arteriovenous hemodiafiltration: an optimal therapy for acute renal failure in an intensive care setting. *Aust NZ J Med* **20**: 237–242.

Bellomo, R., Martin, H., Parkin, G., Love, J., Keazley, Y., Boyce, N. (1991) Continuous arteriovenous haemodiafiltration in the critically ill: influence on major nutrient balances. *Intensive Care Med* **17**: 399–402.

Bellomo, R., Parkin, G., Love, J., Boyce, N. (1992a) Management of acute renal failure in the critically ill with continuous hemovenous hemodiafiltration. *Renal Failure* **14**: 183–186.

Bellomo, R., Mansfield, D., Rumble, S., Shapiro, J., Parkin, G., Boyce, N. (1992b) Acute renal failure in critical illness. Conventional dialysis versus acute continuous hemodiafiltration. *ASAIO J* **38**: M654–M657.

Bellomo, R., Parkin, G., Love, J., Boyce, N. (1992c) Management of acute renal failure in the critically ill with continuous veno-venous hemodiafiltration. *Renal Failure* **14**: 183–186.

Bellomo, R., Mansfield, D., Rumble, S., Shapiro, J., Parkin, G., Boyce, N. (1993a) A comparison of conventional dialytic therapy and acute continuous hemodiafiltration in the management of acute renal failure in the critically ill. *Renal Failure* **15**: 595–602.

Bellomo, R., Tipping, P., Boyce, N. (1993b) Continuous venovenous hemofiltration with dialysis removes cytokines from the circulation of septic patients. *Crit Care Med* **21**: 522–526.

Bellomo, R., Seacombe, J., Daskalakis, M., Farmer, M., Wright, C., Parkin, G., Boyce, N. (1997) A prospective comparative study of moderate versus high protein intake for critically ill patients with acute renal failure. *Renal Failure.* **19**: 111–120.

Berger, R., Adams, L. (1989) Nutritional support in the critical care setting. *Chest* **96**: 139–150.

Bidani, A., Tzounakis, A.E., Cardenas, V.J., Zwischenberger, J.B. (1994) Permissive hypercapnia in acute respiratory failure. *JAMA* **272**: 957–962.

Bischel, M.D., Orrell, F.L., Scoles, B.G., Mohler, J.G., Barbour, B.H. (1973) Effects of microemboli blood filtration during hemodialysis. *Trans Am Soc Artif Intern Organs* **19**: 492–497.

Bischel, M.D., Scoles, B.G., Mohler, J.G. (1975) Evidence for pulmonary microembolization during hemodialysis. *Chest* **67**: 335–337.

Blake, P.G., Sombolos, K., Abraham, G., Weissganten, J., Pemberton, R., Chu, G.L., Oreopoulos, D.G. (1991) Lack of correlation between urea kinetic indices and clinical outcome in CAPD patients. *Kidney Int* **39**: 700–706.

Bocci, V. (1991) Interleukins: clinical pharmacokinetics and practical implications. *Clin Pharmacokinet* **21**: 274–284.

Bouffard, Y., Viale, J-P., Annat, G., Guillame, C., Percival, C., Bertrand, O., Motin, J. (1986a) Pulmonary gas exchange during hemodialysis. *Kidney Int* **30**: 920–923.

Bouffard, Y., Viale, J.P., Annat, G. *et al.* (1986b) Pulmonary gas exchange during hemodialysis. *Kidney Int* **30**: 920–927.

Bouffard, Y., Viale, J.P., Annat, G., Delafosse, B., Guillanne, G., Motin, J. (1987) Energy expenditure in the acute renal failure patient mechanically ventilated. *Intensive Care Med* **13**: 401–404.

Bourne, J.R., Teschan, P.E. (1983) Computer methods, uremic encephalopathy and adequacy of dialysis. *Kidney Int* **24**: 496–506.

Braun, N., Giolai, M., Rosenfeld, S., Banzhaff, W., Fretchner, R., Weinstock, C., Erley, C., Muller, G.A., Warth, H., Northoff, H., Risler, T. (1993)

Clearance of interleukin 6 during continuous veno-venous hemofiltration in patients with septic shock. A prospective controlled study. *J Am Soc Nephrol* **4**: 336 [abstract].

Canand, B., Cristol, J.P., Klouch, K., Berand, J.J., Cailar, G.D., Ferrierre, M., Grolleau, R., Mion, C. (1991) Slow continuous ultrafiltration: a means of unmaking myocardial functional reserve in end-stage cardiac disease. *Contrib Nephrol* **93**: 79–85.

Carlton, G.C., Campfield, P.B., Goldiner, P.L., Turnbull, A.D. (1979) Hypoxemia during hemodialysis. *Crit Care Med* **7**: 497–501.

Cerra, F.B. (1987) Hypermetabolism, organ failure and metabolic support. *Surgery* **101**: 1–6.

Chenoweth, D.E., Cheung, A.K., Henderson, L.W. (1983) Anaphylatoxin formation during hemodialysis: effects of different dialyzer membranes. *Kidney Int* **24**: 764–769.

Chew, S.L., Lins, R.L., Daelemans, R., De Boer, M.E. (1993) Outcome in acute renal failure. *Nephrol Dial Transplant* **8**: 101–107.

Clark, W.R., Mueller, B.A., Alaka, K.J., Macias, W.L. (1994) A comparison of metabolic control by continuous and intermittent therapies in acute renal failure. *J Am Soc Nephrol* **4**: 1413–1420.

Collins, A.J., Ma, J.M., Umen, A., Keshaviah, P. (1994) Urea index and other predictors of hemodialysis patient survival. *Am J Kid Dis* **23**: 272–282.

Conand, B., Garved, L.J., Christol, J.P., Aubas, S., Berand, J.J., Mion, C. (1988) Pump assisted continuous veno-venous hemofiltration for treating acute uremia. *Kidney Int* **33** (Suppl. 24): 5154–5156.

Coraim, F.J., Coraim, H.P., Ebermann, R., Stellwag, F.M. (1986) Acute respiratory failure after cardiac surgery: clinical experience with the application of continuous arteriovenous hemofiltration. *Crit Care Med* **14**: 714–718.

Coraim, F., Trubel, W., Ebermann, R., Wolner, E. (1991) Elimination of myocardial depressant substances by hemofiltration in patients with cardiogenic shock. *Circ Shock* **34**: 117 [abstract].

Craddock, P.R., Fehr, J., Brigham, K.L., Kronenberg, R.S., Jacob, HS. (1977) Complement and leukocyte-mediated pulmonary dysfunction in haemodialysis. *N Engl J Med* **296**: 769–774.

Daly, J.M., Reynold, J., Sigal, R.K., Shou, J., Liberman, M.D. (1990) Effects of dietary protein and amino acids on immune function. *Crit Care Med* **18**: S86–S93.

Davenport, A., Will, E.J., Davison, A.M., Swindells, S., Cohen, A.T., Miloszewski, K.J.A., Losowsky, M.S. (1989a) Changes in intracranial pressure during haemofiltration in oliguric patients with grade IV hepatic encephalopathy. *Nephron* **53**: 142–146.

Davenport, A., Will, E.J., Davison, A.M., Swindells, S., Cohen, A.T., Milozewski, K.J.A., Losowsky, M.S. (1989b) Changes in intracranial pressure during machine and continuous haemofiltration. *Int J Artif Organ* **12**: 439–444.

Davenport, A., Finn, R., Goldsmith, H.J. (1989c) Management of patients with renal failure complicated by cerebral oedema. *Blood Purif* **7**: 203–209.

Davenport, A., Will, E.J., Davison, A.M. (1990) Paradoxical increase in arterial hydrogen ion concentration in patients with hepatorenal failure given lactate-based fluids. *Nephrol Dial Transplant* **5**: 342–346.

Davenport, A., Will, E.J., Davison, A.M. (1993a) Effect of renal replacement therapy on patients with combined acute renal and fulminant hepatic failure. *Kidney Int* **43** (Suppl. 41): S245–S251.

Davenport, A., Will, E.J., Davidson, A.M. (1993b) Improved cardiovascular stability during continuous modes of renal replacement therapy in critically ill patients with acute hepatic and renal failure. *Crit Care Med* **21**: 328–338.

Deitch, E.A., Dazhong, X., Qi, L., Specian, R.D., Berg, R.D. (1992) Protein malnutrition alone and in combination with endotoxin impairs systemic and gut-associated immunity. *J Parent Enteral Nutr* **16**: 25–31.

Delmez, J.A., Windus, D.W. St Louis Nephrology Study Group (1992) Hemodialysis prescription and delivery in a metropolitan community. *Kidney Int* **41**: 1023–1028.

Depner, T.A. (1993) Pitfalls in quantitating hemodialysis. *Semin Dial* **6**: 127–133.

Depner, T.A. (1994) Assessing adequacy of hemodialysis: urea modeling. *Kidney Int* **45**: 1522–1535.

Depner, T., Rizwan, S., Cheer, A., Wagner, J. (1991a) Peripheral urea disequilibrium during hemodialysis is temperature-dependent. *J Am Soc Nephrol* **2**: 321–325.

Depner, T.A., Rizwan, S., Cheer, A.Y., Wagner, J., Eder, L.A. (1991b) High venous urea concentration in the opposite arm: a consequence of hemodialysis-induced compartment disequilibruim. *J Am Soc Artif Intern Organs* **37**: 141–143.

Dieber, L., Kozol, R., Wilson, R.F., Mahajan, S., Abu-Hamdan, D., Thomas, D. (1993) Gastric intramucosal acidosis in patients with chronic kidney failure. *Surgery* **113**: 520–526.

Dinarello, C.A. (1990) Cytokines and biocompatibility. *Blood Purif* **8**: 208–213.

Elwyn, D.H. (1980) Nutritional requirements of adult surgical patients. *Crit Care Med* **8**: 9–20.

Endou, K., Kamijima, J., Kakubari, Y., Kirkawada, R. (1978) Hemodynamic changes during dialysis. *Cardiology* **63**: 175–187.

European Society of Intensive Care Medicine Expert Panel (1991) The use of the pulmonary artery catheter. *Intensive Care Med* **17**: I–VIII.

Fisher, C.J., Opal, S.M., Dhainaut, J.-F., the CB 0006 Sepsis Syndrome Study Group. (1993) Influence of an anti-tumor necrosis factor monoclonal antibody on cytokine levels in patients with sepsis. *Crit Care Med* **21**: 318–327.

Frankenfield, D.C., Reynolds, H.N., Wiles, C.E., Badellino, M.M., Siegel, J.N. (1994) Urea removal during continuous hemofiltration. *Crit Care Med* **22**: 407–412.

Fuerst, P., Zimmerman, L., Bergstroem, J. (1976) Determination of endogenous middle molecules in normal and uremic body fluids. *Clin Nephrol* **5**: 178–187.

Garza-Quintero, R., Ortega-Lopez, J., Stein, J.H., van Katachalam, M.A. (1987) Alanine protects rabbit proximal tubules against anoxic injury in vitro. *Am J Physiol* **258**: F1075–F1083.

Gasche, Y., Pascual, M., Suter, P., Favre, H., Chevrolet, J.-C., Schifferli, J.A. (1996) Complement depletion during haemofiltration with polyacrylonitrile membranes. *Nephrol Dial Transpl* **11**: 117–119.

Gattinoni, L., Feriani, M. (1993) Acid–base derangements in acute renal failure. In: Pinsky, M.R., Dhainaut, J.-F.A. (eds) *Pathophysiologic Foundations of Critical Care*. Battimore: Williams & Wilkins.

Geronemus, R., Schneider, N. (1984) Continuous arteriovenous hemodialysis: a new modality for treatment of acute renal failure. *Trans Am Soc Artif Intern Organs* **30**: 610–613.

Gilli, P., De Bastiani, P. (1983) Cognitive function and regular dialysis treatment. *Clin Nephrol* **19**: 188–192.

Gomez, A., Wang, R., Unruh, H., *et al.* (1990) Hemofiltration versus left ventricular dysfunctiton during sepsis in dogs. *Anesthesiology* **73**: 671–685.

Gotch, F.A., Krueger, K.K. (eds) (1975) Adequacy of dialysis. *Kidney Int* **7** (Suppl. 2): S1–S263.

Gotch, F.A., Yarian, S., Keen, M. (1990) A kinetic survey of US hemodialysis prescriptions. *Am J Kidney Dis* **15**: 511–515.

Gotloib, L., Barzilay, E., Shustak, A., Wais, Z., Jaichenko, J., Lev, A. (1986) Hemofiltration in septic ARDS. The artificial kidney as an artificial endocrine lung. *Resuscitation* **13**: 123–132.

Graziani, G., Badalamenti, S., Bordone, G., Como, G., Grignani, S., Noto, A., Tetta, C., Lubatti, L., Iapichino, G. (1993) The renal removal of cytokines in sepsis. Preliminary report. In: *Proceedings of the 3rd International Satellite Symposium on ARF, Halkidiki*, p. 660.

Groeneveld, A.B.J., Tran, D.D., van der Meulen, J., Nauta, J.J.P., Thijs, L.G. (1991) Acute renal failure in the medical intensive care unit: Predisposing, complicating factors and outcome. *Nephron* **59**: 602–610.

Grootendorst, A.F., van Bommel, E.F.H., van der Hoven, B., van Leengoed, L.A.M.G., van Osta, A.L.M. (1992) High volume hemofiltration improves right ventricular function in endotoxin induced shock in the pig. *Intensive Care Med* **18**: 235–240.

Grootendorst, A.F., van Bommel, E.F.H., van Leengoed, L.A.M.G., van Zanten, A.R.H., Huipen, H.J.C., Groeneveld, A.B.J. (1993) Infusion of ultrafiltrate from endotoxemic pigs depresses myocardial performance in normal pigs. *J Crit Care* **8**: 161–169.

Gutierrez, A., Alvestrand, A., Wahren, J., Bergstrom, J. (1990) Effect of in vivo contact between blood and dialysis membranes on protein catabolism in humans. *Kidney Int* **38**: 487–494.

Hakim, R. (1990) Assessing the adequacy of dialysis. *Kidney Int* **37**: 822–832.

Hakim, R.M. (1993) Clinical implications of hemodialysis membrane biocompatibiliy. *Kidney Int* **44**: 484–494.

Hakim, R.M., Lowrie, E.G. (1982) Hemodialysis associated neutropenia hypoxemia: the effect of dialyzer membrane materials. *Nephron* **32**: 32–39.

Hakim, R.M., Schafer, I.A. (1985) Hemodialysis-associated platelet activation and thrombocytopenia. *Am J Med* **78**: 575–580.

Hakim, R., Depner, T.A., Parker, T.F. (1992a) In-depth review: adequacy of hemodialysis. *Am J Kidney Dis* **20**: 107–123.

Hakim, R., Wingard, R.L., Lawrence, P., Parker, A., Schulman, G. (1992b) Use of biocompatible membranes improves outcome and recovery from acute renal failure. *J Am Soc Nephrol* **3**: 367.

Hakim, R., Breyer, J., Ismail, N., Schulman, G. (1994a) Effects of dose of dialysis on morbidity and mortality. *Am J Kid Dis* **23**: 661–669.

Hakim, R., Wingard, R.L., Parker, R.A. (1994b) Effect of the dialysis membrane in the treatment of patients with acute renal failure. *N Engl J Med* **331**: 1338–1342.

Henrich, W.L. (1993) Arteriovenous or venovenous continuous therapies are not superior to standard hemodialysis in all patients with acute renal failure. *Seminars Dial* **6**: 174–176.

Henrich, W.L., Woodard, T.D., McPaul, J.J. (1982) The chronic efficacy and safety of high dialysate: double crossover study. *Am J Kidney Dis* **2**: 349–353.

Himmelfarb, J., Lazarus, M., Hakim, R. (1991) Reactive oxygen species production by monocytes and polymorphonuclear leukocytes during dialysis. *Am J Kidney Dis* **3**: 271–276.

Hoerl, W.H., Heidland, A. (1984) Evidence for the participation of granulocyte proteinases on intradialytic catabolism. *Clin Nephrol* **21**: 314–322.

Hoffman, J.N., Faist, E., Deppisch, R., Inthorn, D. (1994) Hemofiltration in human sepsis: elimination of immuno modulatory factors. *Intensive Care Med* **20**: S12 [Abstract].

Howdieshell, T.R., Blalock, W.E., Bowen, P.A., Hawkins, M.L., Hess, C. (1992) Management of post-traumatic acute renal failure with peritoneal dialysis. *Am Surg* **58**: 378–382.

Humphrey, H., Hall, J., Sznajder, I. (1990) Improved survival in ARDS patients associated with a reduction in pulmonary capillary wedge pressure. *Chest* **97**: 1176–1180.

Jeejeebhoy, K.N. (1992) Nutrition in critical illness. In: Civetta JM, Taylor RW, Kirby RR (eds) *Critical Care*, 2nd edition, pp. 1093–1117. Philadelphia: J.B. Lippincott.

Johnson, N.R., Bischel, M.D., Boylen, C.T., Mohler, J.G. (1970) Hypoxemia and hyperventilation in chronic hemodialysis. *Clin Res* **19**: 145–149.

Kaplow, L.S., Foffinet, J.A. (1968) Profound neutropenia during the early phase of hemodialysis. *JAMA* **203**: 1135–1137.

Keller, E., Bonorden, P.R., Lucking, H.P., Böhler, J., Schollmeyer, P. (1991) Continuous arteriovenous hemodialysis: experience in twenty-six intensive care patients. *Contrib Nephrol* **93**: 47–50.

Keshaviah, P., Nolph, K., Van Stone, J. (1989) The peak concentration hypothesis: a urea kinetic approach to comparing the adequacy of continuous ambulatory peritoneal dialysis (CAPD) and hemodialysis. *Perit Dial Int* **9**: 257–260.

Kierdorf, H. (1991) Continuous versus intermittent treatment: clinical results in acute renal failure. *Contrib Nephrol* **93**: 1–12.

Kierdorf, H., Kindler, J., Sieberth, H.G. (1986) Nitrogen balance in patients with acute renal failure treated by continuous haemofiltration. *Nephrol Dial Transplant* **1**: 72–77.

Kirkendol, P.L., Pearson, J.E., Bower, J.D., Holbertt, R.D. (1978) Myocardial depressant effects of sodium acetate. *Cardiovasc Res* **12**: 127–136.

Kirschbaum, B., Galishoff, M., Reines, H.D. (1993) Lactic acidosis treated with continuous hemodiafiltration and regional citrate anticoagulation. *Crit Care Med* **20**: 349–353.

Kishimoto, T., Yamagami, S., Tanaka, H., Ohyama, T., Yamamoto, T., Yamakawa, M., Nishino, M., Yoshimoto, S., Malkawa, T. (1980) Superiority of haemofiltration to haemodialysis for treatment of chronic renal failure: comparative studies between haemofiltration and haemodialysis on dialysis disequilibrium syndrome. *J Artif Organ* **4**: 86–93.

Kjellstrand, C.M., Rosa, A.A., Shidemann, J.R. (1980a) Hypotension during hemodialysis: osmolality fall is an important pathogenic factor. *Trans Am Soc Artif Intern Organs* **3**: 11–14.

Kjellstrand, C.M., Rosa, A.A., Shideman, J.R. (1980b) Hypotension during dialysis: osmolality fall is an important pathogenetic factor. *ASAIO J* **3**: 11–18.

Kjellstrand, C., Ulan, R., Odar-Cederlof, I., Ericsson, F., Skroder, R., Jacobson, S. (1991) All derived K_t/V overestimate and increasingly deviate from the true K_t/V as dialysis speed is increased and dialysis time shortened. *J Am Soc Nephrol* **2**: 332–337.

Klapproth, J., Castell, J., Geigh, T., Andaus, T., Heinrich, PC. (1989) Fate and biological action of human recombinant interleukin I beta in the rat *in vivo*. *Eur J Immunol* **19**: 1485–1490.

Knaus, W.A., Draper, E.A., Wagner, D.P., Zimmerman, J.E. (1985) APACHE II: a severity of disease classification system. *Crit Care Med* **13**: 818–829.

Knaus, W.A., Wagner, D.A., Draper, E.A., Zimmermam, J.E., Bergner, M., Bastos, P.G., Sirio, C.A., Murphy, D.T., Lotring, T., Damiano, A., Horrell, F.E. (1991) The APACHE II prognostic system. Risk predictions of hospital mortality for critically ill hospitalized adults. *Chest* **100**: 1619–1636.

Korchik, U.P., Brown, D.C., De Master, E.G. (1978) Hemodialysis induced hypotension. *Int J Artif Organs* **1**: 151–155.

Kramer, P., Wigger, W., Rieger, J., Matthaei, D., Scheler, F. (1977) Arteriovenous hemofiltration: a new and simple method for treatment of overhydrated patients resistant to diuretics. *Klin Wochenschr* **55**: 1121–1122.

Kveim, M., Nesbakken, R. (1975) Utilization of exogenous acetate during hemodialysis. *Trans Am Soc Artif Int Organs* **21**: 138–142.

Laggner, A.N., Druml, W., Lenz, K., Schneeweiss, B., Grimm, G. (1991) Influence of ultrafiltration/hemofiltration on extravascular lung water. *Contrib Nephrol* **93**: 65–70.

La Greca, G., Dettori, P., Biasioli, S., Fabris, A., Feriani, M., Pinna, V., Pisani, E., Ronco, C. (1980) Brain density studies during dialysis. *Lancet* **ii**: 582.

La Greca, G., Biasioli, S., Chiaramonte, S., Dettori, P., Fabris, A., Ferianni, M., Pinna, V., Pisani, E., Ronco, C. (1982) Studies on brain density in hemodialysis and peritoneal dialysis. *Nephron* **31**: 146–150.

Laird, N.M., Berkey, C.S., Lowrie, E.G. (1983) Modeling success or failure of dialysis therapy: the National Cooperative Dialysis Study. *Kidney Int* **23** (Suppl. 13): S101–S106.

Lange, H.W., Aeppli, D.M., Brown, D.C. (1987) Survival of patients with acute renal failure requiring dialysis after open heart surgery: early prognostic indicators. *Am Heart J* **113**: 1138–1143.

Lauer, A., Saccaggi, A., Ronco, C., Belledonne, M., Gladman, S., Bosch, J. (1983) Continuous arteriovenous hemofiltration in the critically ill patient. *Ann Intern Med* **99**: 455–460.

Lee, P., Matson, J.R., Pryor, R.W., Hinshaw, L.B.H. (1993) Continuous arteriovenous hemofiltration therapy for staphylococcus aureus-induced septicemia in immature swine. *Crit Care Med* **21**: 914–924.

Le Febre, J.M. Spanner, E. Heidenheim, A.L. Lindsy, R.M. (1991) K_t/V patients do not get what the physician prescribes. *ASAIO Trans* **37**: M132–M133.

Le Gall, J.-R., Lemeshow, S., Saulnier, F. (1993) A new simplified acute physiology score (SAPS II) based on a European/North American multi-center study. *JAMA* **270**: 2957–2963.

Lemeshow, S., Teres, D.,Klar, J., Spitz Avrunin, J., Gehlbach, S.H., Rapoport, J. (1993) Mortality probability models (MPM II) based on an international cohort of intensive care unit patients. *JAMA* **270**: 2478–2486.

Leski, M., Niethammer, T., Wyss, T. (1979) Glucose enriched dialysate and tolerance to maintenance hemodialysis. *Nephron* **24**: 271–276.

Lewis, E.G., O'Neill, W.M., Dustman, R.E., Beck, E.C. (1980) Temporal effects of hemodialysis on measures of neural efficiency. *Kidney Int* **17**: 357–363.

Lien, J., Chan, V. (1985) Risk factors influencing survival in acute renal failure treated by hemodialysis. *Arch Intern Med* **145**: 2067–2069.

Lindsay, R.M., Henderson, L.W. (1988) Adequacy of dialysis. *Kidney Int* **33** (Suppl. 24): S92–S99.

Linsay, R., Heidenheim, A.P., Spanner, E., Kortas, C., Blake, P.G. (1994) Adequacy of hemodialysis and nutrition – important determinants of morbidity and mortality. *Kidney Int* **45**: S85–S91.

Lowrie, E.G., Laird, N.M., Parker, T.F., Sargent, JA. (1981) Effect of the hemodialysis prescription on patient morbidity. Report from the National Cooperative Dialysis Study. *N Engl J Med* **305**: 1176–1181.

Lowrie, E.G., Laird, N.M. (eds) (1983) Cooperative dialysis study. *Kidney Int.* **23** (Suppl. 13): S1–S122.

Luger, A., Kovarik, J., Stummvoll, H-K., Urbanska, A., Luger, TA. (1987) Blood-membrane interaction in hemodialysis leads to increased cytokine production. *Kidney Int* **32**: 84–88.

Luke, R.G. (1981) Uremia and the BUN. *N Engl J Med* **305**: 1213–1215.

Manns, M., Sigler, M.H., Teehan, B.P., Frees, Dixit, K. (1994) Effects of intermittent hemodialysis on residual renal function in critically ill patients with acute renal failure. *Int J Artif Organs* **17**: 442 [abstract].

Marsh, J.T., Brown, W.S., Wolcott, D., Laudsverk, J., Niessenson, A.R. (1986) Electrophysiological indices of CNS function in hemodialysis and CAPD. *Kidney Int* **30**: 957–963.

Marshall, J.C. (1994) Infection and the host septic response: implications for clinical trials of mediator antagonism. In: Vincent, J.-L. (ed.) *1994 Yearbook of Intensive Care and Emergency Medicine*, pp. 3–13. Heidelberg: Springer-Verlag.

Matsubara, S., Okabe, C., Ouchi, K., Miyazaki, Y., Yajima, Y., Suzuki, H., Otsuki, M., Matsuno, S. (1990) Continuous removal of middle molecules by hemofiltration in patients with acute liver failure. *Crit Care Med* **18**: 1331–1336.

Mault, J.R., Dechert, R.E., Bartlett, R.H., Swartz, R.D., Ferguson, S.K. (1982) Oxygen consumption during hemodialysis for acute renal failure. *Trans Am Soc Artif Intern Organs* **28**: 510–513.

McDonald, B.R., Mehta, R.L. (1991) Decreased mortality in patients with acute renal failure undergoing continuous arteriovenous hemodialysis. *Contrib Nephrol* **93**: 51–56.

Nies, A.S., Robertson, D., Stone, W.J. (1979) Hemodialysis hypotension is not the result of uremic peripheral autonomic neuropathy. *J Lab Clin Med* **94**: 395–401.

Nimmo, G., Grant, I.S., Mackenzie, S.J. (1991) Lactate and acid base changes in the critically ill. *Postgrad Med J* (Suppl 1): S56–S61.

Nimmo, G.R., Mackenzie, S.J., Walker, S., Nicol, M., Grant, I.S. (1993) Acid–base response to high volume haemofiltration in the critically ill. *Nephrol Dial Transpl* **8**: 854–857.

Ogden, D.A.A. (1978) A double blind crossover comparison of high and low sodium dialysis. *Proc Clin Dial Transpl Forum* **8**: 157–161.

Oh, M.S., Uribarri, J., Del Monte, M.L., Friedman, E.A., Carroll, H.J. (1970) Consumption of CO_2 in metabolism of acetate as an explanation for hypoventilation and hypoxemia during hemodialysis. *Proc Clin Dial Transpl Forum* **9**: 226–231.

Ossenkoppele, G.J., ven der Meulen, J., Bronsveld, W., Thijs, L.G. (1985) Continuous arteriovenous hemofiltration as an adjunctive therapy for septic shock. *Crit Care Med* **13**: 102–104.

Owen, W.F., Lew, N.L., Lui, Y., Lowrie, E.G., Lazarus, J.M. (1993) The urea reduction ratio and serum albumin concentration as predictors of mortality in patients undergoing hemodialysis. *N Engl J Med* **329**: 1001–1006.

Parker, T.F., Husni, L., Huang, W., Lew, N., Lowrie, E.G., Dallas Nephrology Associates (1994) Survival of hemodialysis patients in the United States is improved with a greater quantity of dialysis. *Am J Kid Dis* **23**: 670–680.

Patterson, R.W., Nissenson, A.R., Miller, J., Smith, R.T., Narins, R.G., Sullivan, S.F. (1981) Hypoxemia and pulmonary gas exchange during hemodialysis. *J Appl Physiol* **50**: 259–264.

Pattison, M.L., Lee, S.M., Ogden, D.A. (1988) Continuous arteriovenous hemodiafiltration: an aggressive approach to the management of acute renal failure. *Am J Kid Dis* **11**: 43–47.

Pessina, G.P., Pacini, A., Bocci, V., Maioli, E., Naldini, A. (1987) Studies on tumor necrosis factor (TNF). II: Metabolic fate and distribution of human recombinant TNF. *Lymphokine Res* **6**: 35–43.

Pingleton, S.K., Harmon, G.S. (1987) Nutritional management in acute respiratory failure. *JAMA* **257**: 3094–3099.

Reynolds, H.N., Borg, U., Belzberg, H., Wiles, C.E. (1991) Efficacy of continuous arteriovenous hemofiltration with dialysis in patients with renal failure. *Crit Care Med* **19**: 1387–1394.

Ritz, E., Deppisch, R., Nawroth, P. (1994) Toxicity of uraemia – does it come of age? *Nephrol Dial Transpl* **9**: 1–2.

Romaldini, H., Rodriguez-Roisiss, R., Lopez, F.A., Ziegler, T.W., Bencowitz, H.Z., Wagner, P..D. (1984) The mechanisms of arterial hypoxemia during hemodialysis. *Am Rev Respir Dis* **129**: 780–784.

Ronco, C. (1993) Dialysis delivery vs. dialysis prescription. *Int J Artif Organs* **16**: 628–635.

Ronco, C., Burchardi, H. (1993) Management of acute renal failure in the critically ill patient. In: Pinsky, M.R., Dhaunaut, J.F.A. (eds) *Pathophysiobiologic Foundations of Critical Care*. Baltimore: Williams and Wilkins.

Ronco, C., Feriani, M., Chiaramonte, S. *et al.* (1990) Impact of high blood flows on vascular stability in hemodialysis. *Nephrol Dial Transpl* **1** (Suppl. 5): 109–114.

Ronco, C., Conz, P., Bosch, J.P., Lew, S., La Greca, G. (1994a) Assesment of adequacy in peritoneal dialysis. *Adv Renal Repl Ther* **1**: 15–23.

Ronco, C., Conz, P., Agostini, F., Bosch, J.P., Lew, S., La Greca, G. (1994b) The concept of adequacy in peritoneal dialysis. *Perit Dial Intern* **14** (Suppl. 3): S93–S98.

Ronco, C., Bosch, J.P., Lew, S. *et al.* (1994c) Adequacy of continuous ambulatory peritoneal dialysis. Comparison with other dialysis techniques. *Kidney Int.* **48**: S18–24.

Rosa, A.A., Shideman, J., Kjellstrand, C.M. (1980) Dialysis symptoms and stabilization in long-term dialysis, practical application of the CUSUM plot. *Arch Intern Med* **140**: 804–810.

Sargent, J.A. (1990) Shortfalls in the delivery of dialysis. *Am J Kidney Dis* **15**: 500–510.

Schaefer, G.E., Dolring, C., Sodemann, K., Russ, A., Schroeder, H.M. (1991) Continuous arteriovenous and venovenous hemodialysis in critically ill patients. *Contrib Nephrol* **93**: 23–28.

Schiffl, H., Lang, S.M., Koenig, A., Strasser, T., Haider, M.C., Held, E. (1994) Biocompatible membranes in acute renal failure: prospective case-controlled study. *Lancet* **344**: 570–572.

Schneditz, D., Kaufman, A.M., Polaschegg, H.D., Levin, N.W., Dangirdas, J.T. (1992) Cardiopulmonary recirculation during hemodialysis. *Kidney Int* **42**: 1450–1456.

Schoots, A., Mikkers, F., Cramers, C., de Smet, R., Ringoirs, S. (1984) Uremic toxins and the elusive middle molecules. *Nephron* **38**: 1–8.

Schulman, G., Fogo, A., Gung, A., Bad, R.K., Hakin, R. (1991) Complement activation retards resolution of acute ischemic renal failure in the rat. *Kidney Int* **40**: 1069–1074.

Sherman, R.A., Rubin, M.P., Cooly, R.P., Eisinger, R.P. (1985) Amelioration of hemodialysis-associated hypotension by the use of cool dialysate. *Am J Kidney Dis* **5**: 124–127.

Slutsky, A.S. (1994a) Consensus conferencence on mechanical ventilation. Part I. *Intensive Care Med* **20**: 64–79.

Slutsky AS (1994b) Consensus conference on mechanical ventilation. Part II. *Intensive Care Med* **20**: 150–162.

Smit, J.C., Gareth Jones, J. (1993) Oxygen saturation during hemodialysis. *Renal Failure* **15**: 239–245.

Spiegel, D.M., Ullian, M.E., Zerbe, G.O., Berl, T. (1991) Determinants of survival and recovery in acute renal failure patients dialysed in intensive care unit. *Am J Nephrol* **11**: 44–47.

Stein, B., Pfenninger, E., Gruenert, A., Schmitz, J.E., Deller, A., Kocher, F. (1991) The consequences of continuous hemofiltration on lung mechanics and extravascular lung water in a porcine endotoxic shock model. *Intensive Care Med* **17**: 293–298.

Stevens, P.E., Riley, B., Davies, S.P., Gower, P.E., Brown, E.A., Kox, W. (1988) Continuous arteriovenous hemodialysis in critically ill patients. *Lancet* **ii**: 150–152.

Strasser, T, Schiffl, H. (1991) Generation of leukotriene B 4 by hemodialyser membranes: a novel index of biocompatibility. *Klin Wochenschr* **69**: 808–812.

Swartz, R.D., Valk, T.W., Brain, A.J.P., Hsu, C.H. (1980) Complications of hemodialysis and peritoneal dialysis in acute renal failure. *Trans Am Soc Artif Intern Organs* **3**: 98–101.

Teschan, P.E., Ginn, H.E., Bourne, J.R., Ward, J.W., Hammel, B., Nunally, J.C., Musso, M., Vaughn W.K. (1979) Quantitative indices of clinical uremia. *Kidney Int* **15**: 676–697.

Toback, F.G. (1977) Amino acid enhancement of renal regeneration after acute tubular necrosis. *Kidney Int* **12**: 193–198.

Toback, F.G., Dadd, R.C., Maier, E.R., Havener, L.J. (1983) Amino acid administration enhances renal protein metabolism after acute tubular necrosis. *Nephron* **33**: 238–243.

van Bommel, E.F.H., Hesse, C.J., Jutte, N.H.P.M., Zietse, R., Brunning, H.A., Weimar, W. (1995) Cytokine kinetics (TNF-α, IL-β, IL-6) during continuous hemofiltration: a laboratory and clinical study. *Contrib Nephrol* **116**: 62–75.

Vandenbogaede, J.F., Vanholder, R.C., Everaert, J.A., Vogelaers, D.P., Colardyn, F.A., Ringoir, S.M., Clement, D.L. (1988) Cardiac output changes during hemodialysis with ultrafiltration. *Clinical Nephrol* **29**: 88–92.

Vanholder, R.C., Ringoir, S.M. (1992) Adequacy of dialysis: a critical analysis. *Kidney Int* **42**: 540–558.

Vas, S.Q. (1985) Peritonitis. In: Nolph, K.D. (ed.) *Peritoneal Dialysis* 2nd edition. Boston: Martinus Nijhoff.

Velez, R.L., Woodard, Hessrich, W.L. (1984) Acetate and bicarbonate hemodialysis in patients with and withhold autonomic dysfunction. *Kidney Int* **26**: 59–65.

Voerman, H.J., Strack van Schijndel, R.J.M., Thijs, L.G. (1994) Continuous arteriovenous hemodiafiltration in critically ill patients. *Crit Care Med* **18**: 911–914.

Von Hartizch, B., Eaton, J.W., Buselmeier, T.J., Kjellstrand, C.M. (1974) Dialysis disequilibrium: a manifestation of impaired tissue oxygenation. *Trans Am Soc Artif Intern Organs* **20**: 373–377.

Weissman, C., Heyman, A.I. (1987) Nutritional care of the critically ill patient with respiratory failure. *Crit Care Clin* **3**: 185–203.

Wendon, J., Smithies, M., Sheppard, A., Bullenk Tiuker, J., Bihari, D. (1989) Continuous high-volume veno-venous hemofiltration in acute renal failure. *Intensive Care Med* **15**: 358–363.

Wheeler, D.C., Feehally, J., Walls, J. (1986) High risk acute renal failure. *Q J Med* **61**: 977–984.

Winney, R.J., Kean, D.M., Best, J.J.K., Smith, M.A. (1986) Changes in brain water with haemodialysis. *Lancet* **ii**: 1107–1108.

5

Gastrointestinal Function in Critical Illness

Geoff J. Dobb, Simon Atkinson

INTRODUCTION

The everyday language of ill health contains many references to the gastrointestinal tract. Although to be 'sick' is a blanket term applied to all illness, it also has specific reference to the gut. A major reason for this is the gut's response to physiological stimuli. Sympathetic drive and catecholamine release divert blood away from the gut, giving rise to a sensation of nausea. Parasympathetic stimuli cause hypotension, bradycardia and diarrhoea.

The 'bloody flux' noted in medieval times reaffirmed the long-standing conviction that the gastrointestinal tract could be relied upon to harbour and discharge all that was corruption. A less moralistic approach to the gut evolved with the development of the scientific method and the concept that organ function was related to anatomical structure. Descriptions of the vascular system by Harvey were seen to apply to all organ systems and made possible the study of the gut as an organ and not as a repository of evil. The emergence of chemistry as a separate discipline and its relationship to anatomy led to nutrition and gut function being put on a scientific footing. The nineteenth century saw progress in understanding of gastrointestinal physiology with the discovery of the acidic nature of stomach contents and the observations of Beaumont (1825) on changes in mucosal hyperaemia using a gastrostomy created by accidental trauma.

In 1908, Eli Metchinikoff, a pioneer of immunology, suggested that the passage of organisms from the gut into the systemic circulation was a source of significant ill health and this view was given much added impetus by Sir Arbuthnot Lane (1915). His theory of auto-intoxication by the colon helped to inspire the practise of total colectomy for a multitude of conditions. This fashion formed part of the theme for George Bernard Shaw's play *The Doctor's Dilemma* (1915).

The view that the gastrointestinal tract makes a significant contribution to sepsis by allowing lumenal pathogens access to the systemic circulation remains current.

Multiple Organ Failure in Critical Illness

Baue (1975) first described the 'multiple, progressive or sequential systems failure' of a number of organs precipitated by a variety of conditions. Common factors in the development of global organ failure were shock and sepsis.

The first descriptions of patients with multiple organ failure (MOF) (Eiseman *et al.*, 1977; Fry *et al.*, 1980) emphasized its high mortality, often in association with uncontrolled sepsis. Mainstays in treatment were, and to a large extent still are, adequate fluid resuscitation, inotropic support of the cardiovascular system, oxygenation, renal support and a search for any source of infection coupled with appropriate antibiotic therapy.

Often regular microbial cultures of blood and all portals of entry prove negative, and a policy of diagnostic laparotomy to drain or exclude occult septic intra-abdominal foci has been advocated (Polk and Shields, 1977; Ferraris, 1983). Advances in imaging and percutaneous drainage techniques combined with powerful antimicrobial agents has meant that an increasing proportion of these open surgical explorations are also negative (Hinsdale and Jaffe, 1984). The presence of all the features of sepsis in the absence of proven infection has been termed non-bacterial clinical sepsis. The effect of any inflammatory insult giving rise to a clinical picture similar to that seen in proven infection, but which has not yet progressed to MOF has been termed the 'sepsis syndrome' (Bone *et al.*, 1989) or the systemic inflammatory response syndrome (SIRS) (Bone *et al.*, 1992).

Energy requirements increase to maintain the associated clinical signs and the increased work of breathing. MOF exaggerates this response, with progression to a global catabolic state (Cerra, 1987). The consensus conference (Bone *et al.*, 1992) that provided a definition of SIRS also redefined MOF in recognition that, although definitions of organ failure (Knaus *et al.*, 1985) were in use, there was a continuum of organ dysfunction. The conference advocated the use of the term multiple organ dysfunction syndrome (MODS).

The Pathogenesis of Multiple Organ Dysfunction

The clinical features common to almost all patients with MODS suggest that, despite different initiators, it has common promoters. After a major inflammatory insult, homeostatic stability often continues for some time. If early resolution does not occur then progression to a generalized inflammatory response may result with or without proven infection. Peripheral vasodilatation and decreased blood pressure is accompanied by a reflex tachycardia and an increase, when there is sufficient reserve, in cardiac output. The hyperdynamic cardiovascular response does not necessarily perfuse all vascular beds adequately, and a high cardiac output may be associated with evidence of poor tissue perfusion, including metabolic acidosis and hyperlactataemia.

The aetiology of progression from a systemic inflammatory response to full-blown MODS is of considerable interest. There appear to be a restricted number of clinical settings in which it occurs, namely persistent *focal* inflammation with or without infection (e.g. abscesses, necrotic tissue from trauma, burns, infarction) or persistent *generalized* inflammation, again with or without infection (e.g. bacteraemia, fulminant hepatic failure, malignant hyperpyrexia). Gastrointestinal dysfunction in the intensive care unit commonly occurs in the context of multiple organ dysfunctions (Dobb, 1990), with a highly significant correlation between gastrointestinal dysfunction and cardiovascular, respiratory or renal failure.

The consistency of response to these many different stimuli suggests common mediators.

Endotoxin

The effects of endotoxin on experimental animals resemble those of Gram-negative sepsis, producing a generalized inflammatory response. This has been confirmed in man (Morrison and Ulevitch, 1978; Suffredini *et al.*, 1989). Endotoxin concentrations may be increased, at least transiently, in clinical episodes of sepsis and MOF (van Deventer *et al.*, 1988; Brandtzaeg *et al.*, 1989; Parsons *et al.*, 1989; Danner *et al.*, 1991). The concept that endotoxin may initiate a pathway to generalized inflammation led to consideration of its likely portal of entry into the systemic circulation. In the absence of an obvious focus of infection, e.g. urinary sepsis, peritonitis or aspiration pneumonia, the largest mass of Gram-negative organisms, and therefore endotoxin, is the gastrointestinal tract, making the gastrointestinal tract a prime suspect as a source for the development of systemic sepsis.

Cytokines

Although endotoxin is a major initiating factor, a generalized inflammatory response may also be caused by Gram-positive or fungal infection. Complex networks, rather than cascades, modulate these responses. Endotoxin and other molecules activate the alternative complement pathway with production of C3a and C5a, neutrophil stimulation and release of arachidonic acid derivatives (Reines *et al.*,

1982), free radicals and lysosomal enzymes. Factor XII of the coagulation cascade may be activated both by endotoxin and products of Gram-positive bacterial cell walls to trigger the intrinsic coagulation pathway (Glauser *et al.*, 1991).

Most interest, however, has concentrated on the central role of the macrophage cell line in the response to endotoxin. Macrophages can clear endotoxin, but also control the effects of endotoxin through cellular mediators – the cytokine network.

Tumour necrosis factor

Endotoxin-stimulated macrophages can produce tumour necrosis factor (TNF) (Beutler and Cerami, 1987), interleukin-1 (IL-1) (Dinarello, 1984), interleukin-6 (IL-6) (Kishimoto, 1989), interleukin-8 (IL-8) (Rolfe *et al.*, 1991), platelet activating factor (PAF) (Elstad *et al.*, 1994) and interferons (Mone and Lefkowitz, 1992). Lipopolysaccharide (LPS) binds directly to macrophage surface membrane receptors (Hampton *et al.*, 1988), but its potency to stimulate release of TNF is greatly increased when complexed with the acute phase protein LPS-binding protein (LPB). These complexes are a ligand for macrophage CD-14 receptors (Wright *et al.*, 1990). The pivotal role of TNF as a cytokine in sepsis was established by Beutler *et al.* (1985) when they showed that a polyclonal serum raised against TNF was effective in preventing death from endotoxin in mice. These findings were confirmed in primates using a monoclonal antibody (Tracey *et al.*, 1987), and mice unable to synthesize TNF are resistant to the effects of endotoxin (Beutler *et al.*, 1986).

Its appearance in the plasma of human volunteers after endotoxin administration (Michie *et al.*, 1988) and the finding that levels in broncheolar lavage predict mortality in acute respiratory distress syndrome (ARDS) (Millar *et al.*, 1989) demonstrate its importance as a mediator in sepsis. Administration of TNF mimics the inflammatory response to sepsis, leading to the suggestion that it is the cytokine response to endotoxin and other antigens that is responsible for the profound and, if prolonged, deleterious effects of the inflammatory response.

Other inflammatory mediators

Almost all the mediators produced in response to immunostimulation have effects on vascular endothelium (Bone, 1991), not only by increasing vascular permeability but also by directly stimulating endothelial cells.

It seems likely, therefore, that the inflammatory cascade mediated by the macrophage cell line, endothelial cells, cytokines, complement and the coagulation proteases is essential for normal immune function and clearing antigens. It is only when the inflammatory response is inappropriate and uncontrolled that it results in end-organ dysfunction.

THE ROLE OF THE GASTROINTESTINAL TRACT IN THE PATHOGENESIS OF MULTIPLE ORGAN DYSFUNCTION

Efforts to determine the role of the gastrointestinal tract in MODS have concentrated on the effect of low flow states on the splanchnic circulation, the translocation of organisms and molecules from the lumen to the splanchnic circulation, and the relationship between their presence in the portal circulation and appearance systemically. It is suggested that the gut and liver may, in certain circumstances, be considered as 'net producers' of cytokines (Fong *et al.*, 1990).

Splanchnic Ischaemia

The splanchnic circulation receives about 30% of cardiac output and contains approximately a third of the total blood volume (Porter *et al.*, 1989).

Modulation of gut blood flow

Autonomic modulation of gut blood flow is mediated through the adrenergic supply (Gershon and Erde, 1980; Banks *et al.*, 1985) to smooth muscle of precapillary resistance vessels and vasoconstriction of postcapillary vessels. Experimental studies have shown that the effect of both noradrenaline and adrenaline released from the adrenals is similar. However, the net effect of sympathetic stimulation on intestinal blood flow is complicated by effects on bowel motility and secretion (Jacob *et al.*, 1983), making such experimental studies a poor model for human shock.

Splanchnic vessels are more sensitive to the vasoconstrictor effects of vasopressin and angiotensin II than are systemic vessels (Gunther *et al.*, 1980; Said, 1983). Both these hormones are released in response to systemic hypotension. When an angiotension converting enzyme inhibitor, captopril, is given during an experimental model of haemorrhagic shock, blood flow to the small intestine, pancreas, liver and spleen (but not the stomach) is enhanced (Cullen *et al.*, 1994).

A number of other humoral factors are involved in control of splanchnic vasomotor tone, including the gastrointestinal peptides, vasoactive intestinal peptide and cholecystokinin, and the arachidonic acid metabolites (Porter *et al.*, 1989). This 'non-occlusive' splanchnic ischaemia is particularly marked in the low flow states associated with cardiogenic and hypovolaemic (Gilmour *et al.*, 1980) shock. Despite the major vessels remaining patent the relative vasoconstriction may result in mucosal necrosis in both the small and large bowel (Bailey *et al.*, 1987).

The effect and interaction of the local inflammatory and other mediators already described is particularly complex. Many of the arachidonic acid derivatives, including some prostaglandins, leukotrienes and thromboxane, cause splanchnic vasoconstriction and are important mediators of mesenteric vascular constriction in response to bacteraemia (Gosche *et al.*, 1994).

Vasoconstriction leads to ischaemia with acidosis, increased local carbon dioxide tension, decreased oxygen tension, local hyperkalaemia and release of adenosine. All these factors promote vasodilatation. The discovery of endothelium-derived relaxing factor (EDRF) in 1980 by Furchgott and Zawadzki and the subsequent realization that this factor was the evanescent free radical nitric oxide (NO) (Ignarelo *et al.*, 1987; Palmer *et al.*, 1987) has led to much interest on the effects of immune mediators on vascular tone. NO is synthesized from the amino acid L-arginine by NO synthase, and causes vascular smooth muscle relaxation by the activation of guanylate cyclase and subsequent formation of the intracellular messenger cyclic guanosine monophosphate (cGMP) (Moncada *et al.*, 1991). Recent work has shown that nitric oxide plays an important role in maintaining basal splanchnic microvascular vasodilator tone. The splanchnic arteriolar vasoconstriction and hypoperfusion during bacteraemia are exacerbated when a NO synthase inhibitor is given (Spain *et al.*, 1994).

Endothelin appears to be another molecule responsible for the control of vascular tone and is a potent vasoconstrictor (Miyauchi *et al.*, 1990). In sepsis, vascular tone plays an important role in microcirculatory control, and significant shunting and tissue hypoxia may occur, despite a hyperdynamic circulation.

Intestinal ischaemia

The changes induced by haemorrhagic shock, trauma, burns, sepsis and other systemic inflammatory responses cause intestinal ischaemia (Turnage *et al.*, 1994). During experimental haemorrhagic shock, gut oxygen delivery decreases to as little as 30% of the initial value, while oxygen consumption remains unchanged. Peritonitis causes a smaller decrease in gut oxygen delivery, but this is accompanied by increased oxygen consumption. In both cases mucosal ischaemia is reflected by a mucosal intracellular acidosis (Antonsson and Haglund, 1995). During peritonitis, impaired oxygen extraction or utilization also contribute to the intramucosal acidosis, perhaps because oxidative phosphorylation is impaired by endotoxin (Schaefer *et al.*, 1991).

The concept of early hyperdynamic and late hypodynamic stages of sepsis has been questioned (Fink, 1989). It is not uncommon for septic patients to have normal or increased cardiac output until either recovery or death (Parker *et al.*, 1984) and splanchnic perfusion may be preserved (Dahn *et al.*, 1987) during sepsis. It has, therefore, been suggested that any splanchnic ischaemia occurring in septic states derives from an imbalance between increases in oxygen demand and increases in perfusion. This has been termed 'relative ischaemia' (Falk *et al.*, 1985; Fink, 1989).

In the intestinal villi a central arteriole only branches when it gets to the top of the villus with blood flowing back to the base of the villus through subepithelial capillaries and vessels. This creates a counter-current arrangement which favours the maintenance of oxygenation at the base of the villus at the expense of the tip. The 'hairpin' loops of the countercurrent exchange mechanism in the villi are particularly sensitive to reductions in perfusion pressure, even when villous blood flow remains unchanged. Lundgren and Haglund (1978) suggested that a reduction in the velocity of flow through these loops leads to an increased time available for extravascular oxygen shunting, and consequently, to lower oxygen tensions at the tips of the villi. This implies that, even if total splanchnic blood flow is preserved, a reduction in perfusion pressure combined with the increased metabolic demands of the gut in sepsis may be enough to render areas of the splanchnic microcirculation hypoxic.

Effect of resuscitation and treatment

Resuscitation tends to restore splanchnic perfusion, although there is evidence that crystalloid fluid resuscitation does not fully restore splanchnic blood flow after haemorrhage or endotoxaemia (Scannell *et al.*, 1992; Kreimeier *et al.*, 1993). Nevertheless, conditions causing intestinal reperfusion injury can occur. This intestinal injury is associated with systemic inflammation and with remote organ injury involving the lungs, liver and kidneys (Turnage *et al.*, 1994). The local injury process is summarized in Figure 5.1.

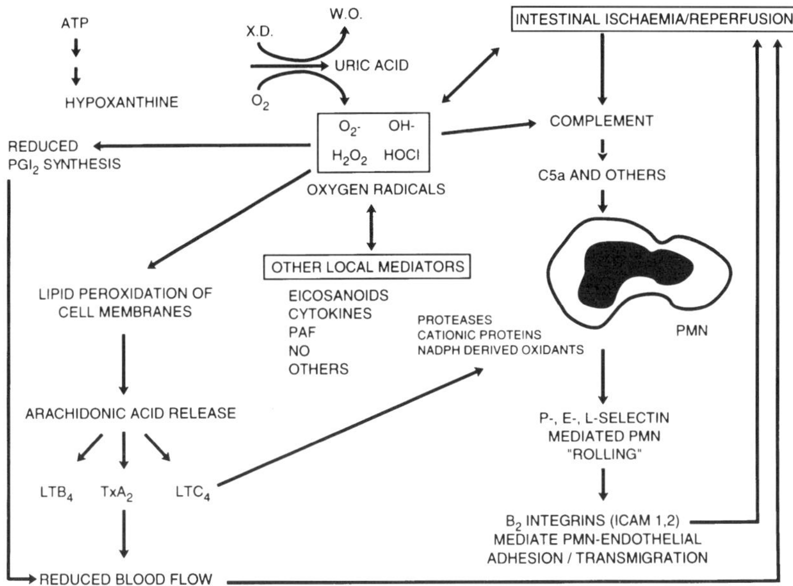

Figure 5.1. Mediators of ischaemia–reperfusion injury include oxygen derived free radicals, complement, cytokines, neutrophils and the other mediators summarized here (modified from Dobb, 1996).

Detailed studies in sheep have shown that dobutamine, noradrenaline, dopamine, dopexamine and salbutamol have no significant effect on blood flow to the stomach or the small or large bowel (Bersten *et al.*, 1992), despite significant increases in cardiac index with all the sympathomimetics. In septic sheep (Bersten *et al.*, 1992), blood flow to the stomach and bowel is increased, but decreased as a percentage of cardiac output. The circulation is less sensitive to the effects of sympathomimetics during sepsis, all sympathomimetics appearing to have similar effects on gut blood flow. Sepsis decreases blood flow to the pancreas. Salbutamol is the only sympathomimetic to reverse the decrease in pancreatic blood flow caused by sepsis. Importantly, however, the authors of this study caution that '. . . it cannot be assumed that changes in organ blood flow induced by the infusion of sympathomimetics will be converted into nutritional flow at the micro-regional level'.

Studies in critically ill patients, however, do show differences between sympathomimetics in their effect on mucosal ischaemia, as assessed by gastric tonometry. During hyperdynamic sepsis (Marik and Mohedin, 1994), infusion of dopamine to maintain mean arterial pressure greater than 75 mmHg decreases gastric intramucosal pH

(pH_i), whereas using noradrenaline to maintain the same arterial pressure increases the pH_i. In patients meeting the criteria for the systemic inflammatory response syndrome, low-dose dopamine (2.5 mg/kg/min) has no effect on pH_i or other indices of splanchnic blood flow, but dopexamine (1 mg/kg/min) increases pH_i and appears to have a selective vasodilating effect on splanchnic vessels. Other work suggests that a redistribution of blood flow within the gut wall which favours the mucosa occurs in response to β-adrenergic receptor stimulation. Whether such an effect has a significant impact on patient outcome has still to be shown.

Structural effects of intestinal ischaemia

Reperfusion injury is only really significant in the mucosa and is greater after partial than total gut ischaemia (Park *et al.*, 1990). Ischaemic injury of sufficient severity to cause injury to deeper parts of the gut wall will be such that no additional damage can occur on reperfusion. Thus, with increasing ischaemic injury there is a progression (Table 5.1) to full-thickness infarction of the gut, as found at autopsy in some patients who have died after severe prolonged hypotension. The full-thickness injuries may be punctate, or discrete areas not involving the full circumference.

At the other end of the range of structural damage, the most minimal is lifting of the epithelial cells at the tip of the villi. As ischaemia becomes more severe or prolonged, epithelial cells are lost from the sides of the villi until the villus core is exposed and disintegrates. The pattern of injury is related to the vascular anatomy of the villi described earlier. However, once adequate oxygen delivery is restored, anatomical recovery can be rapid. In rats mucosal repair is evident just 18 hours after 90 minutes of warm total ischaemia (Park and Haglund, 1992).

Table 5.1 Progression of gut injury caused by increasing severity of ischaemic insults

- Increased capillary permeability
- Increased mucosal permeability
- Superficial injury to the mucosa
- Transmucosal injury
- Full-thickness injury of bowel wall

CHANGES TO GUT FUNCTION IN CRITICAL ILLNESS

Some of the changes in gut function that occur during critical illness are summarized in Table 5.2. While these changes are in part associated with shock, the effects of inflammatory mediators, decreased gut blood flow and the drugs needed by critically ill patients are also significant.

Splanchnic hypoperfusion has been implicated in stress ulceration, intestinal haemorrhage, failure of gastric acid secretion (Stannard *et al.*, 1988), acalculus cholecystitis, ischaemic hepatitis and, more rarely, pancreatitis (Astiz *et al.*, 1993).

Of most interest, however, is the effect of ischaemia on the integrity of the gastrointestinal tract. Separation of the contents of the gut lumen from the portal circulation depends upon intact and functioning mucosal cells and it has been postulated that loss of this integrity leads to ingress of organisms and endotoxin, which contributes to the development and maintenance of multiple organ failure (Meakins and Marshall, 1986).

Nutrient Absorption

Nutrient absorption is a complex process that is dependent on passive and active absorption, the break down of nutrients by enzymes released from the stomach, bowel and pancreas, and gut motility. Factors leading to reduced nutrient absorption include:

- a reduction in the affinity or number of enterocyte transporter proteins;
- reduced blood flow, impairing the export of absorbed substrate across the basolateral membrane of the enterocyte;
- increased enterocyte turnover because of damage to those at the top of the villus (less mature cells have decreased absorptive ability).

Table 5.2   Examples of functional impairment of the gastrointestinal tract during critical illness

- Failure of gastric acid secretion
- Impaired digestive enzyme secretion
- Impaired nutrient absorption
- Decreased gut motility
- Cholestasis
- Increased intestinal permeability
- Translocation of bacteria or endotoxin

For example, shock has been shown to reduce intestinal amino acid absorption (Sodeyama *et al.*, 1992). A significant reduction in amino acid absorption persists after resuscitation to restore both arterial pressure and splanchnic blood flow, suggesting there is delayed recovery of amino acid intestinal active transport.

Gut Barrier Function

The barriers to invading pathogenic micro-organisms are:

- Intraluminal defences: gastric acidity, gut motility, intraluminal digestive enzymes, secreted immunoglobulin.
- Mucosal defences: association with normal flora, mucus layer in the glycocalyx, tight intercellular junctions between enterocytes, escalation of enterocytes along the villi until they are extruded at the tip.
- Gut associated lymphoid tissue: lymphocytes make up about 20% of the intestinal mucosa.
- Macrophages: 70% of the body's macrophages are found in the gut, peritoneum and hepatic reticuloendothelial system.

Bacterial translocation

Simple evidence for translocation of intact organisms arose from finding ingested pathogens such as *Listeria monocytogenes* in the circulation of infected patients (Fleming *et al.*, 1985). Also, after oral ingestion of *Candida albicans*, the organism was isolated from blood and urine a number of hours later (Krause *et al.*, 1969). The potential for translocation appears to be reduced by the presence of normal intestinal flora in appropriate numbers, so called 'colonization resistance' (van der Waaij *et al.*, 1972). Conversely, changes to the gut flora caused by antibiotics may increase translocation.

It seems likely that bacterial translocation is occurring to some extent all the time in health, accounting for the large amounts of lymphoid tissue in the gastrointestinal tract itself, the mesentery and organs receiving portal blood, i.e. the spleen and liver. Interest has centred on the extent to which the response to injury causes translocation to increase and the rate at which organisms appear in the portal and systemic circulation.

Translocation of bacteria and endotoxin appears to involve a complex interaction between enterocytes and macrophages (Saadia *et al.*, 1990) and failure of the gut-associated lymphoid tissue. The process has been documented in numerous experimental studies using animal models of shock, trauma and sepsis (Fink, 1991). In man, simple intestinal obstruction causes translocation to mesenteric lymph nodes recovered at laparotomy (Deitch, 1989), and after burn injury (Fukushima *et al.*, 1992; Manson *et al.*, 1992) an increase in translocation of bacteria occurs and permeability increases at a molecular level (Ziegler *et al.*, 1988). The high incidence of positive blood cultures in patients admitted to trauma units with shock (Border *et al.*, 1987; Rush *et al.*, 1988), provides further weight to the concept of splanchnic ischaemia promoting translocation. There is also some evidence from sampling of the portal circulation that bacterial contamination in shock and sepsis is not uncommon (Mainous *et al.*, 1991), although clearly it does not always occur (van Deventer *et al.*, 1988) and its significance is uncertain. For example, 212 portal blood cultures taken from 20 patients with trauma were negative for gut bacteria and endotoxin, even though six subsequently developed multiple organ failure (Moore *et al.*, 1991). In another clinical study (Moore *et al.*, 1992), blood cultures were taken from 132 acutely injured patients needing an urgent laparotomy for trauma. Blood cultures were positive in 32% of patients with shock, but the majority (73%) of organisms isolated were Gram positive rather than enteric. There also appeared to be little correlation between isolation of bacteria from mesenteric lymph nodes and the clinical course. On the other hand, all the patients with enteric bacteraemia and shock died. Also, in severe haemorrhagic pancreatitis there is evidence (Luiten *et al.*, 1995) that the organisms infecting the necrotic tissue originate from the gut.

The overall clinical significance of bacterial translocation in critical illness has, therefore, still to be determined. Because of the treatment implications (Luiten *et al.*, 1995), the characterization of the circumstances under which bacterial translocation from the gut is clinically important is an important issue that needs to be resolved by critical care research.

Gastrointestinal permeability

Tests of intestinal permeability are not part of routine clinical practice. Differential molecular absorption tests are research methods used to assess gastrointestinal integrity. The range of different molecules for these tests allows testing of the different pathways through the gastrointestinal wall. These permeation pathways are governed by complex pore and fluid dynamics as well as by a number of physical laws (Travis and Menzies, 1992). For the purpose of considering how the probe molecules reach the circulation the pathways used can be broadly divided into groups.

A probe molecule used to assess permeability should be bio-chemically inert, cross intestinal epithelium by non-mediated diffusion and be recoverable in the urine after an oral dose. The proportion of the oral dose recovered, used as a measure of permeability, will be affected by variations in gastric emptying, transit times and renal clearance. If the ratio of two different sized molecules is used the non-mucosal confounding factors will apply to both. Changes in the ratio will imply a difference in permeation of one molecule compared to the other.

Increased intestinal permeability has been demonstrated in patients with burns (LeVoyer *et al.*, 1992), haemorrhagic shock and trauma (Roumen *et al.*, 1993). These studies have used lactulose, ethylene diamine tetra-acetic acid (EDTA), polyethyleneglycol and other non-metabolized molecules as markers of increased intestinal permeability. Because the marker molecules are too large to cross cell membranes, an increase in their intestinal permeability is the sum of their migra-tion between cells (paracellular permeation), through ulcerations and across epithelial extrusion zones at the villus tip. The intercellular tight junction complex, or zona occludens, is a dynamic gate that opens and shuts in response to physiological, chemical and toxic influences (Madara, 1989). The maximum channel size of the junctional complex allows the passage of molecules with hydrodynamic molecular radii up to 1.1 nm. This channel size is too small for bacteria or endo-toxin, but is large enough to allow the passage of bacterially derived small peptides or small dietary antigens that are normally confined to the intestinal lumen. Immediately under the tight junctions are intra-epithelial lymphocytes. These respond to antigens by secreting interferon-γ, which increases the permeability of the intestinal mucosa by stimulating contraction of enterocyte actin–myosin, which in turn is coupled to and opens the tight junctions. Interferon-γ also activates macrophages to release inflammatory mediators, which further increase local mucosal and capillary permeability.

Lactulose and mannitol are the molecules most commonly used for permeability tests because they are readily available and not difficult to measure. Lactulose relies largely on paracellular transport. Mannitol probably permeates by both transcellular and paracellular routes (Dawson *et al.*, 1988). Following absorption there may be some loss of mannitol by cellular absorption and metabolism. L-Rhamnose, often used in combination with lactulose, is thought to permeate by a transcellular route. Simultaneous administration with other markers has also been used to assess differences between mediated and non-mediated transport. D-Xylose and 3-*O*-methyl-D-glucose provide a means of estimating the degree of mediated transport impairment that may occur in injured gastrointestinal epithelium (Travis and Menzies, 1992).

Isotope tests such as [^{51}Cr]EDTA have some advantages, including relative ease of measurement. However, unless combined with a carbohydrate probe, these tests suffer the disadvantages of a single marker and those of using radioisotopes. Polyethylene glycols of different molecular size have also been used. There remains some debate about the route of permeation of these molecules, and the amount recovered in the urine following intravenous administration varies substantially (Philipsen *et al.*, 1988).

Many conditions other than critical illness can affect gut permeability to probe molecules. These include coeliac disease (Bjarnason *et al.*, 1983a), inflammatory bowel disease (Bjarnason *et al.*, 1983b) and most of the nutritional enteropathies such as tropical sprue. The non-gastrointestinal inflammatory conditions, rheumatoid arthritis and seronegative arthropathies are associated with increased permeability, possibly caused by the ingestion of non-steroid anti-inflammatory drugs (NSAIDs) (Bjarnason *et al.*, 1991). Other drugs shown to change permeability include the cytotoxic drugs, 5-fluorouracil (Siber *et al.*, 1980) and methotrexate, as well as radiotherapy.

Intestinal permeability has now been investigated extensively in order to determine the conditions and factors that influence it. Speculation that loss of integrity of the gastrointestinal tract is related to the development of MODS stimulated a number of these permeability studies. Harris *et al.* (1992) measured lactulose/mannitol ratios in patients admitted to their intensive care unit, and found that increases in intestinal permeability were common in these patients but appeared not to be related to disease severity or sepsis. Patients undergoing cardiopulmonary bypass have been shown to have impairment of translumenal transport mechanisms and increases in permeability (Ohri *et al.*, 1993). These changes related to time on bypass and a reduction in gastric mucosal blood flow. The effect of sepsis is complicated by the effects of sepsis itself on the gastrointestinal tract. Endotoxin promotes bacterial translocation and increases permeability in animal models (Deitch *et al.*, 1987; Deitch and Berg, 1987; Fink *et al.*, 1991) and humans (O'Dwyer *et al.*, 1988), although it is not clear if this is as a result of the hypotensive effects of endotoxin (Navaratnam *et al.*, 1990) or is caused by mediator formation.

Evidence for changes in permeability caused by inflammatory mediators is conflicting. TNF does not affect transepithelial resistance or mannitol flux in intestinal epithelial monolayers (Madara and Stafford, 1989), but does increase mannitol permeability in renal epithelial (Mullin and Snock, 1990) and endothelial cells in vitro. It also reduces D-xylose absorption in a mouse model (Singh *et al.*, 1993). Platelet activating factor increases the blood to lumen passage of [^{51}Cr]EDTA in rats and causes mucosal cell damage (Wallace *et al.*, 1987). Given the interrelationships of splanchnic ischaemia, translocation of bacteria and endotoxin, and cytokine production, it is unsurprising that there is no clear cause and effect relationship. It is apparent, however, that the gastrointestinal barrier is a dynamic structure and that even during health there is likely to be translocation. The effect is only significant if normal clearing mechanisms are impaired.

Much of the gastrointestinal tract and associated structures have an immune function. The Peyer's patches of the small intestine, the mesenteric lymph node complexes and the 'backstop' provided by the Kupffer cells of the liver provide cellular structures for immunological protection from the lumenal contents of the gut. However, it still must be emphasized that intestinal permeability, as demonstrated by marker molecules, correlates poorly with sepsis of gut origin or multiple organ failure (Roumen *et al.*, 1993).

MONITORING GUT ORGAN FUNCTION

Attempts to modify the contribution of the gastrointestinal tract to the development of MODS would require accurate and early diagnosis of deteriorations in gut function. Available methods include estimation of hepatic and intestinal blood flow, assessment of gastrointestinal tract integrity and tests of liver function.

Monitoring the Splanchnic Circulation

In acute mesenteric vascular occlusion the sudden onset of an acute abdomen with pain, tenderness, and perhaps gastrointestinal haemorrhage and circulatory collapse are symptoms and signs indicating a severe intra-abdominal catastrophe requiring surgery. Chronic occlusive splanchnic ischaemia is suggested by the history and confirmed by angiography. In contrast, non-occlusive ischaemia has, until recently, been difficult to diagnose because local signs are not specific and because specific investigations have not been available. Clinical evidence of splanchnic ischaemia, abdominal distension, intolerance of enteral nutrition and 'stress ulceration' (Marrone and Silen, 1984), implies that injury has already occurred. Intervention at this stage can only rescue damaged mucosa, not prevent it.

Measures of hepatic and intestinal blood flow have been developed but, with some exceptions, they remain research methods. They can be divided into techniques that measure blood flow directly, total hepatic blood flow (portal and arterial), fractionated blood flow to distinguish between intestinal and hepatic circulations and indirect techniques. Some techniques are experimental and unlikely to have clinical application.

Direct techniques include the collection and measurement of venous outflow, electromagnetic flow probes (Granger and Bulkley, 1981), and pulsed Doppler flowmetry (Haywood *et al.*, 1981; Payen *et al.*, 1989). More commonly, and with greater potential clinical application, the hepatic clearance of a number of different substances has been used to obtain an estimate of total hepatic blood flow. The Fick principle allows estimation of the blood flow through an organ if the concentration of marker molecule before and after the organ and its uptake are known. Suitable markers are those that are rapidly and exclusively metabolized or excreted by the organ. Clearly, the uptake of any molecule by an organ reflects not only blood flow but also the function of the metabolic pathway supporting the extraction. If this pathway is impaired, then decreased clearance may not reflect similar reductions in blood flow (Skak and Keiding, 1987).

Substances that have been used for liver blood flow estimation include indocyanine green (Wiegand *et al.*, 1960; Caesar *et al.*, 1961), galactose (Henderson *et al.*, 1982), sorbitol (Zech *et al.*, 1988) and ethanol. Radiolabelled molecules extracted by the hepatic reticulo-endothelial system ($[^{32}P]$chromic phosphate, $[^{99m}Tc]$sulphur colloid) have also been used. Measurement of intestinal blood flow by itself has required considerable ingenuity. Once again, modified forms of the Fick principle have been tried: aminopyrine clearance (Sack and Spenney, 1982), inert gas clearance (Gharagozloo *et al.*, 1984) and hydrogen clearance (Ashley and Cheung, 1984). Rates of entrapment of radioactive microspheres can be used experimentally to estimate intestinal intramural blood flow (Dregelid *et al.*, 1986). Laser Doppler flowmetry can measure blood flow in gastric mucosal capillaries directly (Kvietys *et al.*, 1985; Ohri *et al.*, 1993), but the gastric mucosa must be visualized by endoscopy and the technique is thus unsuitable for routine clinical use.

Total blood flow rates to a tissue do not, however, always indicate the adequacy of oxygen and substrate delivery. Oxygen tension, haemoglobin concentration and, in most tissues, perfusion pressure are also important. Anatomical changes at the level of the microcirculation, which are likely in the critically ill, including shunting, variations in endothelial morphology and diffusion distances, affect tissue oxygen availability. Oxygen concentrations in the tissues do not, in themselves, indicate that cellular metabolic demands are being met. When there is metabolic stress the opening up of vascular channels, shifts in oxygen dissociation curves and changes in intracellular metabolic pathways may enable reductions in tissue pO_2 to be accommodated, despite hypoxaemia.

Evidence of inadequate tissue oxygenation provided by the products of anaerobic metabolism would be more useful, particularly ATP/ADP, lactate and hydrogen ion concentrations. The latter two are routine measurements in systemic blood, but represent global tissue events (Vincent *et al.*, 1981) rather than those in a single organ or tissue. Direct determination has been attempted in splanchnic tissues in animal models (Antonsson *et al.*, 1990).

Gastrointestinal lumenal tonometry

These devices rely on the ability of dissolved tissue gases to reach an equilibrium in fluid within a lumen. This principle applies to any gas, but is particularly suited for CO_2 estimation because of its solubility and its tension across tissues. The fluid pCO_2 within a hollow viscus can be assumed to represent the pCO_2 within tissues lining that viscus, i.e. its mucosa. If the bicarbonate concentration is assumed to be that of the arterial blood supplying those tissues, then by using a modified form of the Henderson–Hasselbalch equation a value for the tissue pH can be derived. The products of anaerobic metabolism reduce tissue pH and this is reflected in the tonometric pCO_2.

After tissue pO_2 had been measured in the mucosa of isolated loops of intestine (Dawson *et al.*, 1965), Fiddian-Green and colleagues extended the technique. By measuring pCO_2 in a saline-filled balloon permeable to CO_2 within the gut lumen, it has been possible to demonstrate a useful estimate of intramucosal pH (pH_i). This has been validated in the ileum by direct tissue pH measurement in an animal model (Antonsson *et al.*, 1990). The method shows that ileal mucosal H^+ concentration increases after an endotoxin-induced reduction in superior mesenteric artery (SMA) flow (Fink *et al.*, 1989) in an animal model of sepsis. After SMA occlusion in dogs tonometric measurement of ileal intramucosal pH showed marked acidosis (Grum *et al.*, 1984). This was confirmed later for rectal, colonic, jejunal and duodenal measurements (Schonholz *et al.*, 1989). Similar results were obtained in a model of haemorrhagic shock (Hartman *et al.*, 1991).

As it has proved convenient in clinical practice to use a silicone balloon filled with saline inserted nasogastrically to provide the isolated lumen, it remains a source of concern that, as yet, there is no validation of gastric intramucosal pH measured tonometrically with direct tissue pH measurement.

However, Fiddian-Green and others have accrued considerable clinical evidence for the use of this technique. The risk of stress ulceration (Fiddian-Green *et al.*, 1983) and complications after cardiac surgical procedures (Fiddian-Green and Baker, 1987) are related to low gastric intramucosal pH. Similarly, pH_i is highly predictive of outcome after admission for both surgical intensive care unit (ICU) (Gys *et al.*, 1988) and multidisciplinary ICU patients (Doglio *et al.*, 1991; Maynard *et al.*, 1994). A more direct link between low tissue pH measured tonometrically, intestinal ischaemia and episodes of sepsis from gut-derived organisms was shown by Fiddian-Green in patients after aortic aneurysm surgery (Fiddian-Green and Gantz, 1987).

Potential benefits of monitoring gastric pH_i have also been assessed. Gutierrez *et al.* (1992) compared the technique with the already established measures of oxygen transport and consumption after suggestions that increased V_{O_2} and D_{O_2} improve survival in high-risk surgical patients (Shoemaker *et al.*, 1988). They found that pH_i correlated well with both measures. In cardiac surgical patients during cardiopulmonary bypass, Landow *et al.* (1991) demonstrated good correlation between hepatic venous lactate levels and pH_i.

There are some concerns about the technique. As already mentioned, despite validation by direct measurement of tissue pH in the ileum, the absence of this confirmation in the stomach means that this relationship has to be assumed. Also, assuming that arterial bicarbonate is an appropriate measure of tissue bicarbonate has been questioned, particularly if the organ in question is generating lactic acid, i.e. is ischaemic (Fiddian-Green, 1989). Moreover, the alkaline tide produced during acid secretion by the gastric mucosa may invalidate this assumption. The neutralization of gastric acid to duodenal bicarbonate may result in lumenal CO_2 generation and a higher tonometric pCO_2. For these reasons, the administration of H_2-receptor antagonists has been advocated, and there is evidence that, at least in healthy human volunteers, this overcomes a source of underestimation of pH_i (Heard *et al.*, 1991). In clinical practice this finding has to be balanced against potential risks associated with H_2 antagonists (gastric colonization and nosocomial pneumonia) and, while the pH_i estimates are lower without H_2 antagonists, the effect is consistent and therefore can be allowed for by modification of the normal range (Parviainen *et al.*, 1996). There is also the potential for artifact to be introduced by H_2 antagonists, through interference with histamine-mediated homoeostatic processes that influence mucosal blood flow (Nishizaki *et al.*, 1994). To increase the reliability of CO_2 tonometry measurements, the use of a phosphate buffer (Knichwitz *et al.*, 1994) or 4% succinyl-ated gelatin (Gelofusine) has been advocated in place of saline (Riddingon *et al.*, 1994) as the solution. More recent studies have suggested that air is a suitable medium for CO_2 tonometry and can provide a more responsive system (Lahtienen *et al.*, 1996).

Of equal importance to technical problems associated with gastric tenometry is the criticism that the pH_i reflects only systemic changes in the systemic acid–base balance. In a study of 20 patients, Boyd *et al.* (1993) found that the correlation between base deficit and pH_i was such that they recommended that information could be obtained more easily and reliably from routine blood gas analysis. While there is no doubt that pH_i will be low when there is a significant metabolic acidosis, it is the presence of covert splanchnic ischaemia in an apparently resuscitated patient that has the greatest clinical relevance.

In summary, experimental studies show that the pH_i is a good indicator of gut ischaemia, and clinical studies have shown it to be of value in predicting complications in critically ill patients (Silverman, 1991; Maynard *et al.*, 1993). Other clinical studies, however, have high-lighted problems with this method of estimating pH_i (Desai *et al.*, 1993). It also appears that pH_i correlates poorly with total splanchnic flow or oxygen delivery after cardiac surgery (Uusaro *et al.*, 1995), perhaps because there is maldistribution of blood flow rather than because of a problem with measuring the pH_i. These findings suggest that the methods for detecting intestinal ischaemia need some further refine-ment. The relative importance of splanchnic blood flow and mucosal ischaemia also needs to be defined.

Total splanchnic blood flow

The most commonly used tests relating indirectly or directly to total splanchnic blood flow can be divided into those largely associated with liver function and those related to total liver blood flow.

Common clinical tests of liver function include measures of hepato-cyte synthesis (albumin, coagulation factors), hepatocyte metabolism (bilirubin) and enzyme release by hepatocytes and canalicular epithelium (AST, ALT, ALP, γ-GT). These tests are often abnormal in critical illness, but provide little discrimination for early liver dysfunction caused by changes in liver blood flow. Measurements of liver blood flow may provide a more sensitive indicator of a drift towards multiple organ failure. These measures rely on almost com-plete metabolism or excretion of a substance by a relatively small amount of functioning liver, and therefore they are initially only affected by flow rate. Indocyanine green clearance has become the standard molecule used for measuring hepatic clearance. Pollack *et al.* (1979) reported that indocyanine green plasma disappearance rates were markedly different in survivors and non-survivors admitted with trauma. Galactose and sorbitol clearances have also been tried with some success, but have not been used in the critically ill. The extent to which these clearances are affected by liver function remains unclear, but there is little doubt that hepatic extraction is not 100% and there is often some extrahepatic metabolism and renal excretion.

Lignocaine–monoethylglycinexylidide (MEGX) conversion has been suggested as a sensitive test of liver function that may also reflect small changes in liver blood flow (Maynard *et al.*, 1992a). A bolus of lignocaine is rapidly metabolized by cytochrome p450-mediated *N*-deethylation (Pieper and Rodman, 1986) to a number of substances, including MEGX. This is easily measurable in the peripheral blood after 15 minutes. Early identification of liver dysfunction at the mitochondrial level is presumed to reflect splanchnic ischaemia, and reports in critically ill patients suggest that use of lignocaine–MEGX conversion provides better discrimination than ICG or other tests of liver function (Maynard *et al.*, 1992b). In hepatic transplantation, this test was a better predictor of donor initial function and primary non-function than were indocyanine green and galactose clearances, AST, and bilirubin (Burdelski *et al.*, 1987, 1988). Also, differentiation between normal and pathological histology was better with this test. The influence of liver blood flow is not yet clear (Huet and Villeneuve, 1983), but the test appears to be sensitive enough to describe any functional deficit that might be caused by splanchnic ischaemia.

GASTROINTESTINAL ORGAN SUPPORT

It is likely that different parts of the gut require varying methods of organ support. These methods attempt to reverse a particular aspect of gut organ dysfunction. Treatment of critically ill patients should always include prompt and rapid resuscitation, and treatment of the underlying cause for severe illness. Other management strategies specific to intestinal function include:

- prevention of intestinal ischaemia;
- maintaining enteral nutrition;
- enhancing parenteral nutrition if enteral nutrition is impossible.

The functional effects of critical illness on the gastrointestinal system are summarized in Table 5.2.

Prevention of Intestinal Ischaemia

Prevention of intestinal ischaemia currently relies principally on measures to increase global oxygen delivery, although there is some evidence that dopexamine causes a favourable redistribution of blood flow to the splanchnic circulation (see above). Increasing global oxygen delivery by blood transfusion has no effect on gastric intramucosal acidosis, whereas some (but not all) studies show that it can be at least partially corrected by infusion of dobutamine or low-dose dopamine (Dobb, 1995). Other work (Maynard *et al.*, 1992b) has shown that dopexamine, an α_1, β_2-agonist, is able to produce splanchnic vasodilatation and also to cause an increase in the pH_{im} of critically ill patients. A similar effect has been observed with prostacyclin (Radermacher *et al.*, 1994). The effects of these vasoactive drugs has implications for the prevention of translocation injuries and the maintenance of perfusion to surgical anastomoses.

As discussed above, a reduced gastric intramucosal pH implies splanchnic ischaemia. Covert splanchnic ischaemia may be revealed by a low gastric intramucosal pH, even if other indicators of tissue hypoperfusion are absent. The use of resuscitation protocols may be able to identify this deficit and go on to reverse it. The multicentre trial by Gutierrez *et al.* (1992) randomized 260 patients to receive either standard ICU resuscitation or resuscitation with a protocol using measurement of pH_i to guide the management of oxygen delivery and changes in treatment. They showed that in patients admitted with a low pH_i the use of this measure to indicate further resuscitative measures, including the use of dobutamine, did not alter outcome. In contrast, outcome was improved in those patients that were admitted with a normal pH_i and whose subsequent management was guided by the protocol. This may be explained by the suggestion that those patients with low pH_i on admission had already sustained a splanchnic ischaemic insult, whereas in those that had a normal pH_i on admission it was avoided by early intervention.

Maintaining Enteral Nutrition

Splanchnic autoregulation is influenced by lumenal nutrition (Shepherd, 1980), but the precise effect in critically ill patients remains unclear. It has been suggested (Haglund and Rasmussen, 1993) that early enteral nutrition may increase splanchnic blood flow but, in the presence of shock, this might conceivably result in a 'steal syndrome', with diversion of blood from other organs to the gut.

Apart from the obvious need to prevent mucosal ischaemia, the importance of other means of mucosal support have been overlooked in the past. This is despite evidence that lumenal sources of nutrition are required for the maintenance of gut integrity.

Improvements in outcome associated with the nutritional support of the preoperatively severely malnourished are not as evident in that population of patients in the ICU who go on to develop multiple organ failure. Attempts to moderate the catabolic state engendered by a marked immune response have focused on providing exogenous sources of energy and substrate for protein synthesis.

Critically ill patients are not usually able to eat a normal diet. Anorexia, nausea, sedation, tracheal intubation and impaired consciousness lead to alternative forms of nutritional support. Nasogastric feeding should be attempted in all ICU patients as soon as possible, unless there are specific contraindications or normal eating is expected to resume within a day or so. Nasogastric feeding supports normal gut function less well than does a mixed diet. Considerable work is now being directed towards developing more 'complete' feeds (Bower *et al.*, 1995). Important components of the normal diet may include fibre, nucleotides, fatty acids, arginine and glutamine. Elemental feeds stimulate pancreatic exocrine secretion less than do complex feeds. Elemental feeds also do not promote intestinal growth factors, and so cause or perpetuate gut atrophy (Playford *et al.*, 1993). Altered gut motility may, however, cause problems with establishing enteral nutrition in critically ill patients.

Gastric stasis

Gastric emptying can be normal even though bowel sounds are absent in mechanically ventilated patients (Shelly and Church, 1987). However, impaired gastric emptying is common in the critically ill (Spapen *et al.*, 1995) and very common in patients with brain injuries (Norton *et al.*, 1988). Cisapride (10 mg, six hourly) added to the nasogastric feed accelerates gastric emptying and reduces the frequency of vomiting (Spapen *et al.*, 1995).

Ileus

Factors associated with ileus in critically ill patients are listed in Table 5.3. The duration of surgery and amount of bowel handling at laparotomy do not correlate with the duration of ileus (Condon *et al.*, 1986), which normally resolves within 2–3 days. Bowel migratory motor complexes are inhibited when the abdominal muscles are divided, and abolished when the peritoneum is opened. High sympathetic activity and plasma catecholamine concentrations contribute to ileus,

Table 5.3   Factors associated with ileus in critically ill patients

- Laparotomy with bowel surgery or handling
- Peritonitis
- Intestinal ischaemia
- Retroperitoneal haemorrhage
- Trauma
- Spinal cord lesion
- General or spinal anaesthesia
- Drugs: opiates, phenothiazines, calcium antagonists, etc.
- Electrolyte abnormalities
- Hypothyroidism

probably by causing splanchnic hypoperfusion. This appears, for example, to be the cause of ileus and other abdominal complications after cardiac surgery (Christenson *et al.*, 1994), and is implicated as the cause of ileus in other patients needing intensive care.

Pseudo-obstruction

Pseudo-obstruction is bowel obstruction with the usual symptoms, signs and radiological appearances but without an apparent mechanical cause (Doradi *et al.*, 1992). Sometimes no specific underlying cause can be identified.

In the ICU, pseudo-obstruction is particularly troublesome in patients who have taken a large overdose of tricyclic antidepressants or phenothiazines, and after early feeding of patients with retroperitoneal pathology (e.g. haematoma after repair of a leaking abdominal aortic aneurysm).

Effects of nutritional failure in the critically ill

Loss of enteral nutrition changes the gut structure and function (Deitch, 1994) with:

- villus atrophy;
- reduced gut mucosal barrier integrity;
- impaired release of gut trophic hormones.

Beneficial effects of enteral feeding include:

- reduced bacterial overgrowth in the proximal gastrointestinal tract;
- reduced frequency of stress ulceration;
- gallbladder emptying.

Transit of food through the gut prevents stasis in the proximal gastro-intestinal tract, which would favour bacterial overgrowth, provides nutrients to support the normal bowel flora and stimulates secretion of immunoglobulin into the bowel lumen. Feeding also stimulates intestinal blood flow and so may prevent mucosal ischaemia, although the effects in patients whose splanchnic blood flow is compromised (e.g. during severe sepsis) is unclear.

Malnutrition also causes atrophy of the gut-associated lymphoid tissue, further weakening gut-barrier function.

A comparison of enteral with parenteral nutrition in high-risk surgical patients in a meta-analysis of eight randomized clinical trials (Moore *et al.*, 1992) shows the frequency of septic complications is halved in patients given enteral nutrition. As already described, some critically ill patients are intolerant of enteral nutrition, but survival is significantly improved when patients are fed enterally (Chang *et al.*, 1987), so all enteral feeding options, including placement of a jejunal feeding tube, should be considered before enteral nutrition is abandoned. Although surgeons are often reluctant to allow enteral nutrition immediately after bowel resection, a small randomized trial suggests that nasojejunal feeding is possible, safe, prevents an increase in gut mucosal permeability and should be more widely used to minimize negative nitrogen balance (Carr *et al.*, 1996).

Re-feeding syndromes

Restarting nutritional support after a period of starvation or pro-longed malnutrition can precipitate severe electrolyte abnormalities, vitamin deficiency syndromes, glucose intolerance and fluid retention (Solomon and Kirby, 1990). After prolonged starvation or parenteral nutrition, villus atrophy and reduced production of digestive enzymes impair nutrient absorption when enteral nutrition is restarted. Over-enthusiastic feeding causes diarrhoea. Starting with small volumes and increasing slowly, with close clinical monitoring, reduces the frequency of complications.

Complications

Enteral feeding is not without problems. Complications of tube displacement and blockage, peritoneal contamination, microbial colonization of the feed, diarrhoea and aspiration have been reported (Delaney *et al.*, 1973; Adams *et al.*, 1986).

Specific nutrients

The process that is thought to lead towards MOF (splanchnic ischaemia, translocation, endotoxaemia, mediator release, the development of hypermetabolism and so on) may be reduced by enteral nutrition, and manipulation of enteral feeding regimens has been suggested as a means of promoting immune system recovery, and possibly even enhancement (Cerra, 1991).

Amino acids

As a possible improvement in both nutritional parameters and clinical status has been associated with the use of modified amino acid formulations in parenteral nutrition (Naylor *et al.*, 1989; Eriksson and Conn, 1989), this has been attempted using the enternal route. In one study, a regimen with a relatively increased amount of branched-chain amino acids was given to malnourished patients with a moderate degree of postsurgical stress (Cerra *et al.*, 1985). This enhanced the effects of enteral nutrition on nitrogen retention and visceral protein mass, but outcome in terms of survival was not reported.

L-*Arginine*

Nitric oxide (NO) has effects on immune function, and this may explain some of the findings of studies with L-arginine supplemented nutrient regimens, given that NO is produced from L-arginine by NO synthase. Graft rejection can be enhanced by dietary arginine, as can survival in experimental models of burn injury and peritonitis (Saito *et al.*, 1987; Barbul, 1990).

Arginine supplementation of feeds is associated with earlier recovery of the T-helper cell (CD4[+]) subset after surgery (Daly *et al.*, 1988).

Glutamine

Glutamine is the most abundant amino acid in plasma and intracellular fluid. It is the principal interorgan carrier of nitrogen between the organs of synthesis (muscle and liver) and then of utilization (gut, lymphocytes and lung). Glutamine is a major metabolic fuel for the enterocytes of the gut mucosa and gut-associated lymphoid tissue (Smith, 1990).

Plasma glutamine concentrations are decreased by surgery, trauma or sepsis and, although not regarded as an essential amino acid, it becomes conditionally essential during severe illness (Wilmore, 1994).

Adverse effects on the function of glutamine-using tissues, including the gut, may be reduced by feeds supplemented with glutamine (Ziegler *et al.*, 1993). Some, but not all, experimental studies have demonstrated a reduction in bacterial translocation when glutamine-supplemented feeds are given, but the addition of large amounts of glutamine to enteral feeds has been limited by its instability to heat. Heat sterilization of feeds causes conversion of glutamine to ammonia and pyroglutamic acid (Grimble, 1993). Nevertheless, enteral feeds supplemented with glutamine are now commercially available. A small randomized trial of glutamine-supplemented feeds found no improvement in survival (54% vs 58% in controls), but there was a significant reduction in hospital costs for the glutamine-supplemented group (Griffiths *et al.*, 1996). Interestingly, the same report describes a significant improvement in patient survival for those patients given glutamine supplemented *parenteral* nutrition compared with standard parenteral nutrition.

It can be speculated that improved outcomes from glutamine-enhanced nutrition should follow from minimization of gut mucosal atrophy (Platell *et al.*, 1993). For intestinal growth factors to be effective, sufficient glutamine must be available. However, the place of glutamine-supplemented enteral feeds and the amount glutamine that might be needed by critically ill patients has still to be defined fully.

ω-3 Polyunsaturated Fatty Acids

The polyunsaturated fatty acids (PUFAs) are structural and functional components of the cell membrane. They exert significant influence on cell–cell interactions and the expression of various mediators. Many fatty acids are synthesized when the body is provided with suitable substrate, but some PUFAs are essential fatty acids (EFAs) and must be provided exogenously. There are two main classes denoted by the position of the first double bond from the terminal end of the fatty acid chain. An ω-6 PUFA, such as linoleic acid, is derived from commonly available vegetable sources and is a precursor to arachidonic acid. The ω-3 PUFAs, such as linolenic and eicosapentaenoic acid (EPA), are less readily found, although cold-water fish are rich sources of EPA. Both groups are precursors to eicosanoids, mediators in immune system–cell interactions. ω-6 PUFAs are converted via arachidonic acid to the eicosanoid series-2 prostaglandins and series-4 leukotrienes, whereas EPA, an ω-3 PUFA, results in the series-3 and series-5 leukotrienes. The ω-6 derivatives are potent immunological mediators and have been shown to suppress T-cell proliferation through PGE_2 and prevent cytokine stimulation of interleukin-2 (IL-2) by endothelial cells. ω-3 PUFAs are incorporated into cells of the immune system if sufficient exogenous EPA is provided, and once the ratio of this to ω-6 PUFAs rises then there is a decrease in the release of dienoic eicosanoids, tumour necrosis factor and IL-1 by the macrophage (Cerra, 1991). Dietary supplementation with ω-3 PUFAs might be expected to affect the response to injury, and there is some evidence for this (Kinsella *et al.*, 1990). Survival after sepsis in an experimental model in rats was increased if a diet using fish oils as the fat source was provided (Cerra *et al.*, 1988).

Nucleotides

Patients receiving total parenteral nutrition after allograft transplantation have better graft survival. This may be because parenteral nutrition is nucleotide-free. Nucleotide-free diets reduce delayed hypersensitivity reactions and have other effects on cellular immunity. It appears that T cells are either unable to synthesize nucleotides or else demands during metabolic stress outstrip supply. The effects of nucleotide depletion on cellular immunity can be reversed and even enhanced by the administration of uracil (Kulkarni *et al.*, 1986).

Nutritional Manipulation

In the past, parenteral nutrition has been favoured for critically ill patients. This tendency was accentuated in the ICU because of the ready availability of central venous access, the fears of aspiration of gastric contents, the overuse of opiates for inappropriate levels of sedation and failure to use enteral, as opposed to gastric, access to the gastrointestinal tract. The argument for a shift away from parenteral nutrition to a more enthusiastic promotion of enteral nutrition is supported not only by reports of the deleterious effects of parenteral nutrition but also by suggestions (Cerra *et al.*, 1991) that manipulation of an enteral feeding regimen in the critically ill patient may be able to influence outcome.

In a randomized clinical trial (Cerra *et al.*, 1991) an enteral feed supplemented with arginine, an ω-3 fatty acid and RNA was compared with a standard feed in patients on a surgical ICU with prolonged hypermetabolism after surgery, trauma or sepsis. The supplemented group showed stimulation of in vitro lymphocyte proliferative responses and reduction in 3-methylhistidine excretion. However, there was no change in the decreased response to intradermal skin test challenge that was present before dietary supplementation, and no change in outcome. A similar study (Daly *et al.*, 1991) in a smaller number of patients undergoing surgery for upper gastrointestinal malignancy demonstrated an earlier return to normal levels of lymphocyte response and increased nitrogen retention. The same effect on cellular immunity was noted by this group in an earlier trial of patients given arginine supplements compared to glycine in an enteral feed (Daly *et al.*, 1988). A preliminary report of a randomized clinical trial of a similar feed (Impact, Sandoz Nutrition Ltd, Berne, Switzerland) also showed no effect on patient survival, although the duration of mechanical ventilation and hospital stay were significantly reduced (Atkinson *et al.*, 1996).

Secretory immunoglobin A (IgA) is a principal component of the gut mucosal immune system and decreased levels in the bile have been found in animals fed intravenously (Alverdy *et al.*, 1985). Glutamine is commonly absent from preparations of parenteral nutrition, and the mucosal atrophy seen with this form of nutritional supplementation is consistent with the suggestion that the intestinal lumen is the primary source of this amino acid, and thus energy, for mucosal cells (Souba *et al.*, 1990). The absence of other fuels, including butyrate and ketone bodies (again normally derived from lumenal contents), may also contribute to the mucosal atrophy. Mucosal atrophy together with any unrecognized splanchnic ischaemia and the subsequent increase in gastrointestinal permeability is thought to be responsible for the endotoxin and bacterial translocation that may occur with parenteral nutrition in the critically ill (Ziegler *et al.*, 1988; Alexander, 1990).

Parenteral nutrition

If enteral nutrition is totally impossible, some nutritional support can be provided parenterally. While this provides little to specifically maintain gut structure or function, there is experimental evidence that enhancing total parenteral nutrition (TPN) with glutamine minimizes changes to intestinal permeability (Hall *et al.*, 1994). Most human studies of glutamine-enhanced TPN have been in bone-marrow transplant patients. Clear benefit has yet to be shown.

The effects of parenteral nutrition in patients with hypercatabolic states are largely restricted to improvement in indices of nutritional status such as nitrogen retention. In a meta-analysis of 11 studies of parenteral nutrition (Detsky et al., 1987) little clinical benefit was noted and effects were only observed in patients that were previously significantly malnourished. A multicentre prospective study of surgical patients receiving total parenteral nutrition before and after surgery again found no significant reduction in morbidity or mortality, but did confirm a reduction in complications in the most severely malnourished group (Buzby, 1991). This group mostly had upper gastrointestinal malignancy, and any effect depended upon significant preoperative and postoperative nutrition for at least 7–10 days.

Parenteral nutrition in the ICU usually implies that the gastro-intestinal tract is not functioning, and this may be the reason why this form of nutrition is associated with adverse outcomes.

Evidence of the benefits of enteral nutrition compared to TPN has been obtained in a uniform group of patients with trauma. A recent meta-analysis (Moore *et al.*, 1992a) of a number of different trials performed in patients who had suffered some form of trauma showed that septic episodes in the ICU were greatly reduced by enteral nutrition. This led to a reduction in ICU stay not seen with parenteral nutrition. Similarly, in a single-centre study (Kudsk *et al.*, 1992), septic morbidity after blunt and penetrating abdominal trauma was markedly reduced in patients fed via the enteral route.

Effect of Nutritional Support on Outcome in the Most Severely Ill

Attempts to show that a dramatic change in outcome in those patients with hypermetabolic multiple organ failure can be effected by either method of nutritional support has not been readily forthcoming. It also remains to be shown whether enteral nutritional manipulation really does have a clinically significant effect. Although one study (Cerra *et al.*, 1988a) of the effect of enteral nutrition on the progression of a hypermetabolic state to multiple organ failure failed to show a significant improvement in mortality rates compared to parenteral nutrition, it is becoming increasingly clear that parenteral nutrition has more deleterious effects than was commonly realized. If access to the absorptive surface of the gut can be achieved, there should be few patients in whom enteral nutrition is not possible.

CONCLUSION

The gut plays a central role in critical illness. Its function is impaired by shock, sepsis and other causes of a generalized inflammatory response.

The pathway from a shock injury, through splanchnic ischaemia, loss of gastrointestinal integrity, portal transfer of an antigen load, hepatic damage and/or excess cytokine release, to an eventual systemic effect with other end-organ damage is rationally attractive. Each of the described phenomena almost certainly do occur, but a correlation between each has yet to be demonstrated.

Similarly, attempts to influence the development and progression of gastrointestinal dysfunction so as to affect outcome have been difficult. It seems likely that adequate splanchnic oxygenation is associated with improved outcome (Gutierrez *et al.*, 1992) but this may reflect a lesser severity of illness in patients who do not have splanchnic ischaemia on admission. Enteral nutrition is important for maintaining gut structure and function, but the changes associated with critical illness, including mucosal ischaemia, gastric stasis, ileus and pseudo-obstruction, can make enteral feeding difficult or impossible. Evidence for effects on *outcome*, rather than indices of immune function and 'septic episodes', by nutrient modification, are difficult to show. Although the role of the gastrointestinal tract in critical illness should not be underestimated, the evidence for a causative link between gut organ failure and the initiation or promotion of the multiple organ dysfunction syndrome remains circumstantial.

Minimization of intestinal ischaemia currently depends on increasing global cardiac output and oxygen delivery, although dopexamine may also increase the proportion of cardiac output going to the gut. Future clinical work should define the relationship between the markers of gut function that are relatively easy to measure (i.e. mucosal permeability and pH_i) and failure of enteral nutrition, systemic inflammatory response and multiple organ failure. More specific means of 'gut resuscitation' may then improve outcome in critically ill patients.

REFERENCES

Adams, M.B., Seabrook, G.R., Quebbeman, E.A., Condon, R.E. (1986) Jejunostomy: a rarely indicated procedure. *Arch Surg* **121**: 236–238.

Alexander, J.W. (1990) Nutrition and translocation. *J Parent Ent Nutr* **14**: 170S–174S.

Alverdy, J., Hoon Sang Chi, Sheldon, G.F. (1985) The effect of parenteral nutrition on gastrointestinal immunity. *Ann Surg* **202**: 681–684.

Antonsson, J.B., Haglund, U.H. (1995) Gut intramucosal pH and intraluminal Po_2 in a porcine model of peritonitis or haemorrhage. *Gut* **37**: 791–797.

Antonsson, J.B., Boyle, C.B., Kruithoff, K.L., *et al.* (1990) Validation of tonometric measurement of gut intramural pH during endotoxaemia and mesenteric occlusion in pigs. *Am J Physiol* **259**: G519–G523.

Ashley, S.W., Cheung, L.Y. (1984) Measurements of gastric mucosal blood flow by hydrogen gas clearance. *Am J Physiol Gastrointest Liver Physiol* **247**: G339–G345.

Astiz, M.E., Rackow, E.C., Weil, M.H. (1993) Pathophysiology and treatment of circulatory shock. *Crit Care Clin* **9**: 183–203.

Atkinson, S., Sieffort, E., Bihari, D., *et al.* (1996) A randomised controlled clinical trial of the enteral immunonutrition 'Impact' in the critically ill. *Intensive Care Med* **22**: S351.

Bailey, R.W., Bulkley, G.B., Hamilton, S.R., Morris, J.B., Haglund, U.F. (1987) Protection of the small intestine from nonocclusive mesenteric ischaemic injury due to cardiogenic shock. *Am J Surg* **153**: 108–115.

Banks, R.O., Gallaran, R.H., Zinner, M.J., *et al.* (1985) Vasoactive agents in control of the mesenteric circulation. *Fed Proc* **44**: 2743–2749.

Barbul, A. (1990) Arginine and immune function. *Nutrition* **6**: 53–59.

Baue, A.E. (1975) Multiple, progressive, or sequential systems failure. *Arch Surg* **110**: 779–781.

Beaumont, W. (1825) *Medical Recorder* **8**: 14–19.

Bersten, A.D., Hersch, M., Cheung, H., Rutledge, F.S., Sibbald, W.J. (1992) The effect of various sympathomimetics on the regional circulation in hyperdynamic sepsis. *Surgery* **112**: 549–561.

Beutler, B., Cerami, A. (1987) Cachectin: more than a tumour necrosis factor. *New Engl J Med* **316**: 379–385.

Beutler, B., Milsark, I.W., Cerami, A.C. (1988) Passive immunisation against cachectin/tumour necrosis factor protects mice against lethal effects of endotoxin. *Science* **229**: 869–871.

Beutler, B., Krochin, N., Milsark, I.W., Luedke, C., Cerami, A. (1986) Control of cachectin (tumour necrosis factor) synthesis: mechanisms of endotoxin resistance. *Science* **232**: 977–980.

Bjarnason, I., Peters, T.J., Veall, N. (1983a) A persistent defect in intestinal permeability in coeliac disease demonstrated by a ^{51}Cr-labelled EDTA absorption test. *Lancet* i: 323–325.

Bjarnason, I., O'Morain, C., Levi, A.J., Peters, T.J. (1983b) Absorption of ^{51}chromium-labelled ethylenediaminotetraacetate in inflammatory bowel disease. *Gastroenterology* **85**: 318–322.

Bjarnason, I., Felvilly, B., Smethurst, P., Menzies, I.S., Levi, A.J. (1991) Importance of local versus systemic effects of non-steroidal anti-inflammatory drugs in increasing small intestinal permeability in man. *Gut* **32**: 275–277.

Bone, R.C. (1991) The pathogenesis of sepsis. *Ann Int Med* **115**: 457–469.

Bone, R.C., Fisher, C.J., Clemmer, T.P., Slotman, G.J., Metz, C.A., Balk, R.A. (1989) Sepsis syndrome: a valid clinical entity. *Crit Care Med* **17**: 389–393.

Bone, R.C., Balk, R.A., Cerra, F.B,. *et al.* (1992) Definitions for sepsis and organ failure and guidelines for the use of innovative therapies in sepsis. *Chest* **101**: 1644–1655.

Border, J.R., Hasset, J., LaDuca, J., *et al.* (1987) The gut origin states in blunt multiple trauma (ISS = 40) in the ICU. *Ann Surg* **206**: 427–445.

Bower, R.H., Cerra, F.B., Bershadsky, B., *et al.* (1995) Early enteral administration of a formula (Impact) supplemented with arginine, nucleotides and fish oil in intensive care unit patients: results of a multicenter, prospective, randomized clinical trial. *Crit Care Med* **23**: 436–449.

Boyd, O., Mackay, C.J., Lamb, G., Bland, J.M., Grounds, R.M., Bennett, E.D. (1993) Comparison of clinical information gained from routine blood-gas analysis and from gastric tonometry for intramural pH. *Lancet* **341**: 142–146.

Brandtzaeg, P., Kierulf, P., Gaustad, P., *et al.* (1989) Plasma endotoxin as a predictor of multiple organ failure and death in systemic meningococcal disease. *J Infect Dis* **159**: 195–203.

Burdelski, M., Oellerich, M., Lamesch, P., *et al.* (1987) Evaluation of quantitative liver function tests in liver donors. *Transpl Proc* **19**: 3838–3839.

Burdelski, M., Oellerich, M., Raude, E., *et al.* (1988) A novel approach to assessment of liver function in donors. *Transpl Proc* **20** (Suppl. 1): 591–593.

Buzby, G.P. (1991) Perioperative total parenteral nutrition in surgical patients: the Veterans Affairs Total Parenteral Nutrition Cooperative Study Group. *New Engl J Med* **325**: 525–532.

Caesar, J., Shaldon, S., Chiandussi, L., Guevara, L., Sherlock, S. (1961) The use of indocyanine green in the measurement of hepatic blood flow and as a test of hepatic function. *Clin Sci* **21**: 43–57.

Carr, C.S., Ling, K.D.E., Boulos, P., Singer, M. (1996) Randomised trial of safety and efficacy of immediate postoperative enteral feeding in patients undergoing gastrointestinal resection. *Br Med J* **312**: 869–871.

Cerra, F.B. (1987) Hypermetabolism, organ failure and metabolic support. *Surgery* **101**: 1–13.

Cerra, F.B. (1991) Nutrient modulation of inflammatory and immune function. *Am J Surg* **161**: 230–234.

Cerra, F.B., Shronts, R.D., Konstantinides, N.N., *et al.* (1985) Enteral feeding in sepsis: a prospective, randomised, double blind trial. *Surgery* **98**: 632–639.

Cerra, F.B., McPherson, J.P., Konstantinides, F.N., Konstantinides, N.N., Teasley, K.M. (1988a) Enteral nutrition does not prevent multiple organ failure syndrome (MOFS) after sepsis. *Surgery* **104**: 727–733.

Cerra, F.B., Alden, P.A., Negro, F., *et al.* (1988b) Clinical sepsis, endogenous and exogenous lipid modulation. *J Parent Ent Nutr* **12**: 63S-69S.

Cerra, F.B., Lehmann, S., Konstantinides, N., *et al.* (1991) Improvement in immune function in ICU patients by enteral nutrition supplemented with arginine, RNA, and menhaden oil is independent of nitrogen balance. *Nutrition* **7**: 193-199.

Chang, R.W.S., Jacobs, S., Lee, B. (1987) Gastrointestinal dysfunction among intensive care unit patients. *Crit Care Med* **15**: 909–914.

Christenson, J.T., Schmaziger, Maurice, J., Simonet, F., Velebit, V. (1994) Postoperative visceral hypotension the common cause for gastrointestinal complications after cardiac surgery. *Thorac Cardiovasc Surg* **42**: 152–157.

Condon, R.E., Cowles, V.E., Schulte, W.J., Fantizides, C.T., Mahoney, J.L., Sarna, S.K. (1986) Resolution of postoperative ileus in humans. *Ann Surg* **203**: 574–581.

Cullen, J.J., Ephgrave, K.S., Broadhurst, K.A., Booth, B. (1994) Captopril decreases stress ulceration without affecting gastric perfusion during canine hemorrhagic shock. *J Trauma* **37**: 43–49.

Daly, J.M., Reynolds, J., Thom, A., *et al.* (1988) Immune and metabolic effects of arginine in the surgical patient. *Ann Surg* **208**: 512–522.

Dahn, M.S., Lange, P., Lobdel, K., Hans, B., Jacobs, L.A., Mitchell, RA. (1987) Splanchnic and total body oxygen consumption differences in septic and injured patients. *Surgery* **101**: 69–80.

Daly, J.M., Lieberman, M., Goldfine, J., *et al.* (1991) Enteral nutrition with supplemental arginine, RNA and ω-3 fatty acids: a prospective clinical trial. *J Parent Ent Nutr* **15**: 9.

Danner, R.L., Elin, R.J., Hosseini, J.M., Wesley, R.A., Reilly, J.M., Parillo, J.E. (1991) Endotoxemia in human septic shock. *Chest* **99**: 169–175.

Dawson, A.M., Trenchard, G., Guz, A. (1965) Small bowel tonometry: assessment of small gut mucosal oxygen tension in dog and man. *Nature* **206**: 943–944.

Dawson, D.J., Lobley, R.W., Burrows, P.C., Notman, J.A., Malnon, M., Holmes, R. (1988) Changes in jejunal permeability and passive permeation of sugars in intestinal biopsies in coeliac disease and Crohn's disease. *Clin Sci* **74**: 427–431.

Deitch, E.A. (1989) Simple intestinal obstruction causes bacterial translocation in man. *Arch Surg* **124**: 699–701.

Deitch, E.A. (1994) Bacterial translocation: the influence of dietary variables. *Gut* **25**(Suppl 1): S23–S27.

Deitch, E.A., Berg, R. (1987) Endotoxin but not malnutrition promotes bacterial translocation of the gut flora in burned mice. *J Trauma* **27**: 161–166.

Deitch, E.A., Berg, R., Specian, R. (1987) Endotoxin promotes the translocation of bacteria from the gut. *Arch Surg* **122**: 185–190.

Delaney, H.M., Carnevale, N.J., Garvey, J.W. (1973) Jejunostomy by a needle catheter technique. *Surgery* **73**: 786–790.

Desai, V.S., Weil, M.H., Tang, W., Yang, G., Bisera, J. (1993) Gastric intramural $p\text{CO}_2$ during peritonitis and shock. *Chest* **104**: 1254–1258.

Detsky, A.S., Baker, J.P., O'Rourke, K., Goel, V. (1987) Perioperative parenteral nutrition: a meta-analysis. *Ann Intern Med* **107**: 195–203.

Dinarello, C.A. (1984) Interleukin-1. *Rev Infect Dis* **6**: 55–95.

Dobb G. (1990) Multiple organ failure: outcome with intensive care. In: Aochi, O., Amaha, K., Takeshita, H. (eds), *Intensive and Critical Care Medicine*, pp. 28–294. Amsterdam: Excerpta Medica.

Dobb G.J. (1995) Prevention of secondary organ damage. *Current Opinion Anaesthesiol* **8**: 119–125.

Dobb, G.J. (1996) The role of the gut in critical illness. *Current Anaesth Crit Care* **7**: 62–68.

Doglio, G.R., Pusajo, J.F., Egurrola, M.A., *et al.* (1991) Gastric mucosal pH as a prognostic index of mortality in critically ill patients. *Crit Care Med* **19**: 1037–1040.

Doradi, S., Berry, A.R., Kettlewell, M.G.W. (1992) Acute colonic pseudo-obstruction. *Br J Surg* **79**: 99–103.

Dregelid, E., Haukaas, S., Amundsen, S., *et al.* (1986) Microsphere method in measurement of blood flow to wall layers of small intestine. *Am J Physiol Gastrointest Liver Physiol* **250**: G670–G678.

Eiseman, B., Beart, R., Norton, L. (1977) Multiple organ failure. *Surg Gynecol Obstet* **144**: 323–36.

Elstad, M.R., Parker, C.J., Cowley, F.S. *et al.* (1994) CD11b/CD18 integrin and a β-glucan receptor act in concert to induce the synthesis of platelet-activating factor by monocytes. *J Immunol* **152**: 220–230.

Eriksson, L.S., Conn, H.O. (1989) Branched-chain amino acids in the management of hepatic encephalopathy: an analysis of variants. *Hepatology* **10**: 228–246.

Falk, A., Redfors, S., Myrvold, H.E., Haglund, U. (1985) Small intestinal mucosal lesions in feline septic shock; a study on the pathogenesis. *Circ Shock* **17**: 327–337.

Ferraris, V.A. (1983) Exploratory laparotomy for potential abdominal sepsis in patients with multiple-organ failure. *Arch Surg* **118**: 1130–1133.

Fiddian-Green, R.G. (1989) Studies in splanchnic ischemia and multiple organ failure. In: Marston, A., Bulkley, G., Fiddian-Green, R.G., Haglund, U. (eds), *Splanchnic Ischemia and Multiple Organ Failure*, pp. 349–363. London: Edward Arnold.

Fiddian-Green, R.G., Baker, S. (1987) Predictive value of the stomach wall pH for complications after cardiac operations: comparison with other monitoring. *Crit Care Med* **15**: 153–156.

Fiddian-Green, R.G., Gantz, N.M. (1987) Transient episodes of sigmoid ischaemia and their relation to infection from intestinal organisms after abdominal aortic operations. *Crit Care Med* **15**: 835–839.

Fiddian-Green, R.G., McGough, E., Pittenger, G., Rothman, E. (1983) Predictive value of intramural pH and other risk factors for massive bleeding from stress ulceration. *Gastroenterology* **85**: 613–620.

Fink, M.P. (1989) Systemic and splanchnic hemodynamic derangements in the sepsis syndrome. In: Marston, A., Bulkley, G., Fiddian-Green, R.G., Haglund, U. (eds), *Splanchnic Ischemia and Multiple Organ Failure*, pp. 101–106. London: Edward Arnold.

Fink, M.P. (1991) Gastrointestinal mucosal injury in experimental models of shock, trauma and sepsis. *Crit Care Med* **19**: 627–641.

Fink, M.P., Cohn, S.M., Lee, P.C., *et al.* (1989) Effect of lipopolysaccharide on intestinal intramucosal hydrogen ion concentration in pigs: evidence of gut ischemia in a normodynamic model of septic shock. *Crit Care Med* **17**: 641–646.

Fink, M.P., Antonsson, J.B., Wang, H., Rothschild, H.R. (1991) Increased intestinal permeability in endotoxic pigs. *Arch Surg* **126**: 211–218.

Fleming, D.W., Cochi, S.L., MacDonald, K.L., *et al.* (1985) Pasteurised milk as a vehicle for infection in an outbreak of listeriosis. *New Engl J Med* **312**: 404–407.

Fong, Y.M., Marano, M.A., Moldawer, L.L., *et al.* (1990) The acute splanchnic and peripheral tissue response to endotoxin in humans. *J Clin Invest* **85**: 1896–904.

Fry, D.E., Pearlstein, L., Fulton, R.L., Polk, H.C. (1980) Multiple system organ failure: the role of uncontrolled infection. *Arch Surg* **115**: 136–140.

Fukushima, R., Gianotti, L., Alexander, J.W., Pyles, T. (1992) The degree of bacterial translocation is a determinant factor for mortality after burn injury and is improved by prostaglandin analogues. *Ann Surg* **216**: 438–445.

Furchgott, R.F., Zadawski, J.V. (1980) The obligatory role of endothelial cells in the relaxation of arterial smooth muscle by acetylcholine. *Nature* **288**: 373–476.

Gershon, M.D., Erde, S.M. (1980) The nervous system of the gut. *Gastroenterology* **80**: 1571–1594.

Gharagozloo, F., Bulkley, G.B., Zuidema, G.D., O'Mara, C.S., Alderson, P.O. (1984) The use of intraperitoneal xenon for early diagnosis of acute mesenteric ischemia. *Surgery* **95**: 404–411.

Gilmour, D.G., Aitkenhead, A.R., Hothersall, A.P., Ledingham, I.M. (1980) The effect of hypovolaemia on colonic blood flow in the dog. *Br J Surg* **67**: 82–84.

Glauser, M.P., Zanetti, G., Baumgartner, J., Cohen, J. (1991) Septic shock: pathogenesis. *Lancet* **338**: 732–735.

Gosche, J.R., Spain, D.A., Garrison, R.N., Lubbe, A.S., Cryer, H.G. (1994) Differential microvascular responses to cyclooxygenase blockade in the rat small intestine during acute bacteremia. *Shock* **2**: 408–412.

Granger, D.N., Bulkley, G.B. (eds) (1981) *Measurement of Blood Flow: Applications to the Splanchnic Circulation*. Baltimore: Williams & Wilkins.

Griffiths, R.D., Palmer, T.E.A., Jones, C. (1996) Outcome and cost of intensive care patients given glutamine supplemented nutrition. *Intensive Care Med* **22**: S351.

Grimble, G. (1993) Glutamine glutamate and pyroglutamate: facts and fantasies. *Clin Nutr* **12**: 66–69.

Grum, C.M., Fiddian-Green, R.G., Pittenger, G.L., Grant, B.J.B., Rorhman, E.D., Dantzker, D.R. (1984) Adequacy of tissue oxygenation in intact dog intestine. *J Appl Physiol* **56**: 1065–1069.

Gunther, S., Gimbrone, M.A., Alexander, R.W. (1980) Identification and characterization of the high affinity vascular angiotension II receptor in rat mesenteric artery. *Circ Res* **47**: 278–288.

Gutierrez, G., Palizas, F., Doglio, G., *et al.* (1992a) Gastric intramucosal pH as a therapeutic index of tissue oxygenation in critically ill patients. *Lancet* **339**: 195–199.

Gutierrez, G., Bismar, H., Dantzker, D., Silva, N. (1992b) Comparison of gastric intramucosal pH with measures of oxygen transport and consumption in critically ill patients. *Crit Care Med* **20**: 451–457.

Gys, T., Hubens, A., Neels, H., Lawers, L.F., Peters, R. (1988) Prognostic value of gastric intramural pH in surgical intensive care patients. *Crit Care Med* **16**: 1222–1224.

Haglund, U., Rasmussen, I. (1993) Oxygenation of the gut mucosa. *Br J Surg* **80**: 955–956.

Hall, J.C., Heel, K., Barker, R., McCauley, R. (1994) Parenteral nutrition and gut permeability. *Aust NZ J Surg* **64**: 367.

Hampton, R.Y., Golenbock, D.T., Raetz, C.R.H. (1988) Lipid A binding sites in membranes of macrophage tumour cells. *J Biol Chem* **263**: 802–807.

Harris, C.E., Griffiths, R.D., Freestone, N., Billington, D., Atherton, S.T., Macmillan, R.R. (1992) Intestinal permeability in the critically ill. *Intensive Care Med* **18**: 38–41.

Hartman, M., Montgomery, M., Jonsson, K., Haglund, U. (1991) Tissue oxygenation in hemorrhagic shock measured as transcutaneous oxygen tension, subcutaneous oxygen tension, and gastrointestinal intramucosal pH in pigs. *Crit Care Med* **19**: 205–209.

Haywood, J.R., Shaffer, R.A., Fastenow, C., Fink, G.D., Brody, M.J. (1981) Regional blood flow measurement with pulsed Doppler flowmeter in conscious rat. *Am J Physiol, Heart Circ Physiol* **241**: H273–H278.

Heard, S.O., Helsmoortel, C.M., Kent, J.C., Shahnarian, A., Fink, M.P. (1991) Gastric tonometry in healthy volunteers: effect of ranitidine on calculated intramural pH. *Crit Care Med* **19**: 271–274.

Henderson, J.M., Kutner, M.H., Bain, R.P. (1982) First order clearance of plasma galactose: the effect of liver disease. *Gastroenterology* **83**: 1090–1096.

Hinsdale, J.G., Jaffe, B.M. (1984) Re-operation for intra-abdominal sepsis: indications and results in modern critical care setting. *Am Surg* **199**: 31–36.

Huet, P.M., Villenueve, J.P. (1983) Determinants of drug disposition in patients with cirrhosis. *Hepatology* **3**: 913–918.

Ignarello, L.J., Buga, G.M., Wood, K.S., Byrns, R.E. (1987) Endothelium-derived relaxing factor produced and released from artery and vein is nitric oxide. *Proc Natl Acad Sci USA* **84**: 9265–9269.

Jacob, H., Brandt, L.J., Farkas, P., Frishman, W. (1983) Beta-adrenergic blockade and the gastrointestinal system. *Am J Med* **74**: 1042–1051.

Kinsella, J.E., Lokesh, B., Broughton, S., Whelan, J. (1990) Dietary polyunsaturated fatty acids and eicosanoids: potential effects on the modulation of inflammatory and immune cells: an overview. *Nutrition* **6**: 24–44.

Kishimoto, T. (1989) The biology of interleukin-6. *Blood* **74**: 1–10.

Knaus, W.A., Draper, E.A., Wagner, D.P., Zimmerman, J. (1985) Prognosis in acute organ system failure. *Ann Surg* **202**: 685–693.

Knichwitz, G., Mertees, N., Kuhmann, M. (1994) Improvement of intramucosal pH measurements with a phosphate-buffered solution. *Intensive Care Med* **20**: S137.

Krause, W., Matheis, H., Wulf, K. (1969) Fungaemia and funguria after oral administration of *Candida albicans*. *Lancet* **i**: 598–599.

Kreimeier, U., Ruiz-Morales, M., Messmer, K. (1993) Comparison of the effects of volume resuscitation with Dextran 60 vs Ringer's lactate on central hemodynamics, regional blood flow, pulmonary function and blood composition during hyperdynamic endotoxemia. *Circ Shock* **39**: 89–99.

Kudsk, K.A., Croce, M.A., Fabian, T.C., *et al.* (1992) Enteral versus parenteral feeding: effects on septic morbidity after blunt and penetrating abdominal trauma. *Ann Surg* **215**: 503–511.

Kulkarni, A.D., Fanslow, W.C., Rudolph, F.B., Van Buren, C.T. (1986) Effect of dietary nucleotides on response to bacterial infections. *J Parent Ent Nutr* **10**: 169–171.

Kvietys, P.R., Sheperd, A.P., Granger, D.N. (1985) Laser-doppler, H_2 clearance, and microsphere estimates of mucosal blood flow. *Am J Physiol, Gastrointest Liver Physiol* **249**: G221–G227.

Lahtinen, P., Valta, P., Takala, J. (1996) Gas tonometry – evaluation of a new method and comparison with saline tonometry. *Intensive Care Med* **22**: S362.

Landow, L., Phillips, D.A., Heard, S.O., Prevost, D., Vandersalm, T., Fink, M.P. (1991) Gastric tonometry and venous oximetry in cardiac surgery patients. *Crit Care Med* **19**: 1226–1233.

Lane, A. (1915) *The Operative Treatment of Chronic Intestinal Stasis*, 3rd edn. London: Nisbet.

LeVoyer, T., Cioffi, W.G., Pratt, L., *et al.* (1992) Alteration in intestinal permeability after thermal injury. *Arch Surg* **127**: 26–30.

Luiten, E.J.T., Hop, W.C.J., Lange, J.F., Bruining, H.A. (1995) Controlled clinical trial of selective decontamination for the treatment of severe acute pancreatitis. *Ann Surg* **222**: 57–65.

Lundgren, O., Haglund, U. (1978) The pathophysiology of the intestinal countercurrent exchanger. *Life Sci* **23**: 1411–1422.

Madara, J.L. (1989) Loosening tight junctions. Lessons from the intestine. *J Clin Invest* **83**: 1089–1094.

Madara, J.L., Stafford, J. (1989) Interferon-gamma directly effects barrier function of cultured intestinal epithelial monolayers. *J Clin Invest* **83**: 724–727.

Mainous, M.R., Tso, P., Berg, R.D., Deitch, E.A. (1991) Studies of the route, magnitude, and time course of bacterial translocation in a model of systemic inflammation. *Arch Surg* **126**: 33–37.

Manson, W.L., Coenen, J.M.F.H., Klasen, H.J., Horwitz, E.H. (1992) Intestinal bacterial translocation in experimentally burned mice with wounds colonized by *Pseudomonas aeruginosa*. *J Trauma* **33**: 654–658.

Marik, P.E., Mohedin, M. (1994) The contrasting effects of dopamine and norepinephrine on systemic and splanchnic oxygen utilization in hyperdynamic sepsis. *J Am Med Assoc* **272**: 1354–1357.

Marrone, G.C., Silen, W. (1984) Pathogenesis, diagnosis and treatment of acute gastric mucosal lesions. *Clin Gastroenterol* **13**: 635–650.

Marshall, J.C., Cristou, N.V., Meakins, J.L. (1993) The gastrointestinal tract. The 'undrained abscess' of multiple organ failure. *Ann Surg* **218**: 111–119.

Maynard, N.D., Bihari, D.J., Mason, R.C., Baldock, G., McColl, I. (1992a) Assessment of splanchnic oxygenation by tonometry in patients with acute circulatory failure. *Intensive Care Med* **18** (Suppl.2): 235.

Maynard, N.D., Smithies, M.N., Mason, R.C., Bihari, D.J. (1992b) Dopexamine and gastric intramucosal pH in critically ill patients. *Intensive Care Med* **18** (Suppl. 2): A134.

Maynard, N., Bihari, D., Beale, R., *et al.* (1993) Assessment of splanchnic oxygenation by gastric tonometry in patients with acute circulatory failure. *J Am Med Assoc* **270**: 1203–1210.

Maynard, M., Atkinson, S., Smithies, M., Mason, R., Bihari, D. (1994) Relationship between intramucosal pH and outcome at different times following admission to the intensive care unit. *Crit Care Med* **22**: A200.

Maynard, N.D., Bihari, D.J., Dalton, R.M., Smithies, M.N., Mason, R.C. (1995) Increasing splanchnic blood flow in the critically ill. *Chest* **108**: 1648–1654.

Meakins, J.L., Marshall, J.C. (1986) The gastrointestinal tract: the 'motor' of MOF. *Arch Surg* **121**: 197–201.

Metchinikoff, E. (1908) Etudes sur la flore intestinale. *Ann Inst Pasteur* **XXII**: 929–955.

Michie, H.R., Manogue, K.R., Spriggs, D.R., *et al.* (1988) Detection of circulating tumour necrosis factor after endotoxin administration. *New Engl J Med* **318**: 1481–1486.

Millar, A.B., Singer, M., Meager, A., Foley, N.M., Johnson, N.M., Rook, G.A.W. (1989) Tumour necrosis factor in bronchopulmonary secretions of patients with adult respiratory distress syndrome. *Lancet* **ii**: 712–714.

Miyauchi, T., Tomobe, Y., Shiba, R., *et al.* (1990) Involvement of endothelin in the regulation of human vascular tonus. *Circulation* **81**: 1874–1880.

Moncada, S., Palmer, R.M.J., Higgs, E.A. (1991) Nitric oxide: physiology, pathophysiology and pharmacology. *Pharmacol Rev* **43**: 109–142.

Mone, J., Lefkowitz, S.S. (1992) Induction of interferon synthesis and cytotoxicity by murine peritoneal macrophages exposed to glycoprotein ligands. *Acta Virol* **36**: 383–391.

Moore, F.A., Moore, E.E., Poggetti, R., *et al.* (1991) Gut bacterial translocation via the portal vein: a clinical perspective with major torso trauma. *J Trauma* **31**: 629–638.

Moore, F.A., Feliciano, D.V., Andrassy, R.J., *et al.* (1992a) Early enteral feeding, compared with parenteral, reduces post-operative septic complications: the results of a meta-analysis. *Ann Surg* **216**: 172–183.

Moore, F.A., Moore, E.E., Poggetti, R.S., Read, R.A. (1992b) Post-injury shock and early bacteremia. A lethal combination. *Arch Surg* **127**: 893–898.

Morrison, D., Ulevitch, R.J. (1978) The effects of bacterial endotoxins on host mediation systems. *Am J Pathol* **93**: 526–618.

Mullin, J.M., Snock, K.V. (1990) Effect of tumour necrosis factor on epithelial tight junctions and transepithelial permeability. *Cancer Res* **50**: 2172–2176.

Navaratnam, R.L.N., Morris, S.E., Traber, D.L. *et al.* (1990) Endotoxin (LPS) increases mesenteric vascular resistance (MVR) and bacterial translocation (BT). *J Trauma* **30**: 1104–1113.

Naylor, C.D., O'Rourke, K., Detsky, A.S., Baker, J.P. (1989) Parenteral nutrition with branched-chain amino acids in hepatic encephalopathy. *Gastroenterology* **97**: 1033–1042.

Nishizaki, Y., Guth, P.H., Kim, G., Wayland, H., Kaunitz, J.D. (1994) Pentagastrin enhances gastric mucosal defences in vivo: luminal acid-dependent and independent effects. *Am J Physiol* **267**: G94–G104.

Norton, J.A., Ott, L.G., McClain, C. *et al.* (1988) Intolerance to enteral feeding in the brain injured patient. *J Neurosurg* **68**: 62–66.

O'Dwyer, S.T., Michie, H.R., Ziegler, T.R., Revhaug, A., Smith, R.J., Wilmore, D.W. (1988) A single dose of endotoxin increases intestinal permeability in healthy humans. *Arch Surg* **123**: 1459–1464.

Ohri, S.K., Bjarnason, I., Pathi, V., *et al.* (1993) Cardiopulmonary bypass impairs small intestinal transport and increases gut permeability. *Ann Thoracic Surg* **55**: 1080–1086.

Palmer, R.M.J., Ferrige, A.G., Moncada, S. (1987) Nitric oxide release accounts for the biological activity of endothelium-derived relaxing factor. *Nature* **327**: 524–526.

Park, P.O., Haglund, U. (1992) Regeneration of small bowel mucosa after intestinal ischemia. *Crit Care Med* **20**: 135–139.

Park, P.O., Haglund, U., Bulkley, G.B., Falt, K. (1990) The sequence of development of intestinal tissue injury after strangulation ischemia and reperfusion. *Surgery* **107**: 574–580.

Parker, M.M., Shelhamer, J.H., Bacharach, S.L., *et al.* (1984) Profound but reversible myocardial depression in patients with septic shock. *Ann Intern Med* **100**: 483–490.

Parsons, P.E., Worthen, G.S., Moore, E.E., Tate, R.M., Henson, P.M. (1989) The association of circulating endotoxin with the development of the adult respiratory distress syndrome. *Am Rev Respir Dis* **140**: 294–301.

Parviainen, I., Vaisanen, O., Ruokonen, E., Takala, J. (1996) Effect of nasogastric suction and ranitidine on the calculated gastric intramucosal pH. *Intensive Care Med* **22**: 319–323.

Payen, D.M., Fratacci, M.D., Dupuy, P., *et al.* (1989) Portal and hepatic arterial blood flow measurements of human transplanted liver by implanted Doppler probes: interest for early complications and nutrition. *Surgery* **107**: 417–427.

Philipsen, E.K., Batsberg, W., Christensen, A.B. (1988) Gastrointestinal permeability to polyethylene glycol: an evaluation of urinary recovery of an oral load of polyethylene glycol as a parameter of intestinal permeability in man. *Eur J Clin Invest* **18**: 139–145.

Pieper, J.A., Rodman, J.H. (1986) Lidocaine. In: Evans, W.E., Schentag, J.J., Jusko, W.J. (eds), *Applied Pharmacokinetics*, pp. 639–681. Spokane: Applied Therapeutics.

Platell, C., McCauley, R., McCulloch, R., Hall, J.C. (1993) The influence of parenteral glutamine and branched chain amino acids on total parenteral nutrition-induced atrophy of the gut. *J Parent Ent Nutr* **17**: 348–354.

Playford, R.J., Woodman, A.C., Clark, P., *et al.* (1993) Effect of luminal growth factor preservation on intestinal growth. *Lancet* **341**: 866–867.

Polk, H.C., Shields, C.L. (1977) Remote organ failure: a valid sign of occult intra-abdominal infection. *Surgery* **81**: 310–312.

Pollack, D.S., Sufian, S., Matsumoto, T. (1979) Indocyanine green clearance in critically ill patients. *Surg Gynecol Obstet* **149**: 852–854.

Porter, J.M., Sussman, M.S., Bulkley, G.B. (1989) Splanchnic vasospasm in circulatory shock. In: Marston, A., Bulkley, G., Fiddian-Green, R.G., Haglund, U. (eds), *Splanchnic Ischemia and Multiple Organ Failure*, pp. 73–88. London: Edward Arnold.

Radermacher, P., Buhl, R., Kemnitz, J., *et al.* (1994) Prostacyclin improves gastric intramucosal pH in patients with septic shock. *Clin Intensive Care* **4**(Suppl): 9.

Reines, H.D., Halushka, P.V., Cook, J.A., Wise, W.C., Rambo, W. (1982) Plasma thromboxane concentrations are raised in patients dying with septic shock. *Lancet* **ii**: 174–175.

Riddington, D., Venkatesh, K.B., Clutton-Brock, T., Bion, J. (1994) Measuring carbon dioxide tension in saline and alternative solutions: quantification of biasand precision in two blood gas analysers. *Crit Care Med* **22**: 96–100.

Rolfe, M.W., Kunkel, S.L., Standiford, T.J., *et al.* (1991) Pulmonary fibroblast expression of interleukin-8: a model for alveolar macrophage-derived cytokine networking. *Am J Respir Cell Mol Biol* **5**: 493–501.

Roumen, R.M.H., Hendriks, T., Wevers, R.A., Goris, R.J.A. (1993) Intestinal permeability after severe trauma and haemorrhagic shock is increased without relation to septic complications. *Arch Surg* **128**: 453–457.

Rush, F.R., Sori, A.J., Murphy, M.S., Smith, S., Flanagan, J.J., Macheido, G. (1988) Endotoxemia and bacteremia during hemorrhagic shock. *Ann Surg* **207**: 549–554.

Saadia, R., Schein, M., MacFarlane, C., Boffard, K.D. (1990) Gut barrier function and the surgeon. *Br J Surg* **77**: 487–492.

Sack, J., Spenney, J.G. (1982) Aminopyrine accumulation by mammalian gastric glands: an analysis of the technique. *Am J Physiol, Gastrointest Liver Physiol* **250**: G313–G319.

Said, S.I. (1983) Vasoactive peptides. State of the art review. *Hypertension* **5**(Suppl 1): 17–20.

Saito, H., Trocki, O., Wang, S.L., Gonce, S.J., Joffe, S.N. (1987) Metabolic and immune effects of dietary arginine supplementation after burn. *Arch Surg* **122**: 784–789.

Scannell, G., Clark, L., Waxman, K. (1992) Regional blood flow during experimental hemorrhage and crystalloid resuscitation: persistence of low flow to the splanchnic organs. *Resuscitation* **23**: 217–225.

Schaefer, C.F., Biber, B., Lerner, M.R., Jobis-Vandervliet, F.F., Fagraeus, L. (1991) Rapid reduction of intestinal cytochrome-a,a^3 during lethal endotoxemia. *J Surg Res* **51**: 382–391.

Schonholz, S., Pleatman, M., Kasserman, D., Ponsky, J. (1989) Endoscopic tonometric assessment of intestinal perfusion in a canine model. *Gastrointest Endosc* **35**: 425–427.

Shaw, B. (1915) *The Doctor's Dilemma: a Tragedy*. London: Constable.

Shelly, M.P., Church, J.J. (1987) Bowel sounds during intermittent positive pressure ventilation. *Anaesthesia* **42**: 207–209.

Shepherd, A.P. (1980) Intestinal blood flow autoregulation during foodstuff absorption. *Am J Physiol* **239**: H156–H162.

Shoemaker, W., Appel, P., Kram, H., Waxman, K., Lee, T.S. (1988) Prospective trial of supranormal values of survivors as therapeutic goals in high risk surgical patients. *Chest* **94**: 1176–1186.

Siber, G.R., Mayer, R.J., Levin, M.J. (1980) Increased gastrointestinal absorption of large molecules in patients after 5-fluorouracil therapy. *Cancer Res* **40**: 3430–3436.

Silverman, H.J. (1991) Gastric tonometry: an index of splanchnic tissue oxygenation? *Crit Care Med* **19**: 1223–1224.

Singh, G., Chaudry, K.I., Morrison, M.H., Chaudry, I.H. (1993) Tumour necrosis factor depresses gut absorptive function. *Circ Shock* **39**: 279–284.

Skak, C., Keiding, S. (1987) Methodological problems in the use of indocyanine green to estimate hepatic blood flow and ICG clearance in man. *Liver* **7**: 155–162.

Smith, R.J. (1990) Glutamine metabolism and it physiologic importance. *J Parent Ent Nutr* **14**: 40–44.

Sodeyama, M., Kirk, S.J., Regan, M.C., Barbul, A. (1992) The effect of haemorrhagic shock on intestinal amino acid absorption *in vivo*. *Circ Shock* **38**: 153–156.

Solomon, S.M., Kirby, D.F. (1990) The refeeding syndrome: a review. *J Parent Ent Nutr* **14**: 90–97.

Souba, W.W., Herskowitz, K., Salloum, R.M., Chen, M.K., Austgen, T.R. (1990) Gut glutamine metabolism. *J Parent Ent Nutr* **14**: 445–450S.

Spain, D.A., Wilson, M.A., Bar-Natan, M.F., Garrison, R.N. (1994) Role of nitric oxide in the small intestinal microcirculation during bacteremia. *Shock* **2**: 41–46.

Spapen, H.D., Duinslaeger, L., Diltoer, M., Gillet, R., Bossuyt, A, Huyghens LP. (1995) Gastric emptying in critically ill patients is accelerated by adding cisapride to a standard enteral feeding protocol: results of a prospective, randomized, controlled trial. *Crit Care Med* **23**: 481–485.

Stannard, V.A., Hutchinson, A., Morris, D.L., Byrne, A. (1988) Gastric exocrine 'failure' in critically ill patients: incidence and associated features. *Br Med J* **296**: 155–156.

Suffredini, A.F., Fromm, R.E., Parker, M.M., *et al.* (1989) The cardiovascular response of normal humans to the administration of endotoxin. *New Engl J Med* **321**: 280–287.

Tracey, K.J., Fong, Y., Hesse, D.G., *et al.* (1987) Anti-cachectin/TNF monoclonal antibodies prevent septic shock during lethal bacteraemia. *Nature* **330**: 662–664.

Travis, S., Menzies, I. (1992) Intestinal permeability: functional assessment and significance. *Clin Sci* **82**: 477–488.

Turnage, R.H., Guice, K.S., Oldham, K.T. (1994) Pulmonary microvascular injury following intestinal reperfusion. *New Horizons* **2**: 463–475.

Uusaro, A., Ruokonen, E., Takala, J. (1995) Gastric mucosal pH does not reflect changes in splanchnic blood flow after cardiac surgery. *Br J Anaesth* **74**: 149–154.

van der Waaij, D., Berghuis-de Vries, J.M., Lekkerkerk-van der Wees, J.E.C. (1972) Colonisation resistance of the digestive tract and the spread of bacteria to the lymphatic organs in mice. *J Hyg* **70**: 335–342.

van Deventer, S.J.H., ten Cate, J.W., Buller, H.R., Sturk, A., Pauw, W. (1988a) Endotoxaemia: an early predictor of septicaemia in febrile patients. *Lancet* **i**: 601–609.

van Deventer, S.J.H., Knepper, A., Landsman, J., *et al.* (1988b) Endotoxins in portal blood. *Hepato-gastroenterology* **35**: 223–225.

Vincent, J.L., Dufaye, P., Berre, J., Leeman, J., Degaute, J.P., Kahn, K. (1981) Lactate metabolism during circulatory shock. *Crit Care Med* **9**: 234–239.

Wallace, J.L., Steel, G., Whittle, B.J.R., Lagente, V., Vargaftig, B. (1987) Evidence for platelet activating factor as a mediator of endotoxin induced gastrointestinal damage in the rat. *Gastroenterology* **93**: 765–773.

Wiegand, B.D., Ketterer, S.G., Rapaport, E. (1960) The use of indocyanine green for the evaluation of hepatic function and blood flow in man. *Am J Digest Dis* **5**: 427–436.

Wilmore, D.W. (1994) Glutamine and the gut. *Gastroenterology* **107**: 1885–1886.

Wolfe, B.M., Ryder, M.A., Nishikawa, R.A., Halstead, C.H., Schmidt, B.F. (1986) Complications of parenteral nutrition. *Am J Surg* **152**: 93–99.

Wright, S.D., Ramos, R.A., Tobias, P.S., Ulevitch, R.J., Mathison, J.C. (1990) CD14, a receptor for complexes of lipopolysaccharide (LPS) and LPS binding protein. *Science* **249**: 1431–1433.

Zeeh, J., Lange, H., Bosch, J., *et al.* (1988) Steady-state extrarenal sorbitol as a measure of hepatic plasma flow. *Gastroenterology* **95**: 749–759.

Ziegler, T.R., Smith, R.J., O'Dwyer, S.T., Demling, R.H., Wilmore, D.W. (1988) Increased intestinal permeability associated with infection in burn patients. *Arch Surg* **123**: 1313–1318.

Ziegler, T.R., Smith, R.J., Byrne, T.A., Wilmore, D.W. (1993) Potential role of glutamine supplementation in nutrition support. *Clin Nutr* **12**(Suppl 1): S82–S90.

6

The Challenge of Increasing Antibiotic Resistance in Intensive Care

T.J.J. Inglis

INTRODUCTION

Resistance to the first penicillin antibiotics was discovered even before penicillin came into widespread clinical use (Abraham, 1940). From that point on until the 1980s a growing catalogue of resistance mechanisms drove a burgeoning pharmaceutical industry to release a steady stream of novel antibiotics. This was the antibiotic era; a time when infection could be mastered by new antibiotic miracle drugs. Many great infectious scourges of past generations could now be cured by antimicrobial chemotherapy, leading to optimistic predictions of an eventual eradication of infectious disease. The era also had its own heroic myth: the story of penicillin's serendipitous discovery and its first therapeutic failure, due of course to an inadequate supply of antibiotic. However, within 4 years another potential reason for therapeutic failure had arisen; that of acquired antibiotic resistance (Kirby, 1944). Industry responded to the problem of penicillin-resistant staphylococci with penicillinase-resistant antibiotics, but this in turn contributed to the growing importance of Gram-negative infections, particularly in hospital patients from 1960 onwards. Again industry provided an answer, or rather several answers in the form of antibiotics with enhanced activity against Gram-negative bacteria, such as the aminopenicillins, cephalosporins and aminoglycosides. The illusion created by this cycle of antibiotic obselescence and pharmaceutical innovation was that there would always be another agent, whatever new mechanism of antibiotic resistance emerged next.

So what has brought the optimism to an end? Why are leading authorities warning that we are reaching the end of the age of antibiotic miracles (Levy, 1992)? Are they being alarmist by claiming that we are 'running out of therapeutic options' (Lederberg, 1994)?

Antibiotic resistance was first described shortly after the discovery of penicillin, as noted above, but it was not until the appearance of several multiresistant phenotypes in the mid- to late-1980s that earlier warnings about overuse of antibiotics began to find a wider audience. Unlike previous multiresistant strains of bacteria, the new types of resistance were found capable of disabling whole families of antibiotics, in some cases leaving very little choice of therapy. Moreover, some of these forms of resistance could be transmitted between bacteria belonging to different species. A further factor that contributed to increased concern about antibiotic resistance was the occurrence of several outbreaks of multi-drug-resistant tuberculosis that put hospital staff at risk of untreatable disease (Wenger *et al.*, 1995). Examination of other major categories of antimicrobial agent (e.g. antifungals, antivirals, antimalarials) reveals a similar phenomenon; diminishing clinical usefulness caused by antimicrobial resistance.

Faced with ever-shortening commercial lifetimes for new products, the pharmaceutical companies have, understandably, become reluctant to make substantial long-term commitments to antibiotic development. The medical profession is therefore beginning to realize that the industry's reluctance to work on new agents, particularly those with entirely novel mechanisms of action (Wise, 1996), means that reinforcements are unlikely to arrive in time – this is one battle we will have to learn to fight on our own.

EPIDEMIOLOGY OF ANTIBIOTIC RESISTANCE IN INTENSIVE CARE

Currently available surveillance data on antibiotic resistance does not permit a detailed appraisal of resistance and its determinants in the intensive care unit (ICU). The test methodology and choice of test agents varies considerably between microbiology laboratories. Moreover, selection of isolates for sensitivity testing from cultures generated by non-sterile sites such as tracheal secretions can be misleading, and lead to unnecessary antimicrobial therapy (Cunha, 1994). The single largest nosocomial infection surveillance programme, the National Nosocomial Infection Survey (USA) has not collected sensitivity data to date. However, some insight into a few of the more common resistance issues was provided by a recent European point prevalence survey of hospital-acquired infection in ICUs (Vincent *et al.*, 1995). The most commonly reported causes of infection in this survey were Enterobacteriaceae (*Escherichia coli*, *Klebsiella* spp. and *Enterobacter* spp.), *Staphylococcus aureus*, *Pseudomonas aeruginosa*, coagulase-negative cocci and fungi. Sixty per cent of infections and 72% bacteraemias caused by *Staph. aureus* were due to methicillin-resistant strains. Resistance to one or more of gentamicin, ceftazidime, ciprofloxacin or imipenem was present in 65% *P. aeruginosa* isolates. Point prevalence surveys of this kind are susceptible to reporting bias; overreporting common problems, and underemphasizing less common but no less serious problems. Newer patterns of antibiotic resistance that are more difficult to find with standard sensitivity test methods may thus have escaped detection.

Important additions to the list of antibiotic-resistant organisms now found in hospital inpatients include *Acinetobacter baumannii* (formerly *A. anitratus* var. *calcoaceticus*), *Stenotrophomonas* (formerly *Xanthomonas*) *maltophilia*, members of the pseudomonas group, corynebacteria such as *Corynebacterium jeikeium* and enterococci. Some of these have been associated with recent hospital outbreaks of antibiotic-resistant nosocomial infection (Table 6.1). Sadly, many such outbreaks go unreported due to a lack of investigative resources, inconclusive results or a desire to suppress embarrassing news of a breakdown in hospital hygiene. It will be some time before the epidemiology of these less familiar species has been mapped out in the intensive care setting, particularly since recent experience suggests that there may be a complex mixture of endemic and epidemic strains (Seifert *et al.*, 1994).

The acquisition of enteric Gram-negative bacilli (Enterobacteriaceae and *P. aeruginosa*) has received much more attention, since this group of bacteria has been recognized as a potential cause of ICU-acquired infection for many years (Phillips and Spencer, 1965; Casewell and Phillips, 1978). Up to 30% of patients admitted to an ICU have their oropharynx colonized by Gram-negative bacilli, and this figure appears to increase with duration of stay (Johanson *et al.*, 1969; Selden *et al.*, 1971). Severity of underlying illness, the presence of a tracheal tube and prior antibiotic therapy are further predisposing

Table 6.1   Recent outbreaks of antibiotic-resistant nosocomial infection

Organism	Resistance	Setting	Reference
Acinetobacter baumannii	Multiple	ITU	Crowe *et al.* (1995)
Acinetobacter baumannii	Multiple	ICUs	Seifert *et al.* (1994)
Klebsiella pneumoniae	ESBL*	Several	Nouvellon *et al.* (1994)
Klebsiella pneumoniae	ESBL	Several	Meyer *et al.* (1993)
Pseudomonas aeruginosa	Multiple	ICU	Jumaa and Chattopadhyay 1994
Serratia marcescens	ESBL	ICU	Pagani *et al.* (1994)
Enterococcus faecium	vanB[†]	?	Boyce *et al.* (1994)
Mycobacterium tuberculosis	Multiple	HIV unit	Wenger *et al.* (1995)

* Extended-spectrum β-lactamase.
[†] Vancomycin resistant, type vanB.

factors to colonization by Gram-negative bacilli. The speed with which colonization occurs suggests that the origin for these bacteria is the patient's indigenous flora. In the case of bacteria subsequently causing ventilator-associated pneumonia, the evidence favours aspiration into the intubated trachea from an upper gastrointestinal source following gastric bacterial overgrowth (Atherton and White, 1978; du Moulin *et al.*, 1982; Inglis *et al.*, 1993).

Although the above studies did not specifically address the issue of antibiotic resistance in critically ill patients, it is possible to assemble an outline of the type of patient in whom antibiotic resistance is more likely to be encountered. This patient will probably have been in hospital for a prolonged period, and will often have received extensive antibiotic therapy. From personal experience, high APACHE scores, prolonged mechanical ventilation and transfer from another hospital unit are also frequent markers for antibiotic resistance.

In a tertiary referral centre in Singapore, patients transferred into the ICU by Medevac from overseas hospitals often combined all the above risk factors with poor infection control at the point of origin. These patients brought with them combinations of methicillin-resistant *Staph. aureus*, extended-spectrum β-lactamase (ESBL) bearing klebsiellas, multiresistant *Acinetobacter*, and possibly *Candida albicans* as well. Methicillin-resistant *Staphylococcus aureus* (MRSA) infection was a common occurrence in Singaporean patients in the ICU. A small surveillance study demonstrated MRSA in either the anterior nares or groin of 20% patients shortly after admission (Ng and Inglis, unpublished data). The same proportion of patients was colonized with ESBL-bearing klebsiellas in rectal or gastric contents, though some were colonized with only one of these organisms, and some with both. A retrospective analysis of *Staph. aureus* and *Klebsiella* spp. isolated from surgical ICU patients over the preceding year showed that resistant variants of both species were associated with prior antibiotic use, particularly of cephalosporins, and with increasing duration of hospital stay prior to ICU admission. Resistance was detected during two peak periods: immediately after ICU admission, and after a prolonged interval (of over a week) in the ICU. MRSA was first documented in the hospital shortly after it opened in 1985, and rose quickly to around 40% of all *Staph. aureus* isolated (Meers and Leong, 1990). ESBL-bearing klebsiellas probably appeared in Singapore at the same time, according to antibiotic sensitivity data, and by 1993 accounted for almost half of all *Klebsiella pneumoniae* isolated from blood cultures in the hospital (Inglis *et al.*, 1994). The ESBL-bearing strains had also acquired aminoglycoside-modifying enzymes (AMEs) which appeared to be co-transferred with extended-spectrum β-lactamases. The net result was *Klebsiella* species resistant to all penicillins, cephalosporins, monobactams and amino-glycosides available in Singapore. That left only the quinolone and carbapenem antibiotics. By early 1996, ESBL/AME-bearing klebsiellas with high level quinolone resistance were being isolated from small numbers of septicaemic patients. The rise in cephalosporin resistance in the same institution has been linked to a steady increase in usage of third-generation cephalosporins (Kumarasinghe *et al.*, 1992).

Tertiary referral centres in places such as Singapore illustrate the ecological consequences of developing medical technology without corresponding advances in prescribing discipline or hospital hygiene. These centres serve to concentrate antibiotic resistance, promote spread among patients and provide multiple opportunities for exchange of resistance between micro-organisms. However, it would be a misrepresentation to imply that South-East Asia is the only part of the world where poor hospital hygiene contributes to the spread of antibiotic-resistant strains of bacteria. Hands have been repeatedly implicated as a vehicle for the transmission of nosocomial pathogens between patients, yet compliance with hand hygiene practices in ICUs has been shown to be poor in both European and North American centres, especially among senior medical staff (Knittle *et al.*, 1975; Casewell and Phillips, 1977; Albert and Condie, 1981; Sproat and Inglis, 1994).

The hands of staff are not the only vehicle for transmission of anti-biotic-resistant strains. Gastric aspirates can contain several millions of Gram-negative bacteria per millilitre (Inglis *et al.*, 1992a), so that spillage during manipulation of the nasogastric tube could result in major contamination of staff hands, the patient's body surface and surrounding equipment. Respiratory secretions represent a similar potential source of nosocomial pathogens. These are often scattered widely during tracheal suction procedures, as examination of low-lying ICU ceilings will readily demonstrate.

Consideration of the various means of bacterial dissemination within an ICU explains why antibiotic-resistant strains of species such as *A. baumannii* and *P. aeruginosa* can be isolated from so many different sources (Seifert *et al.*, 1994; Crowe *et al.*, 1995), making investigation of a common-source incident a difficult task. Obtaining cultures from possible sources in the patient, staff and intensive care environment may seem to be a simple matter of collecting swabs, but culture results should be seen as no more than a late snapshot of a dynamic ecological process. By the time a preliminary screening exercise has made any contribution to the epidemiological task of identifying the most likely primary source and means of transmission,

Table 6.2   Issues in planning an antibiotic resistance surveillance study

* *Who does the planning?*
  Intensive care physician
  Senior nurse
  Microbiologist

* *Objective of study?*
  Genus, species, and resistance pattern
  Prevalence or incidence?

* *Colonization or infection?*
  Standard definition required
  Use standardized sampling method

* *Which laboratory methods?*
  For initial sensitivity screening
  For confirmation of resistant phenotypes
  For molecular typing methods

* *What clinical outcomes will be measured?*
  Mortality
  Days intubated, ventilated or febrile
  Antibiotic decisions

* *Use of results?*
  Planning presumptive therapy
  Improvements in infection control
  Modification of surveillance methods

colonization and secondary infection may have blurred the microbiological picture. Molecular typing methods are now widely used in
larger centres to help distinguish between otherwise similar isolates,
but these often require a further wait and are only as good as the initial
data and sample collection. In extreme cases it may be several years
before results confirm the initial impression on which the infection
control team based their intervention measures (Snelling *et al.*, 1996).
These considerations should be borne in mind when addressing the
epidemiology of antibiotic resistance in a specific ICU. Important
issues to consider when planning a surveillance study are outlined in
Table 6.2.

MOLECULAR ASPECTS OF ANTIBIOTIC RESISTANCE

The range or spectrum of action of a given antibiotic varies according
to the specific point of action of the antibiotic molecule. Consequently,
every agent in current clinical use has its corresponding group of
intrinsically resistant microbial species. These are the organisms

against which the specific antibiotic can reliably be predicted to have no therapeutically useful action in vivo. It is the acquired form of antibiotic resistance that causes problems for the clinician, by introducing an element of uncertainty when choosing from a diminishing range of suitable antibiotic agents.

Bacteria acquire antibiotic resistance either by spontaneous mutation or by acquisition of DNA from an external source. Development of resistance by spontaneous mutation can occur at high rates in *Staph. aureus* against fusidic acid or rifampicin (Atlas and Turck, 1968; Amirak *et al.*, 1981), but is a less efficient means of acquiring resistance than transfer of DNA between bacteria. The most effective transfer mechanisms involve extrachromosomal fragments of DNA, which can multiply and transfer independent of the parent chromosome. Two major vehicles for bacterial gene transfer are plasmids (circular extrachromosomal fragments of DNA) and transposons (DNA sequences that can insert into or detatch from the bacterial chromosome or a plasmid, sometimes known as 'jumping genes'). Both plasmids and transposons contribute to the continuous process of bacterial genetic reassortment. These different gene-transfer mechanisms provide a route for transmission of antibiotic-resistance genes from an initial locus on the chromosome to distant sites in other species, and even genera. The network of possible routes for gene transfer between bacterial species has proved to be far more complex than initially thought (de Flaun and Levy, 1991). Even transfer of resistance between Gram-positive and Gram-negative bacteria can occur (Trieu-Cuot *et al.*, 1985).

The accumulation of resistance-determining genes by a given strain may result in the acquisition of insertion sequences that modify a specific resistance phenotype, as found in some strains of methicillin-resistant *Staph. aureus* (de Lencastre and Tomasz, 1994). This can result in wide variations in expression of in vitro resistance, making detection difficult for the clinical laboratory unless genetic methods are used. In the case of MRSA, amplification of the *mec A* single gene locus by polymerase chain reaction has been used to confirm the presence of methicillin resistance (Murakami *et al.*, 1991).

Methicillin resistance in *Staph. aureus* involves alteration of a specific penicillin-binding protein (PBP_2) to a new protein with reduced affinity for β-lactam antibiotics (Hartman and Tomasz, 1984). In this case resistance is due to an inability of antibiotic to bind with the bacterial cell wall, rather than to an alteration of the antibiotic molecule itself. Another form of antibiotic resistance due to alteration of the antibiotic target site is high-level quinolone resistance caused by mutational change to bacterial DNA gyrase, which in some bacteria may also confer resistance to the unrelated carbapenem group of antibiotics (Cambau *et al.*, 1995).

A more common bacterial antitherapeutic strategy is alteration of the active site of the antibiotic molecule, as occurs when β-lactamases hydrolyse the β-lactam ring present in penicillins, cephalosporins and related antibiotics. β-Lactamases have been described with a huge variety of substrate specificities (Bush, 1989a, b). These enzymes can be chromosomal or plasmid borne, constitutive or inducible, and narrow or extended spectrum. One of the earliest plasmid-borne β-lactamases was TEM-1, an enzyme that confers resistance to the penicillin and aminopenicillin groups. It may only require a single amino acid substitution at the enzyme's active site to produce a TEM-like enzyme with activity against extended-spectrum cephalosporins such as cefotaxime and ceftazidime (Jiang *et al.*, 1992). These ESBLs are mostly found in Enterobacteriaceae, particularly *Klebsiella* spp. (Sirot *et al.*, 1992). Detection of resistance mediated by ESBLs is hampered in the laboratory by the ability of some strains to escape detection by conventional disk diffusion screening methods, thus necessitating the use of an additional screening test (Jarlier *et al.*, 1988). The prevalence of ESBL-mediated resistance may therefore be underestimated in some centres. This type of resistance has been reported from most developed and many developing countries (Philippon *et al.*, 1994). ESBL-bearing klebsiellas have been reported in a European ICU context (Sirot *et al.*, 1991), and were common in Singapore (Inglis *et al.*, 1994). Another group of β-lactamases associated with infections in intensive care patients are the inducible chromosomal enzymes found in *P. aeruginosa*, *Enterobacter* spp. and *Citrobacter* spp. (Saunders, 1989). β-Lactamase production may only be expressed at clinically detectable levels after prolonged exposure to a potent antibiotic inducer, and may be missed on initial laboratory testing. However, acquisition of additional genes may stabilize resistance by switching on continuous (constitutive) high level β-lactamase production (Lindberg *et al.*, 1985).

Other antibiotic-disabling enzymes of growing importance are the aminoglycoside-modifying enzymes (AMEs); a large family of acetyl-, adenylyl- and phosphotransferases. The AMEs have been known for many years, but are currently gaining renewed attention due to their tendency to add broad-spectrum aminoglycoside resistance to ESBL-bearing bacteria (Fernandez-Rodriguez *et al.*, 1992). The resulting penicillin–cephalosporin–aminoglycoside-resistant phenotype substantially reduces treatment options and is no less capable of causing septicaemia than are fully sensitive strains, as was clear from the experience in Singapore (Inglis *et al.*, 1994).

Bacterial cells appear able to restrict antibiotic access to the cytoplasm by a variety of mechanisms. Some of these, e.g. alterations in outer membrane proteins, have been characterized by molecular research methods, but detection of more than a crude resistance effect is beyond the capability of the average diagnostic laboratory. Moreover, many Gram-negative species combine reduced permeability with other antibiotic-resistance mechanisms including antibiotic-disabling enzymes. The combined effect places a severe limit on therapeutic options. In some nosocomial pathogens, such as *A. baumannii*, multiresistance is so extreme that there may be no effective antibiotic left (Kuah *et al.*, 1994). Recently, concern has been expressed that transferable glycopeptide resistance present in enterococci might be acquired by methicillin-resistant *Staph. aureus*, making MRSA effectively untreatable (Casewell, 1995). The transfer of glycopeptide resistance between enterococci and *Staph. aureus* has already been achieved in vivo (Noble *et al.*, 1992). Although infection caused by vancomycin-resistant *Staph. aureus* has not yet been documented in clinical practice, it may only be a matter of time before the increasingly common, transferable glycopeptide resistance is transmitted to *Staph. aureus* in vivo. Clinical settings with a poor hygiene record, and a concurrence of vancomycin-resistant enterococci and methicillin-resistant staphylococci are likely to be the first in which vancomycin-resistant staphylococci are observed.

Common to all forms of multiresistance is the effect they have on selection of resistance. A single type of resistance means that only the use of an antibiotic belonging to that class can confer a survival advantage on that strain. But when multiresistance is present, the use of any class of antibiotic to which the strain is resistant can select the entire resistance pattern. Thus even the use of amoxycillin would favour selection of ceftazidime- and gentamicin-resistant klebsiellas in Singapore. Moreover, the probability of exchange of resistance genes between bacterial species is likely to be higher when all but antibiotic-resistant bacteria have been removed from the indigenous flora. This 'selection pressure', as it is sometimes known, is in proportion to the number of antibiotics used, their dose and duration of use, and their antibiotic spectrum. It is selection pressure that drives the restless tide of genetic change in the microbial population, and the development of antibiotic resistance represents an adaptive response to aid microbial survival in a hostile environment. *E. coli* takes around 20 minutes to produce a new generation of daughter cells, and therefore around 3 hours, or eight generations, to stabilize a new genotype. It takes a pharmaceutical company years to bring a new agent into use – the odds are not in our favour.

ANTIBIOTIC USE IN THE ICU

Once a specific micro-organism has been implicated in a specific infection and its sensitivities have been determined, the choice of antimicrobial agent is relatively easy. Unfortunately, the nature of intensive care dictates that immediate decisions must be made on the choice of antibiotic long before the laboratory produces any culture-based results. In most instances, laboratory results merely allow fine-tuning of presumptive antimicrobial chemotherapy. If at this late stage the patient has not responded to presumptive therapy, alterations can be made according to sensitivity results. That is not to say that the diagnostic laboratory has no role in the immediate management of the intensive care patient, but it should be clear that its contribution to selection of antibiotic agents is mainly epidemiological. The laboratory should be able to review results from previous patients, on a site-, organism-, and antibiotic-specific basis, particularly if results have been stored on a computer.

Detailed guidelines on antibiotic use in the ICU require specific insight gained from being present at the bedside when therapeutics decisions are made. The antibiotic algorithm developed for a given ICU should at least provide options for major Gram-positive and Gram-negative hospital pathogens, community-acquired infections (during the early phase of intensive care), patients with antibiotic allergy, and a second line of agents reserved for unusually resistant isolates. An algorithm will help ensure consistency in the use of antibiotics within an ICU, and encourage periodic review of resistance patterns which should be performed at least annually. Periodic review of antibiotic use will also be helped by recording: (a) why each new antibiotic has been prescribed, (b) how the effects of treatment will be monitored, and (c) when its use will be reviewed.

A regular and disciplined review of antibiotic use in the ICU will reduce antibiotic selection pressure and make the unit less prone to the development and spread of resistant strains. A programme of rational antibiotic use in the ICU will also highlight the need for a policy on how to change surgical prophylaxis to pre-emptive therapy, or to change presumptive therapy before laboratory results arrive. Therapeutic choices should not include agents used for prophylaxis, nor should prophylactic agents be continued indefinitely as presumptive therapy. Furthermore, agents such as the quinolones, carbapenems or glycopeptides should be reserved for the more resistant species and should not be used either for prophylaxis or for first-line presumptive therapy, unless a high prevalence of multiresistance forces abandonment of other agents.

THE CONTROL OF ANTIBIOTIC RESISTANCE

Once established in a hospital setting, it is difficult completely to eradicate multiresistant bacteria such as MRSA (Boyce, 1989). Restricting use of the antibiotic to which resistance has developed may control an outbreak. The total cessation of all antibiotic therapy successfully eradicated an epidemic strain of resistant *Klebsiella* sp. from a neurosurgical unit (Price and Sleigh, 1970). Many would now regard such measures as unethical, preferring instead to close an ICU to further admissions until the problem is fully under control (Ayliffe *et al.*, 1992).

More than half of patients admitted to an ICU will receive antibiotics at or shortly after admission to the unit (Weinstein and Kabins, 1981). In Singapore and in Leeds, UK, the percentage receiving antibiotics fell just short of 100% in surgical admissions. Such high levels of antibiotic use explain the selection and emergence of resistant strains in individual patients once they have been admitted, but do not explain their transmission from patient to patient or their persistence in the ICU. Dissemination of antibiotic resistance within the ICU requires a breakdown in hospital infection control, such as a failure of hand hygiene, which occurs repeatedly amongst ICU staff (noted above). Good hand hygiene practice should be maintained at all times to prevent the spread of antibiotic-resistant strains within the ICU, and should be stepped up during the management of an outbreak. Other barrier methods of infection control such as use of a side room, disposable aprons, gloves or masks may also be required to interrupt spread between patients (Weinstein and Kabins, 1981). Though only rarely implicated in common-source incidents, the possibility of an environmental or animate (staff or patient) source should always be considered, since elimination of a proven source is essential to prevent recurrence.

Much antibiotic resistance is endemic in intensive care patients, being present in the indigenous flora of the gastrointestinal tract and other body surfaces. Attempts have been made to reduce the impact of this source by conventional infection-control methods and, more recently, with 'selective decontamination' by administering a combination of non-absorbable antibiotics to the mouth and stomach of ICU patients to reduce gastrointestinal Gram-negative flora. It stands to reason that the prolonged use of large quantities of non-absorbable antibiotics against the enteric flora will exert a high level of selection pressure, and eventually bring about the emergence of further antibiotic resistance. One carefully designed study on the consequences of selective decontamination found that, while infections with resistant species did not increase as a result of using prophylactic agents, colonization by resistant bacteria did increase (Saunders *et al.*, 1994). Effective control measures for endogenous-source resistant micro-organisms are limited to maintenance of a high standard of hand hygiene and the use of physical barriers during procedures that require contact with bowel contents, respiratory secretions and gastric aspirates.

Although established multiresistant species such as MRSA no longer justify a 'search and destroy' approach as previously recommended, the appearance of a new type of antibiotic resistance may deserve a programme of enhanced environmental and patient surveillance, an increased emphasis on hand hygiene, and barrier precautions appropriate to the site of infection. The international significance of, for example, vancomycin-resistant MRSA or transmissible quinolone resistance in ESBL-bearing klebsiellas would undoubtedly justify strict source isolation and attempts at eradication from colonized body surfaces. Sadly, not all ICUs have the facilities to support a patient in source isolation, and many have inadequate handwashing facilities for their staff (Inglis *et al.*, 1992b). Recent experience in the prevention of nosocomial transmission of multi-drug-resistant *Mycobacterium tuberculosis* both to staff and other patients (Wenger *et al.*, 1995) may eventually precipitate a general improvement in isolation facilities in ICUs. The high prevalence of pulmonary tuberculosis in South-East Asia combined with widespread concerns about multi-drug-resistant tuberculosis made the provision of negative-pressure ventilation side-wards a priority in our Singapore ICU. Engineering modifications to side rooms were combined with a greater urgency in communicating sputum acid-fast stain results to the unit, in order to reduce the potential risk to other patients and ICU staff.

IS A RATIONAL APPROACH TO ANTIBIOTIC RESISTANCE POSSIBLE?

Grim pronouncements from leading authorities pronouncing the end of the antibiotic era leave little room for optimism. General-practice prescribing and company marketing habits seem far removed from the immediate problem of increasing antibiotic resistance in the ICU. Furthermore, antibiotic formularies, stop orders, restrictive sensitivity resporting and other approaches used in some hospitals have at best been only partly successful. The search for a widely acceptable means of clearing the logjam of antibiotic resistance has been confounded recently by a minority view claiming that 'injudicious use of antibiotics in the general population, if it does indeed occur, shows no epidemiological evidence of harm' (Marcus, 1995). It may be possible to arrive at such a conclusion from a selective reading of the current data, but that argument is no help to intensive care specialists who have to work with the clinical consequences of multiresistant nosocomial pathogens, and the argument is difficult to sustain when confronted with data from outside a North American/European comfort zone (Meers and Leong, 1990; Inglis *et al.*, 1994; Turnidge *et al.*, 1996). The epidemiological incongruities of antibiotic-resistance data are alluded to in a different way by one authority who insists that in the more developed countries the majority of infections remain sensitive to essential first-line antibiotics, while adding that accurate data on the prevalence of resistance to these agents and its impact on public health is lacking (Lorian, 1995). Lorian's proposal to collect data for a short list of antibiotics used against community-acquired pathogens could be adapted to a limited collection of drug–bug combinations in an intensive care setting. Priorities for multicentre data collection are given in Table 6.3.

Attempts to control antibiotic resistance through national guidelines have been the subject of recent criticism (Goldmann *et al.*, 1996). It has been claimed that these rarely have a sustained effect at the point of prescription. Recognizing the impotence of national and international advisory bodies, a group of concerned physicians met to discuss how best inappropriate antibiotic prescription and breakdown

Table 6.3 Priority drug–bug combinations for international surveillance of antibiotic resistance in intensive care

Species	Antibiotic
Escherichia coli *Klebsiella* sp. *Enterobacter* sp. *Serratia* sp. *Citrobacter* sp.	Gentamicin, cefotaxime, ciprofloxacin imipenem, tazobactam
Acinetobacter sp.	As above plus sulphonamide
Pseudomonas aeruginosa	Gentamicin, piperacillin, ciprofloxacin, imipenem
Staphylococcus aureus and coagulase-negative staphylococci	Penicillin, methicillin, erythromycin, fucidic acid, rifampicin, vancomycin
Mycobacterium tuberculosis	Rifampicin, isoniazid, ethambutol, pyrazinamide

of hospital hygiene could be improved. The consensus statement they drew up is a benchmark for hospitals with an antibiotic-resistance problem, and provides a list of practical suggestions that might just work. It is clear that hospital infection control and therapeutics committees must work out a single local strategy together. It is noteworthy that the aforementioned centre with widespread MRSA, ESBL/AME-bearing klebsiellas, and multiresistant acinetobacters had no microbiological input to the therapeutics committee and had not reviewed its antibiotic policy for over 3 years at the time of writing. The scale of the problem may seem overwhelming, but that should not be a reason to ignore the need for control measures. Policy and practice guidelines clearly need to be developed and reviewed at a local level by those with a day-to-day involvement in the use of antibiotics. Probably the greatest challenge of all is to take our concerns about increasing antibiotic resistance and decreasing therapeutic options to those who refer patients for intensive care.

Intensive care units are becoming one of the main flashpoints for complex antibiotic-resistance problems. We need to challenge our colleagues who work outside the ICU to accept collective responsibility for the ecological consequences of antibiotic use. If they remain unwilling to accept that, we will face an increasingly uneven struggle against antibiotic resistance in the years to come.

CONCLUSION

The choice of antimicrobial agents for infections in critically ill patients is often limited by antibiotic resistance. Outbreaks and even endemic colonization due to multiresistant species are well recognized in ICUs. Some bacterial strains present in ICUs have developed a complex pattern of multiple antibiotic resistance, as a result of selection by sustained exposure to potent broad-spectrum antibiotics. The commoner nosocomial pathogens, such as *Staph. aureus* and the enteric Gram-negative bacilli have adopted a wide range of molecular mechanisms that exploit the ecology of the ICU environment. Dissemination of antibiotic-resistant strains from patient to patient then occurs as a result of poor compliance with hand hygiene and other aspects of infection control. In the absence of more effective novel antibiotics, the best hope of meeting the challenge of increasing antibiotic resistance in the ICU lies in a combination of more restrained antibiotic use and substantial improvements in hospital hygiene.

REFERENCES

Abraham, E.P. (1940) An enzyme from bacteria able to destroy penicillin. *Nature* **146**: 837–839.

Albert, R.K., Condie, F. (1981) Hand washing patterns in medical intensive care units. *N Engl J Med* **304**: 146–147.

Amirak, I.D., Li, A.K., Williams, R.J., *et al.* (1981) A fatal infection caused by methicillin-resistant *Staphylococcus aureus* acquiring resistance to gentamicin and fusidic acid during therapy. *J Infect* **3**: 50–58.

Atherton, S.T., White, D.J. (1978) Stomach as source of bacteria colonising respiratory tract during artificial ventilation. *Lancet* **ii**: 968–969.

Atlas, E., Turck, M. (1968) Laboratory and clinical evaluation of rifampicin. *Am J Med Sci* **256**: 47–54.

Ayliffe, G.A.J., Lowbury, E.J.L., Geddes, A.M., *et al.* (1992) *Control of Hospital Infection: A Practical Handbook*, 3rd edition, p. 174. London: Chapman & Hall Medical.

Boyce, J.M. (1989) Methicillin resistant *Staphylococcus aureus*: detection, epidemiology, and control measures. *Infect Dis Clin North Am* **3**: 901–913.

Boyce, J.M., Opal, S.M., Chow, J.W., *et al.* (1994) Outbreak of multidrug resistant *Enterococcus faecium* with transferable *vanB* class vancomycin resistance. *J Clin Microbiol* **32**: 1148–1153.

Bush, K. (1989a) Classification of β-lactamases. Groups 1, 2a, 2b and 2b'. *Antimicrob Agent Chemother* **33**: 264–270.

Bush, K. (1989b) Classification of β-lactamases: Groups 2c, 2d, 2e, 3 and 4. *Antimicrob Agent Chemother* **33**: 271–276.

Cambau, E., Perani, E., Dib, C., *et al.* (1995) Role of mutations in DNA gyrase genes in ciprofloxacin resistance of *Pseudomonas aeruginosa* susceptible or resistant to imipenem. *Antimicrob Agent Chemother* **39**: 2248–2252.

Casewell, M.W. (1995) new threats to the control of methicillin-resistant *Staphylococcus aureus*. *J Hosp Infect* **30** (Suppl.): 465–471.

Casewell, M., Phillips, I. (1977) Hands as route of transmission for *Klebsiella* species. *Br Med J* **2**: 1315–1317.

Casewell M.W., Phillips, I. (1978) Epidemiological patterns of *Klebsiella* colonisation and infection in an intensive care ward. *J Hyg (Lond)* **80**: 295–300.

Crowe, M., Towner, K.J., Humphreys, H. (1995) Clinical and epidemiological features of an outbreak of acinetobacter infection in an intensive therapy unit. *J Med Microbiol* **43**: 55–62.

Cunha, B.A. (1994) Intensive care, not intensive antibiotics. *Heart Lung* **23**: 361–362.

de Flaun, M.F., Levy, S.B. (1991) Genes and their varied hosts. In: Levy, S.B., Miller, R.V. (eds) *Gene Transfer in the Environment*, pp. 1–32. New York: McGraw-Hill Publishing Co.

de Lencastre H & Tomasz A (1994) Reassessment of the number of auxiliary genes essential for the expression of high-level methicillin resistance in *Staphylococcus aureus*. *Antimicrob Agent Chemother* **38**: 2590–2598.

du Moulin, G.C., Hedley-Whyte, J., Paterson, D.G., *et al*. (1982) Aspiration of gastric bacteria in antacid-treated patients: a frequent cause of postoperative colonisation of the airway. *Lancet* **i**: 242–245.

Fernandez-Rodriguez, A., Canton, R., Perez-Diaz, J.C. *et al*. (1992) Aminoglycoside-modifying enzymes in clinical isolates harbouring extended-spectrum beta-lactamases. *Antimicrob Agent Chemother* **36**: 2536–2538.

Goldmann, D.A., Weinstein, R.A., Wenzel, R.P., *et al*. (1996) Strategies to prevent and control the emergence and spread of antimicrobial-resistant microorganisms in hospitals. *JAMA* **275**: 234–240.

Hartman, B.J., Tomasz, A. (1984) Low-affinity penicillin-binding protein associated with β-lactam resistance in *Staphylococcus aureus*. *J Bacteriol* **158**: 513–516.

Inglis, T.J.J., Sproat, L.J., Sherratt, M.J., *et al*. (1992a) Gastroduodenal dysfunction as a cause of gastric bacterial overgrowth in patients receiving mechanical ventilation of the lungs. *Br J Anaesth* **68**: 499–502.

Inglis, T.J.J., Sproat, L.J., Hawkey, P.M., *et al*. (1992b) Infection control in intensive care units: UK national survey. *Br J Anaesth* **68**: 216–220.

Inglis, T.J.J., Sherratt, M.J., Sproat, L.J., *et al* (1993) Gastroduodenal dysfunction and colonisation of the ventilated lung. *Lancet* **341**: 911–913.

Inglis. T.J.J., Kumarasinghe, G., Chow, C., *et al*. (1994) Multiple antibiotic resistance in *Klebsiella* species and other Enterobacteriaceae isolated in Singapore. *Singapore Med J* **35**: 602–604.

Jarlier, V., Nicolas, M.H., Fournier, G., *et al* (1988) Extended broad-spectrum β-lactamases conferring transferrable resistance to newer β-lactam agents in Enterobacteriaceae: hospital prevalence and susceptibility patterns. *Rev Infect Dis* **10**: 867–878.

Jiang, H., Zieg, J., O'Brien, T.F. (1992) Observation of the acquisition of an amikacin resistance gene by an endemic nosocomial plasmid encoding a ceftazidime resistance gene. In: *Program and Abstracts of 32nd Interscience Conference on Antimicrobial Agents and Chemotherapy*, p. 184 (abstract). Washington, DC: American Society for Microbiology.

Johanson, W.G., Pierce, A.K., Sanford, J.P. (1969) Changing pharyngeal bacterial flora of hospitalised patients. Emergence of Gram negative bacilli. *New Engl J Med* **281**: 1137–1140.

Jumaa, P., Chattopadhyay, B. (1994) Outbreak of gentamicin, ciprofloxacin-resistant *Pseudomonas aeruginosa* in an intensive care unit, traced to contaminated quivers. *J Hosp Infect* **28**: 209–218.

Kirby, W.M.M. (1944). Extraction of highly potent penicillin inactivator from penicillin resistant staphylococci. *Science* **99**: 452–455.

Knittle, M.A., Eitzman, D.V., Baer, H. (1975) Role of hand contamination of personnel in the epidemiology of Gram negative nosocomial infections. *J Pediatr* **86**: 433–437.

Kuah, B.G., Kumarasinghe, G., Doran, J., *et al*. (1994) Antimicrobial susceptibilities of clinical isolates of *Acinetobacter baumannii* from Singapore. *Antimicrob Agent Chemother* **38**: 2502–2503.

Kumarasinghe, G., Liew, H.Y., Chow, C., *et al*. (1992) Antimicrobial resistance:

patterns and trends in the National University Hospital, Singapore (1989–1991). *Malay J Pathol* **14**: 95–103.

Lederberg, J. (1994) Quoted in: Garrett, L., *The Coming Plague: Newly Emerging Diseases in a World Out of Balance*, p. 431. New York: Farrar, Strauss & Giroux.

Levy, S.B. (1992) *The Antibiotic Paradox: How Miracle Drugs are Destroying the Miracle.* New York: Plenum Press.

Lindberg, F.L., Westman, L., Normark, S. (1985) Regulatory components in *Citrobacter freundii ampC* β-lactamase induction. *Proc Natl Acad Sci USA* **82**: 4620–4624.

Lorian, V. (1995) The need for surveillance for antimicrobial resistance. *Infect Control Hosp Epidemiol* **16**: 638–641.

Marcus, S. (1995) Paradox of western epidemiology. *Lancet* **346**: 55.

Meers, P.D., Leong, K.Y. (1990) The impact of methicillin and aminoglycoside resistant *Staphylococcus aureus* on the pattern of infection in an acute hospital. *J Hosp Infect* **16**: 231–239.

Meyer, K.S., Urban, C., Eagan, J.A. *et al.* (1993) Nosocomial outbreak of *Klebsiella* infection resistant to late generation cephalosporins. *Ann Int Med* **119**: 353–358.

Murakami, K., Minamide, W., Wada, K. *et al.* (1991) Identification of methicillin-resistant strains of staphylococci by PCR. *J Clin Microbiol* **29**: 2240–2244.

Noble, W.C., Virani, Z., Cree, R.G.A. (1992) Cotransfer of vancomycin and other resistance genes from *Enterococcus faecalis* NCTC 12201 to *Staphylococcus aureus*. *FEMS Microbiol Lett* **93**: 195–198.

Nouvellon, M., Pons, J.L., Sirot, D. *et al.* (1994) Clonal outbreaks of extended-spectrum β-lactamase-producing strains of *Klebsiella pneumoniae* demonstrated by antibiotic susceptibility testing, β-lactamase typing, and multilocus enzyme electrophoresis. *J Clin Micro* **32**: 2625–2627.

Pagani, L., Luzzaro, F., Ronza, P., *et al.* (1994) Outbreak of extended-spectrum β-lactamase producing *Serratia marcescens* in an intensive care unit. *FEMS Immunol Med Microbiol* **10**: 39–46.

Philippon, A., Arlet, G., Lagrange, P.H. (1994) Origin and impact of plasmid-mediated extended-spectrum β-lactamases. *Eur J Clin Microbiol Infect Dis* **13** (Suppl. 1): 17–29.

Phillips, I., Spencer, G. (1965) *Pseudomonas aeruginosa* cross-infection: due to contaminated respiratory apparatus. *Lancet* **ii**: 1325–1327.

Price, D.J.E., Sleigh, J.D. (1970) Control of infection due to *Klebsiella aerogenes* in a neurosurgical unit by withdrawal of all antibiotics. *Lancet* **ii**: 1213–1215.

Saunders, C.C. (1989) The chromosomal β-lactamases. In: Bryan, L.E. (ed.) *Microbial Resistance to Drugs*, pp. 129–144. Berlin: Springer-Verlag.

Saunders, G.L., Hammond, J.M., Potgeiter, P.D., *et al.* (1994) Microbiological surveillance during selective decontamination of the digestive tract (SDD). *J Antimicrob Chemother* **34**: 529–544.

Seifert, H., Boullion, B., Schulze, A., *et al.* (1994) Plasmid DNA profiles of *Acinetobacter baumannii*: clinical application in a complex endemic setting. *Infect Control Hosp Epid* **15**: 520–528.

Selden, R., Lee, S., Wang, W.L.L., *et al* (1971) Nosocomial Klebsiella infections: intestinal colonisation as a reservoir. *Ann Intern Med* **74**: 657.

Sirot, D., de Champs, C., Chanal, C., *et al.* (1991) Translocation of antibiotic resistance determinants including an extended-spectrum beta-lactamase between conjugative plasmids of *Klebsiella pneumoniae* and *Escherichia coli*. *Antimicrob Agent Chemother* **35**: 1576–1581.

Sirot, D.L., Goldstein, F.W., Soussy, C.J., *et al.* (1992) Resistance to cefotaxime and seven other beta-lactams in members of the family Enterobacteriaceae: a three-year survey in Farnce. *Antimicrob Agent Chemother* **36**: 1677–1681.

Snelling, A., Gerner-Smidt, P., Hawkey, P.M., *et al.* (1996) Validation of use of whole-cell repetitive extragenic palindromic sequence-based PCR (REP-PCR) for typing stains belonging to the *Acinetobacter calcoaceticus–Acinetobacter baumannii* complex and application of the method to investigation of a hospital outbreak. *J Clin Microbiol* **34**: 1193–1202.

Sproat, L.J., Inglis, T.J.J. (1994) A multicentre survey of hand hygiene practice in intensive care units. *J Hosp Infect* **26**: 137–148.

Trieu-Cuot, P., Gerbaud, G., Lambert, T., *et al.* (1985) In vivo transfer of genetic information between Gram-negative and Gram-positive bacteria. *EMBO J* **4**: 3583–3587.

Turnidge, J.D., Nimmo, G.R., Francis, G. (1996) Evolution of resistance in *Staphylococcus aureus* in Australian teaching hospitals. *Med J Austral* **164**: 68–71.

Vincent, J.-L., Bihari, D.J., Suter, P.M., *et al.* (1995) The prevalence of nosocomial infection in intensive care units in Europe. *JAMA* **274**: 639–644.

Wenger, P.N., Otten, J., Breeden, A., *et al.* (1995) Control of nosocomial transmission of multidrug resistant *Mycobacterium tuberculosis* among healthcare workers and HIV infected patients. *Lancet* **345**: 235–240.

Weinstein, R.A., Kabins, S.A. (1981) Strategies for prevention and control of multiple drug-resistant nosocomial infection. *Am J Med* **70**: 449–454.

Wise, R. (1996) Global paradox. *Lancet* **348**: 282.

7

Catheter-associated Infections: New Developments in Prevention

Tom S.J. Elliott

INTRODUCTION

Intravascular catheters are now an integral part of the medical management of many patients in the intensive care situation. Over 150 million intravascular catheters, including 5 million central lines (Maki, 1992), are used in the USA per annum. In comparison, in the UK, approximately 200 000 central lines are used annually (Elliott, 1993). The use of intravascular catheters is, however, associated with recognized complications, including air embolism, vessel perforation, haemorrhage and infection. The infections account for a significant morbidity and mortality, with more than half of all nosocomial bacteraemias or candidaemias being associated with intravascular catheters (Elliott, 1988; Maki, 1990). The reported incidence of intravascular catheter-related sepsis is variable, ranging from between zero to greater than 15% (Collingham *et al.*, 1984; Elliott and Faroqui, 1992; Raad and Bodey, 1992).

Patients being managed on intensive care units (ICUs) are at a particularly high risk of developing a catheter-related infection (Pittet *et al.*, 1995). Indeed, in some studies it has been shown that the vast majority of ICU bacteraemias are linked to the use of central venous catheters. Nearly 50 000 bacteraemias associated with central lines occur annually in patients on ICUs in the USA and up to 16 000 deaths have been related to these infections (Mermel, 1994). The reported infection rates vary widely depending on the patient group and their underlying condition, as well as the type of ICU. The infection rates range from a median of 2.1 per 1000 central-catheter-days in respiratory ICUs to over 30 per 1000 central-catheter days in burns patients (National Nosocomial Infections Surveillance System, 1990). In comparison, for similar patients without a central venous catheter in situ, the median rates of bacteraemias per 1000 days was significantly lower.

The incidence of intravascular-catheter-related infections is apparently increasing (Elliott, 1993). More recent, reports to the

Communicable Disease Surveillance Centre (CDSC) from laboratories in England and Wales have demonstrated a rise in notified intravascular-catheter-related bacteraemias. This may be due to several factors, including increased use of these devices, or to a greater clinical awareness of these infections. The generalized acceptance of *Staphylococcus epidermidis* as a major cause of catheter infections, rather than a contaminant, has also probably contributed to this apparent increased rate of infection. There is also likely to be an element of underreporting to the CDSC due to the lack of clear definitions, and the associated difficulty in making a definitive diagnosis. The overall incidence is therefore probably much higher (Elliott, 1993).

In developing a strategy for the prevention of catheter-related sepsis, it is important to diagnose these infections accurately, to recognize the different types of infection that can occur, and to develop suitable audit systems for identifying risk factors. These areas are dealt with in this chapter.

TYPES OF INFECTION ASSOCIATED WITH INTRAVASCULAR-CATHETER-RELATED INFECTIONS

Infections associated with catheters can be divided into two main groups: localized and systemic. The potential sites of infection are shown in Figure 7.1. Localized infections involve the insertion site of the catheter and can be readily diagnosed by the presence of erythema, oedema and exudate, particularly when it is purulent (Figure 7.2). The localized infections may also include thrombophlebitis within the cannulated vessel, as well as a subcutaneous infection

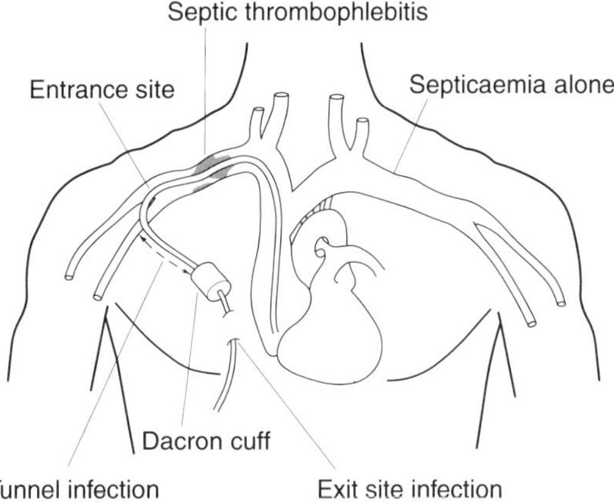

Figure 7.1.   Potential sites of central venous catheter infections.

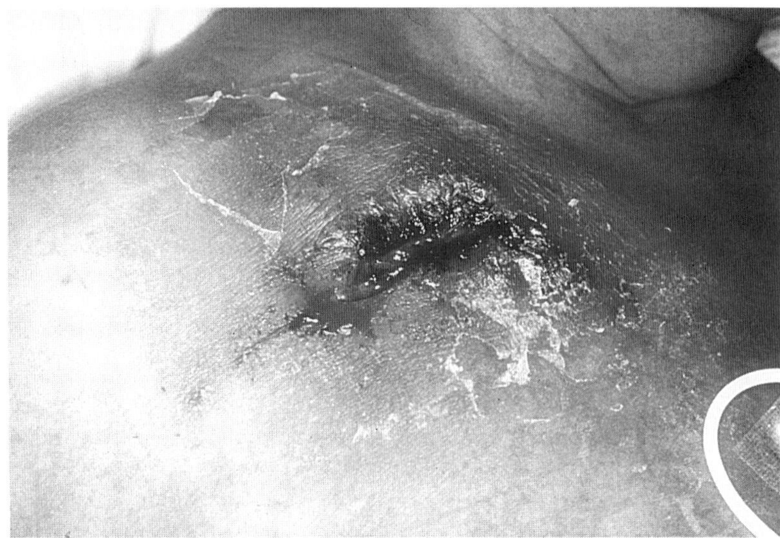

Figure 7.2.   Patient with severe infection at previous central venous catheter insertion site.

associated with tunnelled devices. Spreading cellulitis can also occasionally ensue, particularly when organisms such as β-haemolytic streptococci and *Staphylococcus aureus* are the causative micro-organisms.

A patient may also have a systemic infection associated with an intravascular catheter, resulting from micro-organisms usually colonizing primarily the distal tip. The systemic signs of catheter-related septicaemia may include a low-grade pyrexia ($\leq$38.5°C) with no other obvious focus of infection (Elliott, 1988). Patients may also suffer a transient low-grade pyrexia following flushing of a device. The catheter-related infection may be unresponsive to broad-spectrum antibiotics. This reflects the ability of micro-organisms to survive apparently lethal concentrations of antibiotics when attached to catheter surfaces. (Elliott *et al.*, 1988). However, patients with infections associated with indwelling intravascular catheters may not exhibit any of these clinical signs, and the diagnosis has to be made by exclusion, or based on positive microbiological tests.

Rarely, patients may develop endocarditis, particularly if a device is malpositioned and a septic thrombus forms at the distal end of the catheter, located close to a heart valve. Septic thrombi may also dislodge from catheters, embolize and cause sepsis at distant sites.

ORGANISMS ASSOCIATED WITH INTRAVASCULAR DEVICE INFECTIONS

The commonest organisms associated with intravascular-device-related infections include the coagulase-negative staphylococci and *Staph. aureus*. The numbers of bacteria and fungi associated with catheter-related bacteraemias reported to the CDSC are shown in Table 7.1. Over the past decade, the infections due to Gram-positive bacteria have increased significantly (Goldman and Pier, 1993) The coagulase-negative staphylococci are now the predominant causative organisms of these infections, closely followed by *Staph. aureus*. The incidence of infections caused by coliforms has also increased over the past decade (Elliott, 1993). Since the early 1990s this trend has continued (see Table 7.1). These infections can be severe, leading occasionally to endotoxic shock, with an associated high mortality. It is also of note that the incidence of catheter-related infections caused by *Candida* species is increasing. This may reflect changes in medical practice, which have resulted in a rise of the number of immunocompromised patients with indwelling intravascular catheters. These types of patients are more prone to fungal infections (Elliott, 1996).

Table 7.1 Bacteraemias associated with intravascular lines in England and Wales*

Organism	Year				Total
	1991	1992	1993	1994	
Coagulase-negative staphylococci	1436	1570	1537	1731	6274
Staphylococcus aureus	1058	1148	1296	1462	4964
Streptococcus spp.	225	249	245	252	971
Enterococcus spp.	202	240	307	308	1057
Corynebacterium spp.	66	50	53	46	215
Pseudomonas spp.	174	246	281	279	980
Escherichia coli	160	205	241	290	896
Enterobacter spp.	152	179	175	211	717
Klebsiella spp.	146	164	172	185	667
Proteus spp.	32	42	42	55	171
Acinetobacter spp.	69	94	108	128	399
Yeasts	126	175	146	176	623
Other	138	127	157	167	589
Total	3984	4489	4760	5290	18523

*Data reported to the Public Health Laboratory Service Communicable Disease Surveillance Centre.

This is of particular concern as hospital-acquired candidaemia is associated with a mortality rate of up to 40% and an extended requirement for hospital stay (Wey *et al.*, 1988).

SOURCES OF MICRO-ORGANISMS RESULTING IN CATHETER-RELATED INFECTIONS

There are five routes by which micro-organisms may gain access to intravascular catheters (Figure 7.3): extraluminal, intraluminal, contaminated infusates, haematogenous seeding, and impaction of organisms at the time of insertion (Elliott, 1995). The two principal routes by which organisms gain access to catheters are thought to be extraluminal spread of organisms from the patient's skin at the insertion site, and intraluminal passage via the internal lumen of the device.

Micro-organisms on the patient's skin can migrate from the insertion site down the intracutaneous track on the external catheter surface, resulting in microbial colonization distal to the entry site

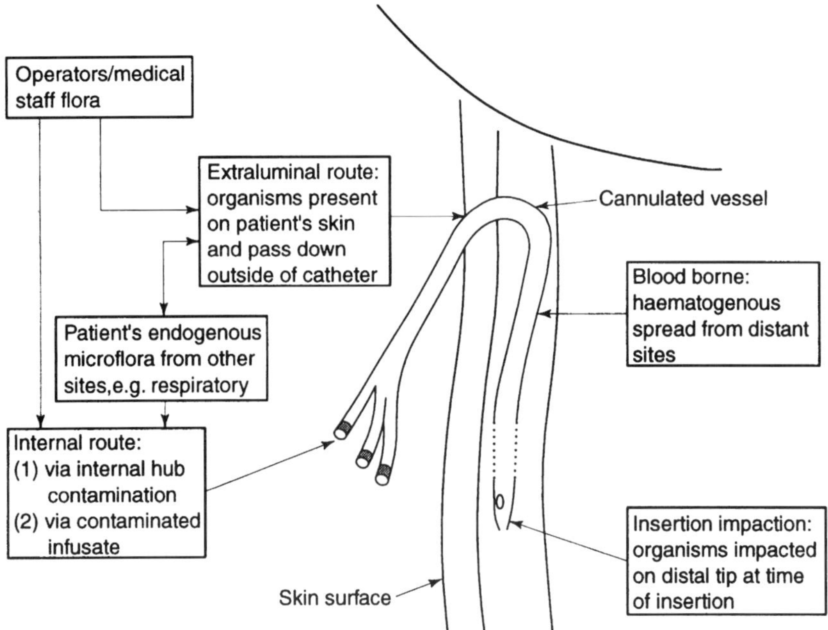

Figure 7.3. Diagrammatic representation of the sources of microbial contamination of central venous catheters.

(Maki, 1990; Raad and Bodey, 1992). It has been claimed that migration down the external surface of the catheter can occur relatively rapidly (Cooper *et al.*, 1988). The commencement of colonization may then act as a focus for the subsequent development of catheter-related bacteraemia, which can progress to septicaemia.

The organisms contaminating the outer part of the catheter may either originate from the patient's skin surface, or from the medical or nursing personnels' hands. Endogenous micro-organisms from other sites of the patient can also contaminate the insertion sites. For example, organisms from the patient's respiratory and gastrointestinal tract may be cross-contaminated into the catheter insertion wound. This may explain why the coliforms account for a significant proportion of catheter-related infections. It has also been demonstrated that certain antiseptics, particularly the iodophor compounds, can become contaminated with organisms, and when applied to the insertion site act as a source of infection (Berkelman *et al.*, 1981).

Micro-organisms may also colonize the catheter hub (Elliott, 1988) and the internal surfaces of the luer connectors (Tebbs *et al.*, 1996). The intermittent opening of a catheter's system, for example, when a luer lock is connected to allow fluids to be given to a patient, may result in internal microbial contamination followed by intraluminal migration. Sitges-Serra and co-workers (Sitges-Serra *et al.*, 1984; Linares *et al.*, 1985) also suggested that colonized hubs were the most common source for catheter-related septicaemia and demonstrated that micro-organisms may migrate along the internal surface of a catheter, resulting in infection. Other workers have also proposed that both intraluminal and extraluminal migration can occur concomitantly, particularly when catheters are in situ for longer than 15 days. It has, however, been suggested that internal catheter surface colonization is of more importance than colonization of the external surface, particularly for long-term catheters. Indeed, Sitges-Serra and Linares (Sitges-Serra *et al.*, 1984; Linares *et al.*, 1985) have advocated taking a swab of the inner surface of the catheter hub for Gram-staining and culture to identify internal contamination before infection subsequently ensues.

Catheter hubs have been cultured in only a few studies and the relative importance of their contamination with micro-organisms is unclear (Goldman and Pier, 1993). In an investigation with pulmonary arterial Swan–Ganz catheters, positive hub cultures were reported in only 7% of patients (Mermel *et al.*, 1991). Similarly, Maki *et al.* (1991a) have demonstrated that hub colonization occurred in up to 5.7% of catheters. More recently, with the use of a specialized absorbant plug, which fitted precisely into the internal luer lumen, allowing complete sampling, up to 23% of hubs were shown to be contaminated with micro-organisms after only 4 days of catheterization (Tebbs *et al.*, 1996). It is therefore likely that the internal route is a major source of micro-organisms causing catheter infections. A strategy therefore needs to be developed to prevent this potential source of microbial contamination from occurring, particularly when opening luer locks.

Contaminated infusions can also occasionally result in catheter-related sepsis. Contamination of the infusate during manufacture or manipulation of the intravenous giving sets when attaching to tubes or opening of stopcocks and other connectors, may all result in catheter colonization and subsequent associated infection (Henderson, 1988) The procedures in place for the aseptic manipulation of infusion systems, together with strict protocols for the preparation of sterile intravascular fluids, have all minimized, but not completely eliminated, this potential source of infection.

Another overlooked potential source of contamination is from the patient's own skin microflora during insertion of the device. It has not been fully explained why micro-organisms that are associated with systemic intravascular sepsis are primarily found at the distal tip of the catheter. It has been suggested that the flow forces of blood around the end of the catheter may encourage microbial attachment at this site. However, in a recent novel study (Elliott, 1995), 30 patients who underwent open cardiac surgery following insertion of a central venous catheter, had the distal tip of their indwelling device sampled in situ. Fifteen per cent of the devices were demonstrated to be contaminated with micro-organisms within 1 hour of implantation of the catheter. The study concluded that organisms had been impacted onto the devices during insertion, despite scrupulous attention to skin preparation, including the application of alcoholic chlorhexidine for more than 2 minutes. The catheter-insertion equipment, including the introducer needle and guidewire, were also contaminated with micro-organisms, confirming these results. It is therefore apparent that improved techniques need to be devised to reduce the likelihood of the skin acting as a potential source of contamination. The results of this study also offer an explanation why many investigators have found a close correlation between the culture results of insertion sites, and catheters (Williams, 1985). Snydman *et al.*, (1982b), for example, demonstrated that similar micro-organisms associated with significant colonization of catheters were also present on the skin site. Maki and Will (1990) reported a close relationship between heavy skin colonization and central-venous-catheter-related infections and bacteraemia. This association may not only be due to organisms gaining access via the external route of the catheters, as claimed by the authors, but also related to impaction at the time of insertion, with an increased risk of this occurring with higher colonization rates at the wound site.

Of the different sources of micro-organisms causing catheter sepsis, it is apparent that the main reservoirs are the hub and skin (DeCicco *et al.*, 1989), and strategies to reduce the numbers of potential pathogens at these sites need to be developed in order to prevent these infections from occurring.

CATHETER COLONIZATION AND INFECTION

Following insertion of an intravascular catheter, a biofilm consisting of host proteins and platelets forms on the polymer's surface within a few hours. Some of the deposits, such as fibronectin, act as specific binding sites for micro-organisms. Once bound to catheters, many micro-organisms, particularly *Staph. epidermidis*, produce a glycocalyx slime which protects the organisms from neutrophil phagocytosis and antibiotic exposure (Figure 7.4). This makes successful treatment of catheter-related sepsis more difficult.

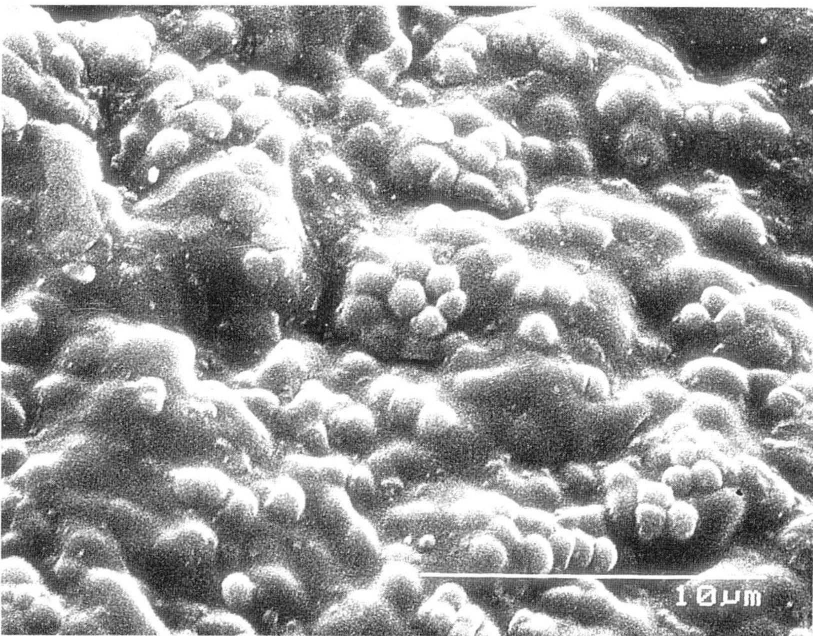

Figure 7.4. Scanning electron microscopy of *Staphylococcus epidermidis* attached to the surface of a central venous catheter. The organism is surrounded by slime.

DIAGNOSIS OF CATHETER-RELATED SEPSIS

The diagnosis of catheter-related sepsis can be considered in two sections: clinical and laboratory investigations.

Clinical Diagnosis

The clinical presentations of catheter-related sepsis have been described above. It is, however, important to have clear definitions of these infections, and an outline is given in Table 7.2. To diagnose a catheter-related infection, the patient's overall clinical condition needs to be taken into account, and consideration always given to any other potential sources of infection or causes of pyrexia.

Microbiological Diagnosis

Blood cultures are a key component of the diagnosis of catheter-related bacteraemias or septicaemias. Adequate volumes of blood

Table 7.2 Clinical symptoms and signs suggestive of a diagnosis of intravascular-catheter-related infection

---

Localized infection at the catheter insertion site

Includes the presence of:
- Erythema
- Oedema
- Purulent exudate

Diagnosis may be supported by positive microbiological results of swabs of purulent exudates, particularly if a single organism is isolated which is a recognized pathogen, such as *Staphylococcus aureus*

Catheter-related septicaemia

Patients may present with one or more of the following:
- Low-grade pyrexia of unknown source
- Pyrexia following flushing of catheter
- Isolation of the same micro-organism from the catheter tip on removal of the device as from blood cultures
- Isolation of the same micro-organism from peripheral venepuncture blood cultures as from the catheter itself, with more organisms being isolated from the latter

Systemic infection may also be found concurrently with localized infection at the site of insertion

---

should be obtained for culture. It has been shown that significant improvements in the yield of micro-organisms can be made when 20–30 ml of blood is cultured. The presence of the same organisms in blood obtained from a peripheral venepuncture and via the catheter is suggestive of device-related sepsis. Quantitative blood cultures can further assist in the diagnosis of catheter-related sepsis. Several studies have demonstrated that if the numbers of organisms obtained from blood cultures through a central venous catheter are greater than those obtained via a separate peripheral venepuncture (by at least 10-fold), this is indicative of catheter-related bacteraemia.

There are several methods for quantifying blood cultures, including the use of pour plates. This involves simply mixing the blood culture with agar, which is then incubated and the numbers of colony-forming units determined. More recently, the introduction of the Isolator® lysis centrifugation system has provided a relatively straightforward method for determining the numbers of organisms in blood. Blood samples are placed in Isolator® tubes containing a lytic agent, which lyse both the white and red blood cells. The sample is centrifuged and then plated onto different media. This system also has the advantage of improving yields from blood cultures. Quantitative cultures obtained via catheters are particularly helpful for the diagnosis of infections associated with devices such as Hickman or Broviac catheters (Douard *et al.*, 1991).

It has also been suggested that swabs taken at the catheter insertion site may be useful in predicting those at risk of infection. Multiplication of micro-organisms at the insertion site may indicate the development of localized or even systemic infection. In clinical practice, however, it is usually only useful to take a swab at the insertion site when there is clear evidence of localized infection. Positive skin cultures may represent the presence of commensals only and can be misleading. Positive culture results of hubs have also been correlated to catheter sepsis (Anaissie *et al.*, 1991). However, the clinical value of surveillance cultures of catheter components, such as hubs, may only reflect contamination, rather than sepsis and again lead to misinterpretations.

If catheter-related sepsis is suspected and the device has to be removed, for example, due to continuing blockage or an infection unresponsive to therapy, it is useful to culture the catheter tip for possible causative organisms. However, care needs to be taken when removing the device to ensure that it is not contaminated during explantation. More recently, it has been demonstrated that if the skin insertion site is not disinfected immediately prior to removal of the device, more organisms may be found on the catheter's surface as compared to those obtained through disinfected skin (Elliott *et al.*, submitted). It is evident that organisms are not only impacted onto catheters at the time of insertion, but they can also contaminate these devices on removal if care is not taken with aseptic technique.

The most widely used method for culturing catheter tips was introduced by Maki *et al.* (1977). In this process, the catheter tip is rolled several times over an agar plate, and after appropriate culture the numbers of colony-forming units determined. It has been suggested that >15 colony-forming units is indicative of catheter-related infections. Snydman *et al.* (1982a) cultured catheter tips from patients on total parenteral nutrition and also found a strong correlation between counts and infection rates. Other workers (Rello *et al.*, 1991) have suggested that a level of 25 colony-forming units is a more sensitive determinant of the presence of catheter-related sepsis.

The roll-plate results do not always allow for clear discrimination to be made between microbial contamination of the catheters on removal, colonization of a device, and true catheter-related sepsis. Similarly, the internal lumen of the catheter, which can be a nidus for infection, is not sampled in the roll-plate technique. Cleri *et al.* (1980) have flushed catheters with broth to determine the numbers of organisms attached to the inner surface, and have found >1000 colony-forming units of various bacteria associated with bacteraemia. The inner surface of a catheter as a focus of infection therefore needs to be considered, particularly when interpreting roll-plate results.

A more recently developed method for determining catheter-related sepsis is the use of a culture brush which is passed down the lumen of the device. The brush is designed to pick up any micro-organisms from the surface of the catheter tip, and on withdrawal is cultured. Preliminary studies suggest that this may be a useful method for culturing the catheter tip (Markus and Buday, 1989). This device may, however, result in organisms being expelled from the catheter in situ, particularly if there is an infected thrombus in the lumen. This system needs further evaluation to determine its potential use in clinical practice.

The use of direct Gram stains (Cooper and Hopkins, 1985) or acridine orange stains (Zufferey *et al.*, 1988) on explanted distal tips of catheters have also been shown to allow rapid diagnosis of a catheter-related infection and the results correlate well with subsequent culture results. These techniques, however, need to be used with caution, as it is important to differentiate between colonization and contamination.

PREVENTION OF INTRAVASCULAR-CATHETER-RELATED INFECTIONS

The methods developed to prevent intravascular-catheter-related infection can be divided into (a) the device and (b) the patient.

The Device

Many modifications have been made to catheters to prevent infection. Some of these are described below.

Tunnelled and cuffed devices

Broviac and Hickman catheters have been designed to reduce microbial migration from the skin down their external surface, by the use of subcutaneous tunnelling and attachment of a catheter cuff. A silver-impregnated collagen cuff has been developed which can be attached to percutaneous central venous catheters at the time of insertion. It is claimed that this cuff provides an antimicrobial barrier and in studies has been shown to reduce catheter colonization (Maki *et al.*, 1988; Flowers *et al.*, 1989), but not necessarily catheter-related infection with prolonged catheterization (Groeger *et al.*, 1993). The role of antimicrobial cuffs needs further evaluation.

The use of totally implanted catheters below the skin may offer even greater protection than cuffs from colonization by micro-organisms (Toltzis & Goldmann, 1990). These also need further clinical assessment.

Surface properties

Several aspects of catheter design have been improved and have resulted in a reduced likelihood of microbial colonization and associated infections. Catheters with a relatively smooth topography have been developed (Figure 7.5), which are less likely to be colonized with micro-organisms (Francois *et al.*, 1996). Similarly, coatings of catheter surfaces, such as with Teflon® or Hydromer®, have been shown to result in a reduced microbial colonization (Tebbs and Elliott, 1994).

Polymers

Polymers used to make catheters have also been designed to be non-thrombogenic, and to avoid host immune response. Further developments are needed in this area, in particular to prevent protein deposition and associated microbial colonization.

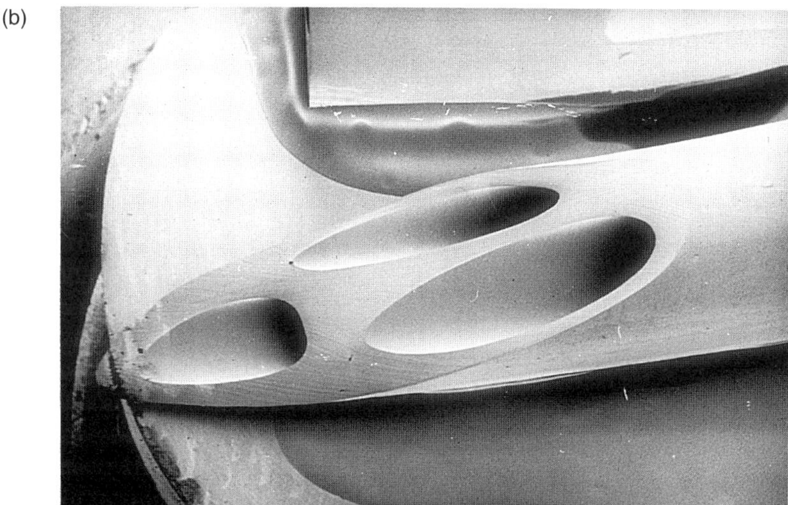

Figure 7.5. Scanning electron micrographs of a catheter (a) with an irregular surface at the distal tip and (b) a smooth triple-lumen catheter (Hydrocath®).

Antimicrobial catheters

Impregnation of antimicrobial agents in catheter materials has been suggested as a possible approach for the prevention of catheter-related sepsis. Catheters have been impregnated with the quarternary ammonium compound benzalkonium chloride, and in laboratory experiments these were shown to reduce microbial colonization for up to 3 weeks (Elliott and Tebbs, 1993a). In preliminary clinical trials, these catheters had no associated sepsis, either localized or systemic (Elliott and Tebbs, 1993b). Other antimicrobial catheters that have been developed include a combination of silver sulphadiazine and chlorhexidine. These catheters have been demonstrated in vitro to retain antimicrobial activity and also to reduce colonization (Mermel, 1994; Bach *et al.*, 1996; Schmitt *et al.*, 1996). In one study, the incidence of catheter-related systemic infection was reduced with this device (Maki *et al.*, 1991b). However, this particular catheter does not have an internal antimicrobial coating and may therefore not prevent hub-related infections.

It is evident that further clinical trials are required to evaluate the efficacy of these types of catheter. Of concern, however, is the development of catheters containing antimicrobials used to treat patients with infections (Janssen *et al.*, 1992). This approach may result in the increased rate of emergence of resistant micro-organisms to these valuable agents, and should be avoided if possible.

The Patient

Insertion site skin preparation

Prior to insertion of an intravascular catheter, it is important that the skin site is adequately disinfected. The patient's skin microflora can act as a source of infection, and therefore careful attention to disinfection is critically important. Chlorhexidine has been found to be a useful skin disinfectant. In a recent prospective, randomized study Maki *et al.* (1991a) reported that the use of 2% aqueous chlorhexidine gluconate before insertion of an intravascular device and every 48 hours thereafter for postinsertion care resulted in a lower rate of device-related infection as compared to the use of 70% alcohol or 10% povidone–iodine. Tincture of iodine (Strand *et al.*, 1993) and 70% isopropanol (Elliott *et al.*, 1988) have also been used as skin preparations, with varying degrees of success at skin disinfection. Care needs to be taken to ensure that the disinfectants used are compatible with the catheter polymer and junction cements.

Aseptic techniques and specialized catheter-care teams

Catheters need to be inserted under careful aseptic conditions (Raad *et al.*, 1994) The principles of aseptic technique include handwashing, the use of sterile gloves, adherence to the well designed catheter site cleansing procedures, and maintenance of an appropriate sterile dressing over the entry site. Procedures such as manipulation of stop locks, connectors and the use of filters should follow strict aseptic techniques with clearly defined protocols. The value of in-line filters is still open to debate particularly as the careful aseptic handling of infusion fluid and administration sets has resulted in intravenous solutions now only rarely being contaminated (Buxton *et al.*, 1979).

Earlier recommendations that administration sets should be changed every 24 hours have now been extended to 48–72 hours (Snydman *et al.*, 1987). This change in policy reflects improvements in aseptic techniques.

Many studies have also suggested that specialized teams should be involved in the insertion and care of catheters, and this has been related to reduced infection rates (Maki, 1992). The cost benefit of such an approach is evident, particularly in high-risk areas.

Prophylactic antibiotics

The prophylactic use of antibiotics to prevent catheter infections has also been suggested (Ransom *et al.*, 1990; Limb *et al.*, 1991). Micro-organisms, once impacted onto catheter surfaces, are, however, able to survive the presence of prophylactic antibiotics (Elliott, 1995). The widespread use of prophylaxis may also encourage the emergence of antimicrobial resistance. It is therefore generally accepted that the use of prophylactic antibiotics is inappropriate.

Sites of insertion

The various insertion sites of catheters have been associated with a differential risk of infection. Catheterization of the internal jugular vein is associated with a significant increased risk of infection compared to subclavian vein insertion (Pinilla *et al.*, 1983; Mermel, 1994). This difference in infection rates may be due to various factors, including differential skin colonization rates. The selection of the insertion site is therefore an important consideration.

Antiseptic ointment at insertion site

Mupirocin ointment, (Bactoban, SmithKline Beecham), when applied to the insertion site of central venous catheters can decrease the skin microbial colonization, and subsequently reduce the colonization of catheters (Hill *et al.*, 1990). Mupirocin resistance is now being reported with methicillin-resistant *Staph. aureus*, which therefore limits this approach of localized topical application. Other types of antimicrobial ointment have been used, including bacitracin and neomycin. These may delay, but do not prevent, cannulae contamination (Zinner *et al.*, 1969). The application of some of these antibiotic ointments is also associated with an increased risk of fungal infection (Flowers *et al.*, 1989). The use of antimicrobial ointments should therefore be restricted. The development of hubs containing reservoirs of antiseptics (e.g. tincture of iodine) (Segura *et al.*, 1990) may, however, offer a future application of this approach of antiseptics around the hub to reduce the potential source of catheter-related infection.

Dressings

The type of dressing used with central venous catheters may also influence the subsequent risk of infection (Baranowski, 1989). Several types of dressing are used for central venous catheters, including gauze and tape, and transparent semi-permeable membranes. Transparent dressings permit regular inspection of the site, adhere relatively well to the skin and provide protection against external contamination. Some transparent dressings promote microbial growth on the underlying skin, which, in turn, is associated with an increased risk of catheter sepsis (Baranowski, 1989; Toltzis and Goldman, 1990). Poor adherence of dressings may also result in several problems, including tunnel formation, which allow micro-organisms access to the insertion site, as has recently been shown with peripheral catheter dressings (Nelson *et al.*, 1996). Dressings also assist in stabilizing the catheter, preventing the pump action of the catheter moving in and out of the skin, which can introduce micro-organisms subcutaneously.

Improved versions of transparent dressings are being produced, with increased moisture vapour transmission rates. Results of studies with new transparent dressings, including Opsite IV 3000, have demonstrated that the skin microflora does not increase excessively when they are in situ, and that there is no apparent increase in the risk of catheter-related infection as compared with gauze and tape dressings (Baranowski, 1989). Opsite and Tegaderm have also recently been shown to have similar properties regarding skin flora around catheter entry sites (Reynolds *et al.*, 1997).

Catheter insertion site care

As part of the care of a device in situ, it is important that the insertion site is inspected on a regular basis for the presence of any symptoms or signs of complications, including infection. With this approach, dressing changes may be performed at regular intervals, allowing cleaning and inspection of the catheter insertion site. Dressings need to be changed at regular intervals, and this is usually carried out every 48 hours in many centres.

Site care may include the application of antiseptic solutions such as iodine (1–2%), 70% isopropanol or chlorhexidine. It is important when applying antiseptics that they are allowed time to have an antimicrobial action. For example, 70% isopropanol should remain on the skin for at least 2 minutes in order to be bactericidal. In some studies, after the application of 70% isopropanol, insertion sites have been treated with povidone iodine.

Needleless connector systems

Several direct access needleless connector systems are available for use with intravenous catheters. They are primarily designed for connections to be made to catheters without having to use a needle. It is currently unclear what risk of infection is associated with these devices. Early reports, however, suggest that there is no increase in risk (Adams *et al.*, 1993; Brown *et al.*, 1997). Prospective, randomized trials are needed.

Catheter patency

Many nursing procedures recommend the flushing of the lumen of intravascular catheters with heparin-containing solutions to maintain patency. The addition of preservatives to heparin flush solutions, such as chlorbutol, may also improve their efficacy, not only by maintaining patency of the device, but also by reducing the risk of infection (Elliott and Curran, 1989). Catheter-related thrombosis and embolism may still occur, despite the use of heparin or low dose warfarin (Mermel, 1994). The addition of sodium metabisulphite to a heparin flush has also been shown to reduce catheter colonization (Freeman *et al.*, 1982). Bacteriostatic saline solutions may also result in a lower risk of infection with long-term tunnelled devices as compared with sterile saline alone (Wiernikowski *et al.*, 1991). The use of antibiotic solutions, including amikacin and vancomycin, to flush devices has also been investigated (Daghistani *et al.*, 1996). However, this approach is likely to result in the emergence of resistant organisms and therefore make subsequent treatment of patients more difficult.

The frequency of reported flushing procedures is variable. Daily flushing is probably the most common approach for central venous catheters (Handy, 1989). Flushing protocols need to reflect frequency of use of a device and the types of infusate. It is important during the flushing procedure to maintain a positive pressure within the device, which will minimize reflux of blood into the catheter. This can be achieved by closing the catheter whilst flushing, before the syringe completely empties. Pressure should also be maintained on the syringe whilst withdrawing it from the injection cap. This will prevent blood entering the catheter tip and subsequently depositing fibrin and fibronectin, which will encourage microbial colonization.

Routine Changing of Catheters

Long-term intravascular catheters are designed to be left in situ for several months. However, there are no standardized recommendations for the optimum time for changing short-term percutaneously placed catheters. A wide variety of policies apply, ranging from routine changes every 3–4 days, to maintaining the catheter in situ until a recognized complication develops. The time at which catheters are changed needs to reflect the patient population and associated risks. However, it is of note that in several trials routine 72 hour catheter exchange did not show any advantages compared to 7-day regime in preventing infections in critically ill patients requiring multiple access (Bonawitz *et al.*, 1991). Infection rates were similar for catheters changed at both 3 and 7 days. This has been confirmed in further studies where routine replacement change of catheters every 3 days did not prevent infection (Cobb *et al.*, 1992).

ELECTRICAL CATHETER

Despite all the current approaches for the prevention of catheter-related sepsis, these infections appear to be increasing (Elliot, 1993). Of concern is the relatively recent emergence of Gram-negative organisms associated with these devices, which are related to more severe infections. In a novel approach to this problem, catheters which conduct low current electrical charge have been demonstrated in vitro to repel organisms or to kill any organisms attached to the polymer surface (Crocker *et al.*, 1992). The mechanism of this appears to be the production of chlorine and hydrogen peroxide due to the electrical current at the catheter surface (Liu *et al.*, 1993). More recently, a silver iontophoretic catheter has been described, and this has also been shown to prevent microbial colonization (Raad *et al.*, 1996). The value of such an approach in the clinical situation still needs to be evaluated, but may offer a relatively simple answer to this problem, without having to resort to antimicrobial agents.

Further approaches to prevent catheter-related sepsis include agents to block the binding of micro-organisms to catheters (Sheth *et al.*, 1983) and the use of heparin-bonded catheters (Mermel *et al.*, 1993). These all need further development and evaluation. It would appear that the use of antimicrobial polymers that do not include agents used for the treatment of infections are the most promising hope on the horizon.

SUMMARY

It is evident that the fundamental aspect of the pathogenesis of organisms associated with intravascular devices is still not clearly understood. Audit programmes (Elliott *et al.*, 1995) to identify risk factors in individual institutions, together with good practice protocols (Elliott *et al.*, 1994) and standardization (Roach *et al.*, 1995) should be introduced.

The skin appears to be the main source of infection associated with catheters. If organisms are impacted at the time of insertion, then improved skin disinfection, such as the application of more than one type of antiseptic, or introduction of catheters without skin contact, need to be considered. The subsequent care of catheters in situ, including skin insertion site, disinfection, and regular inspection, needs to be standard practice. Being aware of the main, albeit non-specific, symptoms and signs of these infections is also important in recognizing this complication of catheter use.

New approaches to the prevention of catheter-related sepsis include catheters that have inbuilt antimicrobial properties, such as the use of benzalkonium chloride. The antimicrobial polymer is a promising development for the increasing problem of catheter-related sepsis.

REFERENCES

Adams, K.S., Zehrer, C.L., Thomas, W. (1993) Comparison of a needleless system with conventional heparin locks. *Am J Infect Control* **21**: 263–269.

Anaissie, E.J., Raad, I., Samouis, G. (1991) Universal colonisation of central venous catheters and low risk of haematogenous seeding. In: *Abstracts of 31st Interscience Conference on Antimicrobial Agents and Chemotherapy.* Washington, DC: American Society for Microbiology.

Bach, A., Schmidt, H., Bottiger, B., *et al.* (1996) Retention of antibacterial activity and bacterial colonisation of antiseptic-bonded central venous catheters. *J Antimicrob Chemother* **37**(2): 315–322.

Baranowski, L. (1989) Central venous access devices: current technologies, uses and management strategies. *J Intravenous Nursing* **16**(3): 167–194.

Berkelman, R..L, Lewin, S., Allen, J.R. (1981) Pseudomonas bacteraemia attributed to contamination of povidone-iodine with *Pseudomonas capacia. Ann Intern Med* **95**: 32–36.

Bonawitz, S.C., Hamel, E.J., Kirkpatrick, J.R. (1991) Prevention of central venous catheter sepsis: prospective randomised trial. *Am J Surg* **57**: 618–623.

Brown, J.D., Moss, H.A., Elliott, T.S.J. (1997) The potential for catheter microbial contamination from a needleless connector. *J Hosp Infect* (in press).

Buxton, A.E., Highsmith, A.K., Garner, J.S., *et al.* (1979) Contamination of intravenous fluid: effects of changing administration sets. *Ann Intern Med* **90**: 764–768.

Cleri, D.J., Corrado, M.L., Seligman, S.J. (1980) Quantitative culture of intravenous catheters and other intravenous inserts. *J Infect Dis* **141**: 781–786.

Cobb, D.K., Highgate, P., Sawyer, R.G., *et al.* (1992) Controlled trial of scheduled replacement of central venous and pulmonary artery catheters. *N Engl J Med* **327**(15): 1062–1068.

Collingham, P.J., Munroe, R., Sorrell, T.C. (1984) Systemic sepsis of intravenous devices: a prospective study. *Med J Aust* **141**: 345–348.

Cooper, G.L., Hopkins, C.C. (1985) Rapid diagnosis of catheter-associated infection by direct gram-staining of catheter segments. *N Engl J Med* **312**: 1142–1147.

Cooper, G.L., Schiller, A.L., Hopkins, C.C. (1988) Possible role of capillary action in pathogenesis of experimental catheter-associated dermal tunnel infections. *J Clin Microbiol* **26**: 8–12.

Crocker, I.C., Liu, W.K., Byrne, P.O., *et al.* (1992) A novel electrical method for the prevention of microbial colonisation of intravascular cannulae. *J Hosp Infect* **22**(1): 7–17.

Daghistani, D., Horn, M., Rodriguez, Z., *et al.* (1996) Prevention of indwelling central venous catheter sepsis. *Med Paediatr Oncol* **226**(6): 405–408.

DeCicco, M., Schiaradia, V., Beronesi, A., *et al.* (1989) Source and route of microbial colonisation of parenteral nutrition catheters. *Lancet* **ii**: 1258–1261.

Douard, M.C., Leverger, G., Paulien, R., *et al.* (1991) Quantitative blood cultures for diagnosis and management of catheter-related sepsis in pediatric hematology and oncology patients. *Intensive Care Med* **17**: 30–35.

Elliott, T.S.J. (1988) Intravascular device infections. *J Med Microbiol* **27**(3): 161–167.

Elliott, T.S.J. (1993) Line-associated bacteraemias. *Communicable Disease Report* **3**: 7.

Elliott, T.S.J. (1995) Are central venous catheters contaminated with microorganisms on insertion? In: *Abstracts of 35th Interscience Conference on Antimicrobial Agents and Chemotherapy*, p. 257. San Francisco: American Society for Microbiology.

Elliott, T.S.J. (1996) Infections following transplantation. In: Klinck, J.R., Lindop, M.J. (eds) *Anaesthesia and Intensive Care for Organ Transplantation.* London: Chapman & Hall (in press).

Elliott, T.S.J., Curran, A. (1989) Effects of heparin and chlorbutol on bacterial colonisation of intravascular cannulae in an in vitro model. *J Hosp Infect* **14**(3): 193–200.

Elliott, T.S.J., Faroqui, M.H. (1992) Infections and intravascular devices. *Br J Hosp Med* **48**(4): 496–503.

Elliott, T.S.J., Tebbs, S.E. (1993a) Intravascular catheters impregnated with benzalkonium chloride. *J Antimicrob Chemother* **32**(6): 905–906.

Elliott, T.S.J., Tebbs, S.E. (1993b) Intravascular catheter sites and sepsis. *Lancet* **338**: 1219.

Elliott, T.S.J., D'Abrera, V.C., Dutton, S. (1988) The effect of antibiotics on bacterial colonisation of vascular cannulae in a novel in-vitro model. *J Med Microbiol* **26**(3): 229–235.

Elliott, T.S.J., Faroqui, M.H., Armstrong, R.F., *et al.* (1994) Guidelines for good practice in central venous catheterisation. *J Hosp Infect* **28**: 163–176.

Elliott, T.S.J., Faroqui, M.H., Tebbs, S.E., *et al.* (1995) An audit programme for central venous catheter-associated infections. *J Hosp Infect* **30**: 181–191.

Elliott, T.S.J., Moss, H.A., Tebbs, S.E., *et al.* (1997) A novel approach to investigate a source of microbial contamination of central venous catheters. *Eur J Clin Microbiol* (in press).

Flowers, III, R.H., Schwenzer, R.J., Kopel, R.J., *et al.* (1989) Efficacy of an attachable subcutaneous cuff for the prevention of intravascular catheter related infection. *J Am Med Assoc* **261**: 878–883.

Francois, P., Vaudaux, P., Nurdin, N., *et al.* (1996) Physical and biological effects of a surface coating procedure on polyurethane catheters. *Biomaterials* **17**(7): 667–678.

Freeman, R., Holden, M.P., Lyon, R., *et al.* (1982) Addition of sodium meta-biosulfite to left atrial catheter infusate as a means of preventing bacterial colonisation of the catheter tip. *Thorax* **37**: 142–144.

Goldman, D.A., Pier, G.B. (1993) The pathogenesis of infections related to intravascular catheterisation. *Clin Microbiol Rev* **6** (2): 176–192.

Groeger, J.S., Lucas, A.B., Coit, D., *et al.* (1993) A prospective randomized evaluation of the effect of silver impregnated subcutaneous cuffs for preventing tunnelled chronic venous access catheter infections in cancer patients. *Ann Surg* **218**: 206–210.

Handy, C.M. (1989) Vascular access devices: hospital/home care. *J Intravenous Nursing* **12**(Suppl.): S10–S18.

Henderson, D.K. (1988) Intravascular device associated infection: current concepts and controversies. *Infect Surg* **4**: 365–400.

Hill, R.L.R., Fisher, A.P., Ware, R.J., *et al.* (1990) Mupirocin for the reduction of colonisation of internal jugular cannulae – a randomised controlled trial. *J Hosp Infect* **15**: 311–321.

Hoffman, K.K., Weber, D.J., Samsa, G.P., *et al.* (1992) Transparent polyurethane film as an intravenous catheter dressing. A meta-analysis of infection rates. *J Am Med Assoc* **267**: 2072–2076.

Janssen, B., Janssen, S., Peters, G., *et al.* (1992) In vitro efficacy of a central venous catheter (Hydrocath) loaded with teicoplanin to prevent bacterial colonisation. *J Hosp Infect* **22**: 93–107.

Limb, S.H., Smith, M.P., Salooja, N., *et al.* (1991) A prospective randomised study of prophylactic teicoplanin to prevent early Hickman catheter-related sepsis in patients receiving intensive chemotherapy for haematological malignancies. *J Antimicrob Chemother* **28**: 109–116.

Linares, J., Sitges-Serra, A., Garan, J., *et al.* (1985) Pathogenesis of catheter sepsis: a prospective study with quantitative and semi-quantitative cultures of catheter hub and segments. *J Clin Microbiol* **21**: 357–360.

Liu, W.K., Tebbs, S.E., Byrne, P.O., *et al.* (1993) The effects of electric current on bacteria colonising intravascular catheters. *J Hosp Infect* **27**(3): 261–269.

Maki, D.G. (1990) Epidemiology and prevention of nosocomial bloodstream infections. In: *3rd International Conference on Nosocomial Infections.* Atlanta: Center for Disease Control, The National Foundation of Infectious Diseases and the American Society for Microbiology [abstract].

Maki, D.G. (1992) Infections due to infusion therapy. In: Bennett, J.V., Brachmen, P.S. (eds) *Hospital Infections*, 3rd edition, pp. 849–898. Boston: Little, Brown.

Maki, D.G., Will, L. (1990) Risk factors for central venous catheter-related infection with an ICU. A prospective study of 345 catheters In: *Abstracts of the 30th Interscience Conference on Antimicrobial Agents and Chemotherapy.* Washington, DC: American Society for Microbiology.

Maki, D.G., Weise, C.E., Sarafin, H.W. (1977) A semiquantitative culture method for identifying intravenous catheter-related infection. *N Engl J Med* **296**: 1305–1309.

Maki, D.G., Cobb, L., Garman, J.K., *et al.* (1988) An attachable silver-impregnated cuff for prevention of infection with central venous catheters. A prospective randomized multi-center trial. *Am J Med* **85**: 307–314.

Maki, D.G., Alvardo, C.J., Ringer, M. (1991a) A prospective randomised trial of povidone–iodine, alcohol and chlorhexidine: prevention of infection associated with central venous and arterial catheters. *Lancet* **338**: 339–343.

Maki, D.G., Wheeler, S.J., Stolz, S.M., *et al.* (1991b) Clinical trial of a novel antiseptic central venous catheter. In: *Abstracts of 31st Interscience Conference on Antimicrobial Agents and Chemotherapy.* Washington, DC: American Society for Microbiology.

Markus, S., Buday, S. (1989) Culturing indwelling central venous catheters in situ. *Infect Surg* **5**: 157–162.

Mermel, L.A. (1994) Prevention of intravascular catheter related infections. *Infect Dis Clin Pract* **3**(5): 391–398.

Mermel, L., Stolz, S., Maki, D.G. (1991) Epidemiology and pathogenesis of infection with Swan-Ganz catheters. A prospective study using molecular epidemiology. *Am J Med* **91**(3B): 197–295S.

Mermel, L.A., Stolz, S.M., Maki, D.G. (1993) Surface antimicrobial activity of heparin-bonded and antiseptic-impregnated vascular catheters. *J Infect Dis* **167**: 920–924.

National Nosocomial Infections Surveillance System (1990) Nosocomial infection rates for inter-hospital comparison. Limitations and possible solutions. *Infect Control Epidemiol* **12**: 609–621.

Nelson, R.R.S., Tebbs, S.E., Richards, N., *et al.* (1996) An audit of peripheral catheter care in a teaching hospital. *J Hosp Infect* **32**: 65–69.

Pinilla, J.C., Ross, D.F., Martin, T., Crump, H. (1983) Study of the incidence of intravascular catheter infection and associated septicaemia in critically ill patients. *Crit Care Med* **11**: 21–25.

Pittet, D., Hulliger, S., Auckenthaler, R. (1995) Intravascular device related infections in critically ill patients. *J Chemother* **7**(Suppl. 3): 55–66.

Raad, I.I., Bodey, G.B. (1992) Infectious complications of indwelling vascular catheters. *Clin Infect Dis* **15**: 197–210.

Raad, I.I., Hohn, D.C., Gilbreath, B.J., *et al.* (1994) Prevention of central venous catheter related infections by using maximal sterile barrier precautions during insertion. *Infect Control Hosp Epidemiol* **15**: 231–238.

Raad, I., Hachem, R., Zermeno, A., Stephens, L.C., Bodey, G.P. (1996) Silver iontophorectic catheter: a prototype of a long-term anti-infective vascular access device. *J Infect Dis* **173**(2): 495–498.

Ransom, M.R., Oppenheim, B.A., Jackson, A., *et al.* (1990) Double-blind, placebo controlled study of vancomycin prophylaxis for central venous catheter insertion in cancer patients. *J Hosp Infect* **15**: 95–102.

Rello, J., Coll, P., Prats, G. (1991) Laboratory diagnosis of catheter-related bacteraemia. *Scand J Infect Dis* **23**: 583–588.

Reynolds, M.S., Tebbs, S.E., Elliott, T.S.J. (1997) Do dressings with increased permeability reduce the incidence of central venous catheter-related sepsis? *Intens Care Crit Care Nurs* (in press).

Roach, H., Larson, E., Cohran, J., *et al.* (1995) Intravenous site care practices in critical care: a national survey. *Heart Lung* **24**(5): 420–424.

Schmitt, S.K., Knapp, C., Hall, G.S., *et al.* (1996) Impact of chlorhexidine-silver sulfadiazine-impregnated central venous catheters on in vitro quantitation of catheter-associated bacteria. *J Clin Microbiol* **34**(3): 508–511.

Segura, M., Alia, C., Valverde, J., *et al.* (1990) Assessment of a new hub design and the semi-quantitative catheter culture method using an in vivo experimental model of catheter sepsis. *J Clin Microbiol* **28**: 2551–2554.

Sheth, N.K., Franson, T.R., Rose, H.D., Buckmeir, F.L.A., Cooper, J.A., Sohnle, P.G. (1983) Colonisation of bacteria on polyvinyl chloride and teflon intravenous catheters in hospitalised patients. *J Clin Microbiol* **18**: 1061–1063.

Sitges-Serra, A., Puig, P., Linares, J., *et al.* (1984) Hub colonization as the initial step in an outbreak of catheter-related sepsis due to coagulase-negative staphylococci during parenteral nutrition. *J Parenteral Enteral Nutr* **8**: 668–672.

Snydman, D.R., Murray, S.A., Kornfield, S.J., *et al.* (1982a) Total parenteral nutrition-related infections. Prospective epidemiologic study using semiquantitative methods. *Am J Med* **73**: 695–699.

Snydman, D.R., Pober, B.R., Murray, S.A., *et al.* (1982b) Protective value of surveillance skin cultures in total parenteral nutrition-related infection. *Lancet* **2**: 1385–1388.

Snydman, D.R., Reidy, M.D., Perry, L.K., *et al.* (1987) Safety of changing intravenous (IV) administration sets containing burettes at longer than 48 hour intervals. *Infect Control* **8**: 113–116.

Strand, C.L., Wajsbort, R.R., Sturmann, K. (1993) Effect of iodophor vs iodine tincture skin preparation on blood culture contamination rate. *J Am Med Assoc* **269**: 1004–1006.

Tebbs, S.E., Elliott, T.S.J. (1994) Modification of central venous catheter polymers to prevent in vitro microbial colonisation. *Eur J Clin Microbiol Infect Dis* **13**: 111–117.

Tebbs, S.E., Ghose, A., Elliott, T.S.J. (1996) Microbial contamination of intravenous and arterial catheters. *Intensive Care Med* **22**(3): 272–273.

Toltzis, P., Goldmann, D.A. (1990) Current issues in central venous catheter infection. *Ann Rev Med* **41**: 169–176.

Wey, S.B., Mori, M., Pfaller, M.A., *et al.* (1988) Hospital acquired candidaemia the attributable mortality and excess length of stay. *Arch Intern Med* **148**: 2642–2645.

Wiernikowski, J.T., Elderthornly, D., Dawson, S., *et al.* (1991) Bacterial colonisation of tunnelled right atrial catheters in paediatric oncology: a comparison of sterile saline and bacteriostatic flush solution. *Am J Paediatr* **13**: 137–140.

Williams, W.W. Infection control during parenteral nutrition therapy. *J Parenteral Enteral Nutr* **9**: 735–746.

Zinner, S.H., Denny-Brown, B.C., Braun, P., *et al.* (1969) Risk of infection with intravenous indwelling catheters: effect of application of antibiotic ointment. *J Infect Dis* **120**: 616–619.

Zufferey, J., Rime, B., Francioli, P., *et al.* (1988) Simple method for rapid diagnosis of catheter-associated infection by direct acridine orange staining of catheter tips. *J Clin Microbiol* **26**: 175–177.

8

Adjusting Analgo-sedation for Mechanical Ventilation

Jörg Rathgeber, Hilmar Burchardi

INTRODUCTION

During the last decade, there has been a fundamental change in our perception of the role of pain and anxiety in critically ill patients. The contribution of pain and anxiety to morbidity, and possibly even to mortality, is now appreciated (Ledingham and Watt, 1983). Therefore, the aim of analgo-sedation in intensive care is not only the relief of pain and anxiety in order to increase the comfort of the patient (and the staff), but also to reduce pain and stress-related complications in the postoperative period, after traumatic injuries and in mechanically ventilated patients. Simultaneously, significant advances in the treatment of critically ill patients have become possible as a result of the availability of better analgesic and sedative agents.

In clinical practice on intensive care units (ICUs), however, pain management and stress reduction are often still not very effective. A survey of critically ill patients conducted after discharge from the ICU revealed that many recall having pain (40%) and anxiety (55%) during their treatment in the ICU (Bion, 1988). Of major importance to the patient's discomfort were endotracheal intubation and the performance of mechanical ventilatory support. Nearly 50% of patients described mechanical ventilation as unpleasant and stressful and, in addition, reported feelings of helplessness, fear and panic (Bergbom-Engberg and Haljamae, 1989). Particularly stressful were difficulties with synchronization, suctioning manoeuvres, their inability to communicate and their fear of equipment failures. The respiratory weaning period in particular was recalled as very stressful. Anxiety was increased by disorientation, desperation regarding the seriousness of their illness and loss of control. Emotional suffering and stress was heightened if therapeutic muscle paralysis was induced without adequate analgesia and sedation.

On the other hand, the development of new modes of ventilatory support, which enable and encourage patients' spontaneous breathing, has influenced the concepts of analgo-sedation in intensive care medicine in a fundamental way. Previously, when the restrictive pattern of totally controlled mechanical ventilation had to be used, deep sedation and even neuromuscular blockade was often mandatory in order to adapt the patient to the ventilator and prevent them from 'fighting' (Marcy and Marini, 1991). New modes of partial ventilatory support, however, enable patients to tolerate mechanical ventilation even at light levels of sedation. At least in Europe, there now seems to be a change in attitude. The objective is to keep the patient free of pain, stress and anxiety, and enable the patient to sleep if undisturbed (Bion and Ledingham, 1987), but not necessarily deeply sedated. This aim is reflected in the recommendations of the recent American consensus conference on mechanical ventilation (Slutsky, 1994a, b). At that conference it was stated that 'it may be desirable to allow spontaneous ventilatory efforts whenever it is possible to do so without incurring an excessive breathing workload or unbalancing the $\dot{V}o_2/Do_2$ relationship'.

BENEFIT OF PARTIAL VENTILATORY SUPPORT

Partial ventilatory support modes such as synchronized intermittent mandatory ventilation (SIMV), pressure support ventilation (PSV) and, in particular, biphasic positive airway pressure (BIPAP)* (Hörmann *et al.*, 1994) and airway pressure release ventilation (APRV) (Downs and Stock, 1987), combine the beneficial effects of both ventilatory support and spontaneous breathing. In contrast to the former pressure-controlled ventilatory modes, BIPAP and APRV allow completely unrestricted spontaneous breathing on both preset pressure plateaux. Since the inspiratory and expiratory valves of the respirator are open virtually all the time, fighting the respirator is excluded. The changes in the BIPAP and APRV levels are strictly time cycled: therefore, the patient and the machine have minimal influence on each other. Thus, unlike volume- or pressure-controlled mandatory ventilation and SIMV, BIPAP/APRV ventilation allows the patient to adapt more adequately to the rapid dynamic changes of ventilatory requirements by increasing or decreasing spontaneous ventilation.

---

*In the USA, BIPAP (biphasic positive airway pressure) should not be confused with BiPAP (bilevel positive airway pressure) which is a trademark for a simple ventilator for assisted ventilation in non-intensive-care patients. BIPAP, however, means unrestricted spontaneous breathing at two different continuous positive airway pressure (CPAP) levels. The patient's respiration is further supported by the volume displacement caused by the difference between the CPAP levels. If there is no spontaneous breathing, the mechanical volume displacement is, effectively, pressure-controlled mechanical ventilation. The duration of both pressure levels can be adjusted separately, enabling a wide variation in ventilatory frequency as well as in *I/E* ratio. As BIPAP allows rather short expiratory times, this method can easily be used in an APRV mode.

The beneficial effects of BIPAP and APRV on pulmonary function compared to conventional volume and pressure controlled ventilatory modes can be attributed to the maintenance of the physiological respiratory pump at all times. Spontaneous breathing within mechanical ventilation may diminish not only the side-effects of positive pressure ventilation by reducing the mechanical support and the intrathoracic pressure; maintenance of the respiratory pump, in particular the movement of the diaphragm, results in an improved efficiency of pulmonary gas distribution (Froese and Bryan, 1974; Hedenstierna *et al.*, 1994). In recent investigations it has been pointed out that spontaneous breathing superimposed on mechanical ventilation is more effective for alveolar recruitment and pulmonary gas exchange in patients with acute respiratory failure than is totally controlled ventilation. In a controlled clinical study in patients suffering from non-obstructive acute lung injury, Sydow *et al.* (1994) demonstrated that, during BIPAP/APRV, gas exchange improves significantly compared to during volume-controlled inverse ratio ventilation (VC-IRV). In a recent experimental study in 12 dogs with oleic acid-induced lung injury Putensen *et al.* (1994) found that even small efforts of spontaneous breathing superimposed on pressure-controlled mechanical ventilation (BIPAP) significantly improve pulmonary gas exchange and systemic circulation. As a consequence, oxygen delivery improves, which is ultimately the overall essential objective of ventilation. These results indicate that at least these modes of partial ventilatory support may offer significant therapeutic advantages for acute respiratory distress syndrome (ARDS) patients by enhancing alveolar recruitment and improving pulmonary gas exchange. This means that, apart from the very few absolute indications for totally controlled ventilation (Table 8.1), most mechanically ventilated, critically ill patients may benefit from partial ventilatory support.

In comparison to former volume-controlled ventilatory modes and even to SIMV, which allows spontaneous breathing only between preset mandatory tidal volumes, BIPAP ventilatory support may offer

Table 8.1   Examples for indications for totally controlled ventilation

- Minimization of oxygen consumption (e.g., severe head injury)
- Elimination of excessive autonomous effects (e.g., tetanus)
- Minimization of work of breathing (e.g., acute decompensation of chronic obstructive pulmonary disease)
- Prevention of excursions of the injured thorax (e.g. flail chest)
- Facilitation of non-physiological ventilatory patterns (e.g., inverse ratio ventilation)

some advantages even in the postoperative period. In particular, after large, long-lasting and traumatizing operations, abnormalities of mechanical pulmonary function and gas exchange consistently occur. They are characterized by marked decreases in vital and inspiratory capacities and a substantial decrease in functional residual capacity (FRC). The restrictions are most pronounced after upper abdominal surgery with a decrease in FRC of approximately 30% below the preoperative level (Craig, 1981). The mechanisms which reduce lung volumes following abdominal and thoracic surgery and thoracic trauma are not completely known, but limited diaphragmatic movement and pain appear to be primary factors (Hedenstierna *et al.*, 1985; Duggan and Drummond, 1987; Dureuil *et al.*, 1987). In the recovery period these deficits improve gradually, returning to preoperative levels within the following 2 weeks. After lower abdominal surgery, or minor or peripheral procedures, the changes in vital capacity and functional residual capacity are smaller, with lung volumes remaining normal or increasing to preoperative levels after a few hours. However, a persistently decreased FRC even after minor surgical intervention is common in elderly patients, the obese and those patients with preoperative cardiopulmonary disease. These patients need ventilatory support until normalization of pulmonary and circulatory functions occurs.

Rathgeber *et al.* (1997) investigated the effects of different ventilatory modes on the duration of intubation, pulmonary gas exchange and the requirement for analgo-sedation in 596 adult patients during the postoperative period following coronary artery bypass graft surgery. In patients ventilated with the BIPAP mode the duration of intubation was significantly shorter than in those patients treated with SIMV/PSV and volume-controlled mandatory ventilation. Following extubation the patients in the synchronized controlled mandatory ventilation (SCMV) group more frequently exhibited signs of ventilatory insufficiency (i.e. increased $P_a\text{CO}_2$) than did the patients in the other groups. Apparently, after extubation, these patients may still have been handicapped by prolonged sedation: nearly 40% of the volume-controlled ventilated patients required additional sedation, whereas this was necessary only in approximately 10% of patients who had an opportunity for intermittent or superimposed spontaneous breathing. In addition, opioids were administered to almost all patients, but the overall consumption was significantly lower in patients who had been able to influence their ventilatory support.

In conclusion, the intended level of sedation for critically ill patients depends not only on the patient's illness, but also on the type and extent of ventilatory support. In a recent American national survey

(Hansen-Flaschen *et al.*, 1991) it was shown that sedative drugs and neuromuscular blocking agents are still widely used in patients requiring mechanical ventilation. This means that myorelaxation (and sedation) is still administered to enable a therapy which is intended not to be tolerated without. New ventilatory modes supporting spontaneous breathing, such as BIPAP and APRV, offer the opportunity to adapt the ventilatory support better and more easily to the patient's needs than do conventional modes of ventilation. As a consequence, the requirement for sedation and analgesia (and of course for myorelaxation) is considerably reduced. Moreover, since spontaneous breathing is no longer considered undesirable, and therefore does not have to be suppressed by strong analgo-sedation, our concept of analgo-sedation potentially alters towards a more active patient, who is free of pain, stress and anxiety, but still co-operative, easy to rouse and is breathing spontaneously (Slutsky, 1994a, b). Spontaneous breathing also preserves patient's cough reflex, which improves clearance of bronchial secretions. Inadequate levels of analgo-sedation will negate the benefits of spontaneous breathing for pulmonary gas exchange and should therefore be avoided whenever possible.

MONITORING ANALGO-SEDATION IN CRITICALLY ILL PATIENTS

The extent of emotional suffering or stress is as individually different as the pathophysiological importance of the related stress response. It is well known that the activation of the sympathetic nervous system with an increase of heart rate, blood pressure and myocardial oxygen consumption is especially deleterious in patients with pre-existing cardiac disease: in particular, patients with cardiac risk factors who have undergone major abdominal or thoracic surgery have a higher incidence of perioperative cardiac morbitidy. In these patients sympathetic reactions with hypertension and elevated heart rates are frequently associated with cardial complications such as myocardial ischaemia, serious arrhythmia, myocardial infarction and cardiac death (Mangano, 1991). Sufficient pain management and stress reduction in critically ill patients is therefore mandatory not only to increase the patient's comfort and to avoid postoperative/traumatic neurosis, but also to reduce life-threatening complications.

However, pain and anxiety are always subjective and cannot be measured directly (Merskey, 1979; Chapman *et al.*, 1985). In addition, it is often difficult to differentiate pain from anxiety, as the latter increases the awareness of pain. This intrinsic subjectivity imposes obvious limitations to any analysis of pain management and control of anxiety in critically ill patients. A wide variety of methods are available for assessing pain. Rating scales are most commonly used. A major strength of this technique, particularly in the critical care setting, is its simplicity: patients simply rate their level of pain relative to a visual, verbal or numerical scale. The most widely accepted of these instruments, the visual analogue scale (VAS), requires patients to rate their pain by locating a point along a line the poles of which represent extremes such as 'no pain' and 'the worst pain I've ever had'. The degree of pain is identified by the distance from the poles. Despite its obvious simplicity, the VAS has been shown to have a high degree of reliability and validity. Nevertheless, even this simple pain scale can often be too difficult to administer to critically ill patients. Moreover, it is not applicable if the patient is not co-operative or is deeply sedated.

Similarly, monitoring of sedation in the ICU is inexact. The parameters most commonly used are the qualitative state of consciousness and assessment of the patient's haemodynamic responses to invasive procedures (e.g. endotracheal suctioning, chest physiotherapy). In most mechanically ventilated patients, a balanced combination of analgesics and sedative drugs is administered to provide pain relief, to control anxiety and to permit sleep. The concept of sedation has to be adapted to each individual patient's requirements, to special therapeutic essentials, to the day/night variations and, last but not least, in order to maintain and even to encourage spontaneous breathing.

One should keep in mind that agitation should not necessarily be interpreted as a lack of sedation, especially in mechanically ventilated patients. In these patients it is more often the result of an insufficient interaction between respirator and patient. This may become obvious in stress reactions, such as hyperventilation, hyperactive autonomic reflexes (hypertension, tachycardia, sweating) and unco-operative responses. If hypoxaemia or other respiratory problems (e.g. obstructed endotracheal tube, pneumothorax) and extrapulmonary causes such as distension of the stomach or the bladder can be excluded, methods of optimizing the ventilatory support should be considered before increasing analgo-sedation.

OBJECTIVES FOR SEDATION AND ANXIOLYSIS

A principal goal is to keep the patient co-operative and easy to rouse, so that he or she can support the measures for mobilization and other physical nursing interventions. It seems desirable to bring the patient into a sitting position regularly in order to enhance lung function and, in particular, to improve clearance of bronchial secretions. This can often be done even if the patient is still ventilated. Of course, all these measures strain the patient considerably and require sedation that is carefully adapted to the actual situation. However, the mental and emotional state of the patient during and after the intensive care period is much better with adapted analgo-sedation than with heavy sedation.

In general, the choice of a specific drug is not conclusive. The individual depth of sedation required varies considerably and also needs to be adjusted to the different situations and the requirements for various interventions. A guideline may be a Ramsay score of 2–3 (Ramsay *et al.*, 1974) (Table 8.2). With this level of sedation the dosage of analgesics can often be easily adapted to an individual patient's needs.

If *benzodiazepines* are used for sedation and anxiolysis, intensive care patients can also benefit from the amnesia and anticonvulsant effects. Until recently, the use of *diazepam* was common (Table 8.3). However, its long elimination half-life (24–40 hours) and that of its active metabolite, *N*-demethyldiazepam (elimination half-life up to 96 hours), may prolong recovery. Particularly in long-term sedation and in the elderly, the risk of accumulation and overdose always exists, particularly when the patient is kept deeply sedated, or has impaired hepatic and renal function (Bodenham *et al.*, 1988), and redistribution from large body depots occur. In principle, short-acting substances such as *midazolam* are preferable to allow rapid adaptation to the

Table 8.2   Quantification of the level of sedation ('Ramsay' score) (Ramsay *et al.*, 1974)

Score	Definition
Awake	
1	Anxious and agitated or restless, or both
2	Co-operative, oriented and tranquil
3	Responding to commands
Asleep	
4	Brisk response to stimulus (light glabellar tap or loud auditory stimulus)
5	Sluggish response to stimulus (light glabellar tap or loud auditory stimulus)
6	No response to stimulus (light glabellar tap or loud auditory stimulus)

Table 8.3   Pharmacology of intravenous sedatives

		Suggested initial dose	
Drug	Elimination half-life	Bolus (mg)	Continuous infusion (mg/kg/h)
Diazepam	24–96 h	2.5–10	*
Midazolam	1–12 h	1–15	0.05–0.3
Propofol	50–70 min	50–200	1.4

* Not recommended.

actual situation, (e.g. therapeutic interventions, neurological examinations, mobilizing measures). It has a rapid onset of action and a relatively short elimination half-life (1–4 hours). However, in critically ill patients, particularly those with impaired hepatic and renal metabolism, its elimination half-life may be prolonged (4–12 hours) (Byrne *et al.*, 1984; Dirksen *et al.*, 1987). In addition, midazolam may cause hypotension, particularly in the presence of hypovolaemia (Adams *et al.*, 1985). The respiratory depression is usually an undesired side-effect in patients with partial ventilatory support. In critically ill patients, sedation is initiated by administration of 0.5–1.0 mg increments of midazolam every 1–3 minutes until the desired level of sedation is achieved. However, there is a wide interindividual variability in requirement; loading doses may vary between 0.1 and 0.5 mg/kg, and maintenance infusion rates range between 0.05 and 0.3 mg/kg/h.

Benzodiazepine-related sedation and respiratory depression are reversible using *flumazenil* (Bodenham and Park, 1989). Because of the short half-life of flumazenil (50 min), reversal of benzodiazepine effects may require a prolonged infusion, but this is rarely indicated. However, flumazenil may allow periodic assessment of neurological status in patients who require prolonged deep levels of sedation, and this drug therefore increases the flexibility and safety of sedation with benzodiazepines.

Propofol is a new intravenous anaesthetic drug formulated in a lipid emulsion, which produces sedation in low doses. Critically ill patients may become hypotensive after bolus injection; this effect seems comparable to that of midazolam (Aitkenhead *et al.*, 1989). Recovery from a single injection or a short infusion is very rapid (5–10 minutes). Doses of 1–3 mg/kg/h effectively sedate most critically ill patients (Newman *et al.*, 1987; Beller *et al.*, 1988), but large individual variations have been reported. Because of its rapid onset and short duration of action, propofol is easy to adapt to the varying requirements of the patient and the therapist (day/night variation, therapeutic/diagnostic interventions). Therefore, propofol is rapidly becoming the most favoured sedative drug in ICUs. However, high costs sometimes limit its use.

Barbiturates have several disadvantages which limit their usefulness as sedatives for critically ill patients, e.g cardiovascular and respiratory depression, loss of thermoregulation in higher doses, induction of hepatic microsomal enzymes, accumulation of drug with repeated doses or infusions, tolerance and possible immune suppression. In addition, barbiturates cause hyperalgesia in subanaesthetic doses. However, repeated applications of small doses in combination with benzodiazepines, propofol or opioids are sometimes useful to increase hypnosis (complementary sedation) or to reduce the total amount of other sedatives.

Clonidine is an agonist at the α_2-adrenergic receptor, which stimulates α_2-presynaptic adrenoceptors and decreases noradrenaline release from sympathetic nerve terminals. Injection of a bolus causes a sustained decrease in blood pressure after a transient increase in pressure. In the postoperative period, clonidine (75–150 µg i.v.) is effective in the treatment of postanaesthetic shivering (Delauney *et al.*, 1993; Joris *et al.*, 1993). Furthermore, clonidine produces anxiolysis, sedation and analgesia, which makes this substance useful in the treatment of withdrawal syndromes (e.g. from alcohol or opioids) and as an adjuvant to conventional analgo-sedation (Jarvis *et al.*, 1992). Clonidine has no effect on cardiac contractility or cardiac output (Flacke *et al.*, 1987), but when given continuously and for long periods, it reduces the responsiveness of peripheral vessels to vasoactive substances and sympathetic stimulation. The resulting haemodynamic effects may sometimes limit the use of clonidine, especially in seriously ill patients.

PREFERRED ANALGESICS IN MECHANICALLY VENTILATED PATIENTS

Analgesia is required in intensive care patients in many situations, not just postoperatively or during painful therapeutic interventions. Analgesia is also required to a certain degree so that the patient will accept the endotracheal and gastrointestinal tubes, tolerate endotracheal aspiration manoeuvres, etc. In co-operative patients, patient-controlled analgesic infusions can be used advantageously. Their use generally reduces the total dose of analgesics and minimizes the risk of excessive sedation.

However, the conventional practice of administering fixed doses of analgesics based on weight often will either result in a significant degree of overdosage or inadequate analgesia in many patients. In addition, it should always kept in mind that sedative agents, namely benzodiazepines, will potentiate analgesic effects as well as having some side-effects, e.g. hypotension and a decrease of respiratory drive. This can be minimized by using the lowest effective dose, slow rates of administration and ensuring adequate circulatory blood volume. Most opioids depend on hepatic transformation before renal excretion. In case of hepatic and/or renal insufficiency, opioids and their metabolites may accumulate considerably during prolonged application. The only effective strategy for avoiding overdosage is regular and intermittent trials of dose reduction or suspension. This can be assessed much more reliably when the sedation level is not too profound.

Morphine remains the most commonly used analgesic in the ICU setting because most clinicians are familiar with its pharmacokinetic and pharmacodynamic properties (Table 8.4). In addition to this, it is inexpensive compared to other opioids. Disadvantages include a relatively slow onset of action and possible release of histamine. In addition, morphine-6 glucoronide, a metabolite with a potency four times greater than that of morphine, accumulates in patients with impaired renal function (Osborne *et al.*, 1986).

Pethidine has a rapid onset of action. Compared to other opioids, its elimination half-life is low. Pethidine is a fairly potent suppressor of postanaesthetic shivering (Claybon and Hirsh, 1980; Pauca *et al.*, 1984; Kurz *et al.*, 1993), which may be of benefit in the immediate postoperative period. An important drawback is that a major metabolite, norpethidine, may accumulate, particularly in patients with impaired renal function (Bodenham *et al.*, 1988).

Fentanyl has a much more rapid onset of action than morphine. After the administration of small doses, its duration of action is short because the drug is rapidly redistributed from the brain to other tissues. When large doses are administered, termination of effect requires elimination. Because its elimination half-life is 2–5 hours, the duration of action of fentanyl is similar to that of morphine. The pharmacokinetics of fentanyl are not significantly altered in the presence of hepatic cirrhosis, and clearance appears to remain normal in cases of renal failure (Bodenham *et al.*, 1988). Fentanyl does not release histamine, and therefore may be the better choice for patients who are haemodynamically unstable or have significant obstructive airway disease.

In comparison to other compounds, *alfentanil* has the most rapid onset and the shortest duration. Its short duration of action is a result of both rapid redistribution from brain to blood and a short elimination half-life (Maitre *et al.*, 1987). Hepatic disease prolongs elimination,

Table 8.4 Pharmacology of intravenous analgesics

Drug	Elimination half-life (h)	Peak effect (min)	Duration of action (min)	Approximate equivalent analgesic dose	Suggested initial dose		
					Bolus	Continuous infusion	PCA bolus
Morphine	2–4	30	120–180	10	2–5 mg	2–10 mg/h	0.5–1.0
Pethidine	3–5	4	60–240	100	25–100 mg	–	5–10
Fentanyl	2–6	4	30–60	0.1	25–100 µg	25–200 µg/h	10–50
Sufentanil	2–3	8	45–60	0.01	2–100 µg	2.5–100 µg/h	2–5
Alfentanil	1–3	1	20–40	0.5	2–3 mg	0.5–6 mg/h	–*
Ketamine	1–3	1	5–15	–	0.5–1 mg/kg	10–30 µg/kg/min	–*

* Not recommended.
PCA, patient controlled analgesia

but renal failure has only a small effect. Because alfentanil does not accumulate, rapid recovery follows discontinuation of therapy.

Sufentanil has a potency about 10 times that of fentanyl. Its onset time is about one-half as long as that of fentanyl. The cardiovascular stability is remarkable. Because of its full effect despite a lower receptor occupancy, which may be an important factor in the avoidance of tolerance, sufentanil may be of benefit in patients requiring long-term administration of analgesics with high potency (Lehmann *et al.*, 1991).

Ketamine is the only intravenous anaesthetic drug that produces analgesia at subanaesthetic doses. Given as a bolus (0.5–1.0 mg/kg), ketamine has a very rapid onset and short duration of action (5–20 minutes). Its elimination half-life ranges from 1–3 hours (White *et al.*, 1982). Additional doses of 0.25–0.5 mg/kg are used for procedures lasting longer than 10–15 minutes. Alternatively, an intramuscular dose of 2–3 mg/kg will provide a similar effect. The drug may accumulate with continued administration. Ketamine is often used in the ICU during short but painful procedures, such as dressing changes in burns patients or for minor debridements. Of advantage is its minor effect on central respiratory drive in subanaesthetic doses. The sympathomimetic effects of ketamine may be beneficial for maintaining circulatory stability in emergency cases or in hypovolaemic patients. Furthermore, because of its specific bronchodilatory effect, ketamine is particularly useful in patients with asthma who require mechanical ventilation. Undesirable effects of ketamine include pulmonary and systemic hypertension, tachycardia and hallucinations, especially in anaesthetic doses. The psychomimetic side-effects can be avoided by combining ketamine with benzodiazepines (e.g. diazepam, midazolam). Because of excessive upper airway secretion, the use of atropine or glycopyrolate is recommended.

DELETERIOUS EFFECTS OF ANALGESICS AND SEDATIVES

The fact that sedatives and analgesics themselves may cause numerous complications related to their effects on the central and autonomic nervous systems should be taken into consideration. In general, opioids alone, and especially in combination with sedatives, impair consciousness and respiratory drive. This requires careful and individual titration according to the patient's actual needs. In contrast, in dyspnoeic patients (e.g. in acute decompensation of chronic obstructive pulmonary disease (COPD)) opioids may sometimes be useful for reducing the excessive respiratory drive in order to facilitate interaction between the patient and the ventilator. Deep analgo-sedation inhibits rigorous coughing and clearance of bronchial secretions, and thus promotes pulmonary complications. Also, the depression of intestinal motility is often a serious problem and complicates the attempts at enteral feeding. Impaired gastrointestinal motility may impede spontaneous breathing and respiratory function due to abdominal distension and elevation of the diaphragm. Moreover, we now know about the essential role of the gut in bacterial translocation and sepsis development. Thus, every attempt must be made to keep intestinal function intact. There is strong evidence that ketamine has no depressive influence on intestinal motility (Grant *et al.*, 1981; Takahashi *et al.*, 1987; Freye and Knüffermann, 1994).

Negative inotropic effects of the drugs as well as their influence on vascular resistance may cause a significant reduction in cardiac output, severe hypotension and myocardial ischaemia. These effects are dose dependent and so the uncritical and excessive use of these agents should be avoided. In addition, they may impede the patient's mobilization, and may mask the occurrence of intercurrent complications (Wheeler, 1993). Treatment of anxiety therefore relies on the appropriate use of sedation, adequate pain control, and frequent communication and reassurance by the critical care staff.

Routinely prescribed fixed combinations of drugs administered continuously (e.g. midazolam, fentanyl) are inadequate, as they further carry the risk of overdosing a different single drug with the corresponding side-effects (e.g. depression of respiratory drive, intestinal motility). Whenever possible, the day/night variations should be preserved.

NEUROMUSCULAR BLOCKADE

Neuromuscular blockade is rarely indicated in ventilated patients, such as during excessive dyspnoea (e.g. in severe status asthmaticus), for facilitating extreme inverse ratio ventilation, in case of profound permissive hypercapnia, or to reduce oxygen consumption in patients with life-threatening arterial oxygenation (see Table 8.1). Even in these situations there is little evidence that muscle paralysis is superior to deep sedation (Hansen-Flaschen *et al.*, 1991) because of the detrimental effects of muscle relaxant drugs on mucociliary clearance. Impairment of the cough reflex and immobilization may promote other complications (e.g. risk of pulmonary aspiration, development of decubitus ulcers, inadvertent nerve compressions, corneal erosions). Patients deprived of normal activity are prone to deep venous thrombi and muscular atrophy. Paralytic agents may also obscure the diagnosis of intercurrent problems such as intra-abdominal complications, seizures and other central nervous system dysfunctions. Furthermore, the degree and the duration of effects of neuromuscular blocking agents are considerably affected by the medical condition and concomitant medications. Thus, the effects of neuromuscular agents are difficult to control unless they are closely monitored (e.g. by train-of-four monitoring), or at least allowed to lapse intermittently. Recently, investigators have pointed out that prolonged neuromuscular blockade may contribute to prolonged muscular weakness and critical illness polyneuromyopathy (Gooch *et al.*, 1991; Op de Coul *et al.*, 1991; Rossiter *et al.*, 1991; Griffin *et al.*, 1992). Furthermore, there is a real danger of underestimating the need for analgesic and sedative agents even for experienced clinicians.

CONCLUSION

New ventilatory modes supporting spontaneous breathing, such as BIPAP and APRV, offer the opportunity to adapt ventilatory support better and more easily to a patient's requirements than do conventional modes of controlled ventilation. Preservation and support of a patient's spontaneous breathing improves pulmonary gas exchange and reduces the stress imposed by mechanical ventilation. The 'invasiveness' of mechanical ventilation is reduced and the patient's comfort is less disturbed. As a consequence, the need for sedation and analgesia is considerably reduced. This may minimize systemic side-effects and complications from analgo-sedation and mechanical ventilation. It may be presumed that weaning from mechanical ventilation is easier if not more rapid. In postoperative situations with short-term ventilatory support these modes facilitate recovery to spontaneous breathing and physiological organ functions.

COMMENTARY   Gilbert Park, *Cambridge*

Drs Rathgeber and Burchardi have written an interesting chapter on this subject. They fully describe the newer ventilation modes and how they might reduce the need for sedative and analgesic drugs. They make the excellent point that the level of sedation needed will depend not only on the disease affecting the patient, but also on the mode of respiratory support used.

Monitoring of sedation and analgesia is difficult. This chapter supports the use of visual analogue scores. Very often, however, patients are too sick to complete them and few ICUs in the UK use them. In this situation the best we have for clinical use is a variety of scales, one of which, the Ramsay scale, is mentioned here. Newer methods such as changes in the electro-cardiogram (ECG) (R–R interval) are being explored now and may be applicable in the future.

The need for a good night's sleep and how it is achieved is mentioned briefly. Drugs are one solution, although the quality of sleep they provide is often poor. Should the mode of ventilation also be changed? Certainly, during weaning from ventilation we often do not wean at night, so that the patient is not disturbed. Whether this is right or wrong is a matter which needs to be explored.

All the standard drugs are mentioned briefly, as are some of the newer ones. When choosing drugs it is best, if at all possible, to find out first what the patient feels and then try to match the drugs to the patient. I emphasize the word 'drugs' because rarely can adequate comfort be obtained with a single drug; pain needs analgesics, anxiety requires benzodiazepines and for night-time sedation a drug like propofol is probably needed. Trying to use only one drug can be dangerous because excessive amounts of the drug may be given, resulting in toxicity from the drug or its solvent. A good example of this is propofol. There are several reports in the literature of excessive amounts of this drug being given with resulting fat overload from the soya bean in which it is dissolved.

The use of barbiturates in combination with other drugs is mentioned as a means of promoting sleep. In the UK, this group of drugs is not used for this purpose because of the risk of addiction as well as the other hazards mentioned by the authors. It would be interesting to see some comparative studies to see if the benefits outweigh the risk.

Clonidine is a drug that is popular in some centres. Although it has been available for many years I do not think it has achieved widespread popularity. This is probably because of the adverse cardiovascular effects described by the authors.

When discussing the opioids, the authors quite rightly mention the active metabolites. However, the mechanism by which supposedly inactive metabolites become active is a subject worthy of mention. Carrupt *et al.* (1991) have described the mechanism for morphine. This might also apply to other drugs with active metabolites, e.g. midazolam (Bauer *et al.*, 1995). The metabolite of pethidine is not an analgesic, but causes fits. As our understanding of these mechanisms and effects increases, we should be able to use these and other drugs more safely and effectively.

Ketamine is also mentioned. This drug is a mixture of isomers and some have the analgesic effects without most of the disadvantages. Manufacturers are looking at producing the less-toxic isomer and this drug then may be of great value in the critically ill.

Deciding which drug(s) to give is only half the story. Greater emphasis needs to be placed on how the drug(s) are given. The authors describe patient-controlled systems and talk about the use of fixed combinations of drugs. However, whether drugs need to be given by continuous intravenous infusion or intermittent bolus dose is an area of controversy. Continuous administration avoids peaks and troughs in effect, but may risk overdosage and may cause tolerance to be reached more quickly. Intermittent bolus injection means that the need for the drug is assessed, but it may have adverse haemodynamic effects.

Neuromuscular blockade is used less now than previously. However, as the authors state, it does still have a place. Unlike the authors I find that once neuromuscular blockers are used oversedation becomes a problem because of the fear of the patient being awake and paralysed. Perhaps this reflects a difference between our ICUs. Because of my experience I stop all infusions of sedative analgesic and muscle relaxants each day, unless this risks harm to the patient, to ensure that the patient can recover from their effects. This avoids accumulation of drugs.

Sedation and analgesia are not easy to do well in the critically ill. Partly this is because there are no easy laboratory tests or numbers to generate. Yet, as the authors state, there are significant risks associated with the use of these drugs. A greater understanding is needed by all clinicians of this area. The explanation given in this chapter of one variable, ventilatory support, may change the way it is used in the future.

REFERENCES

Adams, P., Gelman, S., Reeves, J.G., *et al.* (1985) Midazolam pharmacodynamics and pharmacokinetics during acute hypovolemia. *Anesthesiology* **63**: 140–144.

Aitkenhead, A.R., Willatts, S.M., Parks, G.R., *et al.* (1989) Comparison of propofol and midazolam for sedation in critically ill patients. *Lancet* **ii**: 704–707.

Bauer, T.M., Ritz, R., Harberthur, C., *et al.* (1995) Prolonged sedation due to accumulation of conjugated metabolites of midazolam. *Lancet* **364**: 145–147.

Beller, J.P., Pottecher, T., Lugnier, A., *et al.* (1988) Prolonged sedation with propofol in ICU patients: recovery and blood concentration changes during periodic interruptions in infusion. *Br J Anaesth* **61**: 583–588.

Bergbom-Engberg, I., Haljamae, H. (1989) Assessment of patient's experience of discomforts during respiratory therapy. *Crit Care Med* **17**: 1068–1072.

Bion, J.F. (1988) Sedation and analgesia in the intensive care unit. *Hosp Update* **14**: 1272–1275.

Bion, J.F., Ledingham, I. McA. (1987) Sedation in intensive care - a postal study. *Intensive Care Med* **13**: 215–216.

Bodenham, A., Park, G.R. (1989) Reversal of prolonged sedation using flumazenil in critically ill patients. *Anaesthesia* **44**: 603–607.

Bodenham, A., Shelly, M.P., Park, G.R. (1988) The altered pharmacokinetics and pharmacodynamics of drugs commonly used in critically ill patients. *Clin Pharmacokinet* **14**: 347–355.

Byrne, A.J., Yeoman, P.M., Mace, P. (1984) Accumulation of midazolam in patients receiving mechanical ventilation. *Br Med J* **289**: 1309.

Carrupt, P.A., Testa, B., Bechalany, A., El Tayar, N., Descas, P., Perrissoud, D. (1991) Morphine 6-glucuronide and morphine 3-glucuronide as molecular chameleons with unexpected lipophilicity. *J Med Chem* **34**: 1272–1275.

Chapman, C.R., Casey, K.L., Dubner, R., *et al.* (1985) Pain measurement: an overview. *Pain* **22**: 1–3.

Claybon, L.E., Hirsh, R.A. (1980) Meperidine arrests postanesthesia shivering. Anesthesiology **53**: 180–184.

Craig, D.B. (1981) Postoperative recovery of pulmonary function. *Anesth Analg* **60**: 46–51.

Delaunay, L., Bonnet, F., Liu, N., Beydon, L., Catoire, P., Sessler, D.I. (1993) Clonidine comparably decreases the thermoregulatory thresholds for vasoconstriction and shivering in humans. *Anesthesiology* **79**: 470–474.

Dirksen, M.S.C., Vree, T.B., Driessen, J.J. (1987) Clinical pharmacokinetics of long-term infusion of midazolam in critically ill patients – preliminary results. *Anaesth Intensive Care* **15**: 440–443.

Downs, J.B., Stock, M.C. (1987) Airway pressure release ventilation: a new concept in ventilatory support. *Crit Care Med* **15**: 459–461.

Duggan, J., Drummond, G.B. (1987) Activity of lower intercostal and abdominal muscles after upper abdominal surgery. *Anesth Analg* **66**: 852–855.

Dureuil, B., Cantineau, J.P., Desmonts, J.M. (1987) Effects of upper or lower abdominal surgery on diaphragmatic function. *Br J Anaesth* **59**: 1230–1234.

Flacke, J.W., Bloor, B.C., Flacke, W.E., Wong, D., Dazza, S., Stead, S.W., Laks, H. (1987) Reduced narcotic requirements by clonidine with improved hemodynamic and adrenergic stability in patients undergoing coronary bypass surgery. *Anesthesiology* **67**: 11–19.

Freye, E., Knüffermann, V. (1994) Keine Hemmung der intestinalen Motilität nach Ketamin/Midazolamnarkose. Ein Vergleich zur Narkose mit Enfluran und Fentanyl/Midazolam. *Anaesthesist* **43**: 87–91.

Froese, A.B., Bryan, A.C. (1974) Effects of anesthesia and paralysis on diaphragmatic mechanics in man. *Anesthesiology* **41**: 242–255.

Gooch, J.L., Suchyta, M.R., Balbierz, J.M., *et al.* (1991) Prolonged paralysis after treatment with neuromuscular junction blocking agents. *Crit Care Med* **19**: 1125-1131.

Grant, I.S., Nimmo, W.S., Clements, J.A. (1981) Lack of effect of ketamine analgesia on gastric emptying in man. *Br J Anaesth* **53**: 1321–1323.

Griffin, D., Fairman, N., Coursin, D., *et al.* (1992) Acute myopathy during treatment of status asthmaticus with corticosteroids and steroidal muscle relaxants. *Chest* **102**: 510–514.

Hansen-Flaschen, J.H., Brazinsky, S., Basile, C., *et al.* (1991) Use of sedating drugs and neuromuscular blocking agents in patients requiring mechanical ventilation for respiratory failure. A national survey. *JAMA* **266** (Suppl.): 2870–2875.

Hedenstierna, G., Strandberg, A., Brismar, B., Lundquist, H., Svensson, L., Tokics, L. (1985) Functional residual capacity, thoracoabdominal dimensions, central blood volume during general anaesthesia with muscle paralysis and mechanical ventilation. *Anesthesiology* **62**: 247–254.

Hedenstierna, G., Tokics, L., Lundquist, H., Andersson, T., Strandberg, A., Brismar, B. (1994) Phrenic nerve stimulation during halothane anesthesia. Effects on atelectasis. *Anesthesiology* **80**: 751–760.

Hörmann, Ch., Baum, M., Putensen, Ch., Mutz, N.J., Benzer, H. (1994) Biphasic positive airway pressure (BIPAP) – a new mode of augmented ventilation. *Eur J Anaesthesiol* **11**: 37–42.

Jarvis, D.A., Duncan, S.R., Segal, I.S., Maze, M. (1992) Ventilatory effects of clonidine alone and in the presence of alfentanil in human volunteers. *Anesthesiology* **76**: 899–905.

Joris, J., Banache, M., Bonnet, F., Sessler, D.I., Lamy, M. (1993) Clonidine and ketanserin both are effective treatments for postanesthetic shivering. *Anesthesiology* **79**: 532–539.

Kurz, M., Belani, K.G., Dessler, D.I., Kurz, A., Larson, M.D., Schroeder, M., Blanchard, D. (1993) Naloxone, meperidine, and shivering. *Anesthesiology* **79**: 1193–1201.

Ledingham, I., Watt, I. (1983) Influence of sedation on mortality in critically ill multiple trauma patients. *Lancet* **i**: 1270.

Lehmann, K.A., Gerhard, A., Horrichs-Haermeyer, G., Grond, S., Zech, D. (1991) Postoperative patient-controlled analgesia with sufentanil: analgesic efficacy and minimum effective concentrations. *Acta Anaesthesiol Scand* **35**: 221–226.

Maitre, P.O., Vozeh, S., Heykants, J. (1987) Population pharmacokinetics of alfentanil: the average dose–plasma concentration relationship and interindividual variability in patients. *Anesthesiology* **62**: 3–6.

Mangano, D.T. (1991) Perioperative cardiac morbitity. *Anesthesiology* **72**: 153–158.

Marcy, T.W., Marini, J.J. (1991) Inverse ratio ventilation in ARDS. Rationale and implementation. *Chest* **100**: 494–504.

Merskey, H. (1979) Pain terms: a list with definitions and notes on usage. Recommended by the International Association for the Study of Pain. Subcommittee on Taxonomy. *Pain* **6**: 249–257.

Newman, L.H., McDonald, J.C., Wallace, P.M., Ledingham, I.M. (1987) Propofol infusion for sedation in intensive care. *Anaesthesia* **42**: 929–933.

Op de Coul, A.A.W., Verheul, G.A.M., Leyten, A.C.M., *et al.* (1991) Critical illness polyneuromyopathy after artificial respiration. *Clin Neurol Neurosurg* **93**: 27–33.

Osborne, R.J., Joel, S.P., Slevin, M.L. (1986) Morphine intoxication in renal failure: the role of morphine-6 glucoronide. *Br Med J Clin Res Ed* **292**: 1548–1549.

Pauca, A.L., Savage, R.T., Simpson, S., Roy, R.C. (1984) Effect of pethidine, fentanyl, and morphine on post-operative shivering in man. *Acta Anaesthesiol Scand* **28**: 138–143.

Putensen, C., Räsänen, J., Lopez, F.A. (1994) Ventilation–perfusion distributions during mechanical ventilation with superimposed spontaneous breathing in canine lung injury. *Am J Respir Crit Care Med* **150**: 101–108.

Ramsay, M.A.E., Savege, T.M., Simpson, B.R.J., *et al.* (1974) Controlled sedation with alphaxalone–alphadalone. *Br Med J* **2**: 656–659.

Rathgeber, J., Schorn, B., Falk, V., Kazmaier, S., Burchardi, H. (1997) The influence of controlled mandatory ventilation (CMV), intermittent mandatory ventilation (IMV), and biphasic intermittent positive airway pressure (BIPAP) on duration of intubation and consumption of analgesics and sedatives. A prospective analysis in 596 patients. *Eur J Anaesth* **14**: in press.

Rossiter, A., Souney, P.F., McGowan, S., *et al.* (1991) Pancuronium-induced prolonged neuromuscular blockade. *Crit Care Med* **19**: 1583–1587.

Slutsky, A.S. (1994a) Consensus conference on mechanical ventilation – January 28–30, 1993 at Northbrook, Illinois, USA. Part I. *Intensive Care Med* **20**: 64–79.

Slutsky, A.S. (1994b) Consensus conference on mechanical ventilation – January 28–30, 1993 at Northbrook, Illinois, USA. Part II. *Intensive Care Med* **20**: 150–162.

Sydow, M., Burchardi, H., Ephraim, E., *et al.* (1994) Long-term effects of two different ventilatory modes on oxygenation in acute lung injury. Comparison of airway pressures release ventilation and volume-controlled inverse ratio ventilation. *Am J Respir Crit Care Med* **149**: 1550–1556.

Takahashi, R.N., Morato, G.S., Rae, G.A. (1987) Effects of ketamine on nociception and gastrointestinal motility in mice are unaffected by naloxone. *Gen Pharmacol* **18**: 201–203.

Wheeler, A.P. (1993) Sedation, analgesia, and paralysis in the intensive care unit. *Chest* **104**: 566–577.

White, P.F., Way, W.L., Trevor, A.J. (1982) Ketamine – its pharmacology and therapeutic uses. *Anesthesiology* **56**: 119–123.

9

Pulmonary Embolism

Frederick R. Bode

INTRODUCTION

Venous thromboembolism, which includes venous thrombosis and pulmonary embolism (PE), is a leading cause of morbidity and mortality in intensive care unit (ICU) patients. The estimated incidence of deep venous thrombosis (DVT) of the lower extremities is 1 per 1000 persons per year (Kierkegaard, 1980). In the 1960s, Freiman *et al.* (1965) found evidence of subclinical pulmonary emboli in 64% of consecutive autopsies in patients with various causes of death. More importantly, 50 000 deaths annually in the USA are attributable to fatal PE (Dalen and Alpert, 1975). The mortality rate of untreated venous thromboembolism approaches 30%, but prompt recognition and treatment can reduce this to under 10% (Alpert *et al.*, 1976).

We are only beginning to understand the true incidence of venous thromboembolism in the ICU setting. Rudolph Virchow recognized DVT in 1856 and described the classic triad of vessel wall inflammation, hypercoagulability, and venostasis that underlie all risk factors for venous thrombosis. Essentially all ICU patients have one or more risk factors.

Hirsch *et al.* (1995), in a prospective ultrasound series, detected DVT in 33% of 100 eligible patients admitted over an 8-month study period to a Boston medical ICU. This high rate occurred despite prophylaxis in 61%. Geerts *et al.* (1994) did prospective venographic studies in 349 patients admitted to a trauma unit. Prophylaxis against thromboembolism was not used. DVT was found in 201 (58%) and proximal vein thrombosis was found in 63 (18%).

We are now able to identify other patients at high risk, such as those who have undergone hip surgery. Barnes *et al.* (1989) studied 78 patients with total hip or knee arthroplasty. The preoperative prevalence and postoperative incidence of major DVT were 2.5% and 14.1% of patients, respectively, despite intensive mechanical and pharmacologic prophylaxis. Trottier *et al.* (1995) found acute DVT in 25% of patients with femoral vein catheters, and Horattas *et al.* (1988) found that in 28% of all subclavian catheterizations, venous thrombosis developed, often subclinically. In a prospective surveillance program of 361 major neurosurgical procedures in which the patient received standard DVT prophylaxis, Flinn *et al.* (1989) still found 17 cases of perioperative DVT (4.7%).

The reason for entering the ICU may be a PE, either diagnosed clinically or totally unsuspected as the cause for the patient's change in clinical status. Every patient entering the ICU should be considered at risk of thromboembolism and immediately assessed for prophylaxis and choice of prophylaxis. Prevention is better than cure: avoiding a PE is better for the patient and more cost-effective than diagnosing and treating the event and its aftermath. The current prophylaxis recommendations for both surgical and medical situations are listed in Table 9.1 (Clagett *et al.*, 1995).

Include PE often in your differential diagnosis. Your challenge is to reverse this axiom of medicine: more PEs are diagnosed at autopsy than at the bedside.

DIAGNOSING PULMONARY EMBOLISM

Clinical suspicion of PE is heightened by the presence of DVT, but the clinical diagnosis of DVT is most often inaccurate. In the ICU setting, it is generally agreed that for DVT detection duplex ultrasonography is the diagnostic study of choice. For the diagnosis of PE, a bedside perfusion lung scan is best. Other routinely available laboratory tests have obvious limitations in the diagnostic scrutiny of PE. Arterial hypoxemia in conjunction with respiratory alkalosis is the general rule on arterial blood gases. However, a normal P_aO_2 (McIntyre and Sasahara, 1971) or a normal alveolar/arterial oxygen gradient (The Urokinase Pulmonary Embolism Trial, 1973) do not rule out pulmonary embolism. The principal value of the chest radiograph is to exclude competing diagnoses such as pneumothorax or pneumonia and to help with interpretation of ventilation/perfusion scintigraphy. The electrocardiogram is helpful in ruling out an acute myocardial infarction, but may be abnormal due to PE if there is acute right ventricular overload.

The most common clinical presentation of PE consists of sudden-onset dyspnea, tachycardia, tachypnea, or low-grade fever. Leeper *et al.* (1988) found that dyspnea or tachypnea was present in 96% of subjects with PE and the absence of either of these symptoms argue strongly against a diagnosis of PE. Benotti and Dalen (1985) pointed

Table 9.1   Deep vein thrombosis and pulmonary embolism prophylaxis*

Surgical situations
- In low-risk patients, no specific prophylaxis other than early ambulation is recommended
- ES, LDUH (given 2 h before and every 12 h after operations), or IPC should be used in moderate-risk patients
- LDUH (every 8 h) or LMWH should be used in higher risk patients
- In high-risk general surgery patients who are prone to wound complications such as hematomas and infections, IPC is a good alternative prophylaxis
- In very high-risk surgery patients with multiple risk factors, pharmacologic methods (LDUH, LMWH, or dextran) combined with IPC are most effective. LDUH and LMWH therapy should be started preoperatively and dextran given intraoperatively. IPC should be applied intraoperatively, if possible. Alternatively, perioperative warfarin (INR 2.0–3.0) therapy may be used
- In patients undergoing total hip replacement surgery, postoperative, subcutaneous twice-daily fixed-dose unmonitored LMWH, low-intensity (INR 2.0–3.0) oral anticoagulation heparin (started preoperatively) are the most effective anticoagulant-based prophylaxis regimens. Adjuvant prophylaxis with ES or IPC may provide additional efficacy
- In patients undergoing total knee replacement surgery, postoperative subcutaneous twice-daily fixed-dose unmonitored LMWH is the most effective anticoagulant-based prophylaxis regimen. IPC is the most effective non-pharmacologic prophylaxis regimen and provides a reduction in relative risk comparable to LMWH
- In patients undergoing hip fracture surgery, either preoperative subcutaneous fixed-dose unmonitored LMWH or oral anticoagulation (INR 2.0–3.0) is effective
- Prophylactic inferior vena cava filter replacement should be limited to high-risk patients in whom other forms of anticoagulant-based prophylaxis are not feasible because of contraindications
- IPC with or without ES should be used in patients undergoing neurosurgery. LDUH therapy may be an acceptable alternative. IPC and LDUH may be more effective in combination than individually
- Aspirin is ineffective prophylaxis and should not be used

Medical situations
- In multiple-trauma patients, IPC, warfarin, or LMWH should be used when feasible. Because of the high risk of venous thromboembolism and the inability to apply standard methods of prophylaxis, serial surveillance with duplex ultrasonography may be a successful strategy. In selected very high-risk patients, prophylactic inferior vena cava filter placement may be employed
- LDHU should be used in patients with myocardial infarction. Full-dose anticoagulation is also effective. IPC and possible ES may be useful when heparin is contraindicated
- In patients with ischemic stroke and lower extremity paralysis, LDUH and LMWH are effective. IPC and ES are also probably effective

Table 9.1 *Continued*

- In patients with acute spinal cord injury with paralysis, treatment with adjusted-dose heparin or LMWH is recommended for prophylaxis. Warfarin prophylaxis also may be effective. LDUH, ES, and IPC when used alone are ineffective
- In general medical patients with clinical risk factors for venous thrombo-embolism, particularly those with heart failure or chest infections, LDUH and LMWH are effective
- In patient with long-term indwelling central vein catheters, warfarin, 1 mg daily, should be used to prevent axillary-subclavian venous thrombosis.

ES, Elastic stockings; INR, international normalized ratio; IPC, intermittent pneumatic compression; LDUH, low-dose unfractionated heparin; LMWH, low-molecular-weight heparin.
* Adapted, with permission from Department of Health and Science Policy, Committee on Health and Science Policy (1995) pp. 6–7.

out the subtle manifestation of PE in ICU patients that should heighten suspicion for the diagnosis:

- Worsening arterial hypoxemia and respiratory alkalosis in a spontaneously breathing patient.
- A reduction in arterial carbon dioxide, persistent dyspnea and hypoxemia, despite bronchodilator therapy, in a patient with chronic lung disease and known CO_2 retention.
- Unexplained fever, atelectasis, or pleural-based pulmonary infiltrate.
- Sudden development of pulmonary hypertension in a hemodynamically monitored patient.
- Sudden elevation of central venous pressure.
- Unexplained tachycardia and tachypnea.
- Worsening hypoxemia, hypercapnia, and respiratory acidosis in a sedated patient on controlled mechanical ventilation.

The ICU patient is less likely to present a straightforward history and physical findings of PE. Still, valuable signs of PE may be present on the monitoring devices being used (Schmidt, 1992). An unexplained increase in minute ventilation should lead to prompt consideration of PE. Pulmonary embolism leads to an increase in dead space, and if end-tidal CO_2 is being measured PE causes a detectable fall in end-tidal CO_2 . It may support the suspicion that PE has occurred. When a pulmonary artery catheter is in place, one may see elevation in right atrial, right ventricular, and pulmonary artery pressures following PE. Cardiac output may fall. Whereas the normal relationship of end-diastolic pulmonary artery pressure and the pulmonary artery occlusive pressure (PAOP) is within 5 mmHg, an increase in this difference may suggest pulmonary artery obstruction due to PE. Thus, the wealth of monitoring information available in the ICU setting may point to PE and provide the clinician with the confidence to proceed with more specific diagnostic studies.

If the patient is well enough to go to the nuclear medicine area, ventilation and perfusion lung scanning can be accomplished. Then the revised PIOPED criteria may be used to aid in diagnosis (Table 9.2) (Gottschalk *et al.*, 1993).

The duplex ultrasound study (if done) and the perfusion lung scan results lead to a clear-cut diagnosis or the need for pulmonary angiography. A clinical schema for using these results is given in Table 9.3.

In very ill patients, it may be appropriate to diagnose a *lower extremity DVT* and, if hemodynamically stable PE is suspected, this provides the armamentarium for definitive therapy, since therapy is the same for both. A *low probability scan* finding, in conjunction with a normal lower extremity duplex examination, allows some clinicians temporarily to stop the diagnostic process, initiate prophylaxis, and repeat a lower extremity ultrasound study in 3–5 days.

A *normal perfusion lung scan* effectively rules out the diagnosis of clinically significant pulmonary embolism. A *high probability lung scan* essentially rules in the diagnosis of pulmonary embolism (The PIOPED Investigators, 1990). The only occasion where a high probability lung scan would still require further diagnostic confirmation would be in a situation where it was positive in an area where the patient had previously had a high probability scan and there had been no repeat lung scan months after treatment to show that the previous perfusion defect had returned to normal. We suggest that both *intermediate and low probability scans* simply be labeled as 'indeterminate' (nondiagnostic) and further consideration be given to pulmonary angiography (Mehra and Bode, 1997).

Echocardiographic findings typical for PE would include a dilated, thin-walled, poorly contracting right ventricle, and displacement of the interventricular septum to the left, all compatible with acute increases in pulmonary artery pressure (Goldhaber *et al.*, 1993). Traditionally, it has been recommended that, prior to thrombolytic therapy, the diagnosis of PE must be established via angiography. Current thinking has shifted to earlier use of thrombolytics, even with noninvasive diagnostic confirmation, such as in the setting of a high probability lung scan along with echocardiographic evidence of right ventricular dysfunction where the clinical suspicion of thromboembolism is also high. In summary, contemporary PE thrombolysis

Table 9.2   Revised PIOPED *V/Q* scan criteria*

High probability (≥80%)
- Two or more large mismatched segmental perfusion defects or the arithmetic equivalent in moderate or large + moderate defects[†]

Intermediate probability (20–79%)
- One moderate to two large mismatched segmental perfusion defects or the arithmetic equivalent in moderate or large + moderate defects[†]
- Single matched ventilation-perfusion defect with clear chest radiography[‡]
- Difficult to categorize as low or high, or not described as low or high

Low probability (≤19%)
- Nonsegmental perfusion defects (e.g. cardiomegaly, enlarged aorta, enlarged hila, elevated diaphragm)
- Any perfusion defect with a substantially larger chest radiographic abnormality
- Perfusion defects matched by ventilation abnormality[‡] provided that: (1) there is a clear chest radiograph; and (2) there are some areas of normal perfusion in the lungs
- Any numbers of small perfusion defects with a normal chest radiograph

Normal
- No perfusion defects or perfusion outlines exactly the shape of the lungs seen on the chest radiograph (note that hilar and aortic impressions may be seen and the chest radiograph and/or ventilation study may be abnormal)

---

* The PIOPED Investigators. (1990) p. 2755.
[†] Two large mismatched perfusion defects are borderline for 'high probability'. Individual readers may correctly interpret individual scans with this pattern as 'high probability'. In general, it is recommended that more than this degree of mismatch be present for the 'high probability' category.
[‡] Very extensive matched defects can be categorized as 'low probability'. Single *V/Q* matches are borderline for 'low probability' and thus should be categorized as 'intermediate' in most circumstances by most readers, although individual readers may correctly interpret individual scans with this pattern as 'low probability'.

can be applied without mandatory angiography with a brief infusion via a peripheral vein, with no special additional tests (Goldhaber, 1995).

Pulmonary angiography is the current gold standard for diagnosing PE. Safeguards for a proper study include a detailed precatheterization evaluation, optimal oxygen administration, minimization of the amount of contrast medium (preferably using nonionic media) and the immediate availability of complete resuscitation capabilities. The mortality risk in experienced hands approaches 0.3%, with a morbidity rate of 1–4% (Sasahara *et al.*, 1964). The specific findings for a PE includes filling defects and abrupt vascular cut-off. Other findings that

Table 9.3 Strategy for diagnosing pulmonary embolism

Study	Probability of PE	Next step
Proximal lower extremity DVT by DUS	Unknown without further studies	Begin heparin therapy (this also treats submassive PE)
Normal perfusion scan	<4%	End diagnostic studies. Begin or continue prophylaxis. Continue to monitor for DVT development
High probability V/Q scan; stable patient	>88% (unless history of previous high probability scan with no follow-up scan)	Begin heparin therapy. Echocardiography? Pulmonary angiography
Intermediate V/Q scan (low or intermediate probability); stable patient	10–80%	Pulmonary angiography. Echocardiography?
Echocardiography positive for right ventricular failure and pulmonary hypertension	High	Avoid pulmonary angiography*. Thrombolytic therapy
Persistant hypotension	High	Echocardiography. Thrombolytic therapy. Pulmonary angiography. Surgery

DUS, duplex ultrasonography; DVT, deep vein thrombosis; PE; pulmonary embolism.
* See Goldhaber (1995).

suggest PE include oligemia, delayed filling in the lower zone, asymmetric filling, and a prolonged arterial phase (Sasahara *et al.*, 1964; Bettman, 1987). A pulmonary angiogram is warranted in the following situations (Mehra and Bode, 1997):

- Nondiagnostic noninvasive studies for thromboembolism, especially in patients with pre-existing cardiopulmonary disease.
- Patients deemed at high risk for bleeding complications from anticoagulation.
- Before embolectomy.
- Before thrombolytic therapy, particularly in the setting of right ventricular hemodynamic compromise where lung scanning gives equivocal results.
- Recurrent PE preceding vena caval interruption.

THERAPY

Guidelines for anticoagulation in venous thromboembolism are given in Table 9.4. The guidelines are derived from evidence-based recommendations from the fourth American College of Chest Physicians (ACCP) Consensus Conference on Antithrombotic Therapy (Clagett *et al.*, 1995).

When the diagnosis of pulmonary embolism is suspected, one should immediately obtain a baseline activated partial thromboplastin time (APTT), prothrombin time (PT) and complete blood count (CBC). After checking for contraindications to heparin therapy, begin with heparin 5000 U i.v. and order imaging studies. Patients with DVT or PE should be treated with heparin (i.v., or adjusted-dose s.c.). The heparin dosage should prolong the APTT to a range that corresponds to a plasma heparin concentration range of 0.2–0.4 U/ml. The ACCP has published a quick reference guide for clinicians that allows optimal monitoring and adjusting dosage in venous thromboembolism (Table 9.5) (Department of Health and Science Policy, Committee on Health and Science Policy, 1995).

Heparin-induced thrombocytopenia occurs in 3–30% of patients receiving therapeutic doses (Cines *et al.*, 1980; Magnani, 1993). This

Table 9.4   Guidelines for anticoagulation in venous thromboembolism*

Suspected disease
- Obtain baseline APTT, PT and CBC
- Check for contraindication to heparin therapy
- Give heparin 5000 U i.v. and order imaging study

Confirmed disease
- Rebolus with heparin 5000–10 000 U i.v. and start maintenance infusion at 1300 U/h (heparin 20 000 U in 500 ml D_5W, infused at 33 ml/h)
- Check APTT at 6 h to keep APTT between 1.5 and 2.5 times control (blood heparin level 0.2–0.4 U/ml)
- Check platelet count daily
- Start warfarin therapy on day 1 at 5–10 mg and then administer warfarin daily at estimated daily maintenance dose
- Stop heparin therapy after 4–7 days of joint therapy when INR is 2.0–3.0 without heparin therapy
- Anticoagulate with warfarin for 3 months at an INR of 2.0–3.0 (longer treatment should be given to patients with ongoing risk factors or recurrent thrombosis)

*Used, with permission, from Department of Health and Science Policy, Committee on Health and Science Policy (1995), p. 9.
APPT, activated partial thromboplastin time; CBC, complete blood count; INR, international normalized ratio; PT, prothrombin time.

usually occurs 2 days after therapy is begun and promptly reverses after the drug is stopped. Heparin-induced thrombocytopenia is more common with unfractionated heparin than with low-molecular-weight heparin (Warkentin *et al.*, 1993). To monitor this potential complication, daily platelet counts should be ordered. Dangerous hemorrhagic and arterial thrombolic complications may also develop, as may rare serious complications of heparin therapy, including anaphylaxis, hyperkalemia, and vertebral fractures secondary to osteoporosis after prolonged administration. Heparin may also elevate the serum aminotransferase levels. These tend to peak after 7 days and may decline despite continuous treatment (Dukes *et al.*, 1984).

The action of heparin can be terminated almost immediately by the intravenous injection, milligram per milligram, of protamine sulfate; 10 000 U of heparin is the equivalent to a 100-mg dose. Protamine sulfate should be administered by slow intravenous injection over 1–3 minutes. Adverse reactions include rash, urticaria, bronchospasm, pulmonary hypertension, hypertension, and death. They are more common in diabetic patients who have received protamine insulin and have developed antiprotamine antibodies (Weiss *et al.*, 1989).

Table 9.5   Monitoring and adjusting heparin dosage*[†]

APTT[‡] (s)	Rate change (ml/h)	Dose change (U/24 h)	Additional action	Next APTT
≤45	+6	+5760	Rebolus w/5000 U	4–6 h
46–54	+3	+2880	None	4–6 h
55–85[§]	0	0	None	Next morning[¶]
86–110	−3	−2880	Stop infusion 1 h	4–6 h after restart
>110	−6	−5760	Stop infusion 1 h	4–6 h after restart

* Adapted, with permission, from Department of Health and Science Policy, Committee on Health and Science Policy (1995) p. 10.
[†]Initial dosing; loading, 5000–10 000 U; maintenance infusion, 1300 U/h (APTT in 4–6 h). A starting bolus of 5000–10 000 U i.v. is given followed by i.v. infusion of 1300 U/h (heparin 20 000 U in 500 ml D_5W at approximately 33 ml/h). The concentration of heparin is 40 U/ml. When APTT is checked at 6 h or longer, steady-state kinetics can be assumed. Dosage adjustments are made according to the protocol.
[‡]Normal APTT range with Dade-Actin FS reagent of 27–35 s.
[§]The therapeutic range 55–85 is roughly equivalent to a plasma heparin concentration range of 0.2–0.4 U/ml by protamine titration or to 0.35–0.7 U/ml by inhibition of factor X_a. The therapeutic range will vary with different APTT reagents and coagulation times. Thus, the therapeutic range should be determined in every laboratory.
[¶]During the first 24 h, repeat APTT in 4–6 h. Therafter, monitor APTT daily unless it is outside the therapeutic range.

Many patients can be started on warfarin at the same time that heparin is begun. The heparin therapy should be continued for 5–10 days, overlapping with oral anticoagulation for 4–5 days. The heparin can be discontinued on day 5 or 6 if the prothrombin time is within the therapeutic range (Department of Health and Science Policy, Committee on Health and Science Policy, 1995). Using the international normalized ratio (INR), the correct therapeutic prothrombin time should be an INR of 2.0–3.0. In most laboratories, this recommendation translates to a prothrombin time prolongation to 15–18 seconds (control, 12 seconds). If the patient is on warfarin when prompt control of bleeding is required, hemostatic concentration of factors II, VII, IX, and X can usually be established by the rapid infusion of 500–600 ml of fresh frozen plasma, repeated every 6 hours. Vitamin K is indicated if there is less urgency.

Life-threatening PE offers further therapeutic challenges. Pulmonary embolectomy may be required in a patient who presents with syncope and/or shock. Thrombolytic therapy may also be useful in this situation and is currently being tried in patients with evidence that suggests right ventricular dysfunction with acute pulmonary embolus. The clinical signs of right ventricular dysfunction include tachycardia, right ventricular heave, right-sided gallops, jugular venous distention, and tricuspid regurgitation (Come, 1992). Electrocardiographic evidence includes sinus tachycardia, new incomplete or complete right bundle branch block, and a right ventricular strain pattern. More specific evidence is provided by echocardiographic findings that include right ventricular dilatation, right ventricular hypokinesis, septal flattening, right ventricular thrombi, and/or tricuspid regurgitation.

Thrombolytic therapy should be used in patients who present with acute massive PE with acute cor pulmonale. The effectiveness of thrombolytic agents in such a situation most certainly outweighs the potential risk of therapy. Angiographic conformation of PE is not needed in the setting of a high-probability lung scan along with echocardiographic evidence of right ventricular dysfunction where the clinical suspicion of PE is high (Goldhaber *et al.*, 1993). Thrombolytic drugs can be administered by a brief infusion through a peripheral vein.

The first evidence of a potentially beneficial effect of thrombolytic therapy came from the randomized, open label Urokinase Pulmonary Embolism Trial (UPET) (1973). A later study by Sharma *et al.* (1980) demonstrated that patients treated with thrombolytic therapy had a more complete resolution of pulmonary embolism, with evidence of preserved exercise pulmonary dynamics and less functional disability at 7 years of follow-up.

The development of recombinant tissue plasminogen activator (rTPA) ushered in the era of target-clot-specific thrombolysis with less systemic hematologic aberrations. The potency of rTPA allowed consideration of shorter duration of bolus therapy. Meyer *et al.* (1992), on behalf of the European Cooperative Study Group Investigators, compared 100 mg rTPA given over 2 hours to a regimen of weight-adjusted urokinase administered as a 4400 U/kg bolus followed by 4400 U/kg/h for 12 hours, and followed hemodynamic parameters with a view to assessing pulmonary vascular resistance. However, the initially observed differences failed to persist at 6 hours. Other studies (Goldhaber *et al.*, 1986, 1988) have demonstrated that rTPA provides better clot dissolution, with greater rapidity and safety than urokinase.

More recently, Goldhaber *et al.* (1993) have compared right ventricular function and pulmonary perfusion in a randomized study of rTPA thrombolysis (100 mg over 2 hours followed by heparin) versus heparin therapy. All patients in this trial were hemodynamically stable and only 20% underwent a pulmonary angiogram for definitive diagnosis. This trial concluded that twice as many rTPA-treated patients demonstrated improvement in right ventricular function compared to those receiving heparin alone. More important, however, was the finding that no patients in the rTPA-treated group suffered recurrent embolism, whereas 9% of heparin-treated patients suffered from fatal and nonfatal recurrent events. It should be emphasized that all these patients presented with echocardiographic evidence of right ventricular hypokinesis, which suggests that the presence of echocardiographic right ventricular involvement, even when hemodynamically stable, might signal a high-risk patient who should be considered for thrombolytic therapy. In such a situation, thrombolytic therapy might serve to prevent the precipitation of clinical right ventricular failure resulting from second embolic events. The thrombolytic regimens currently approved by the US Food and Drug Administration are given in Table 9.6 (Department of Health and Science Policy, Committee on Health and Science Policy, 1995).

Pulmonary Embolectomy

Pulmonary embolectomy for acute massive PE is the last therapeutic option. Mattox *et al.* (1982) reported a series of only 39 patients collected during 29 years. Lund *et al.* (1986) reported excellent results with a more 'routine' use of embolectomy in all patients with large PE, regardless of hemodynamic stability. Today, most physicians consider surgical embolectomy only in patients with proven massive

Table 9.6   Thrombolytic therapy*

- *Stop heparin infusion:* start thrombolytic infusion when APTT or TT is ≤1.5 times control
- *Streptokinase:*[†] 250 000 IU loading dose; 100 000 IU/h maintenance
- *Urokinase:*[†] 4400 IU/kg loading dose; 4400 IU/kg/h maintenance (for 12 h)
- *Tissue plasminogen activator (tPA):*[†] 100 mg (56 million IU) over 2 h
- *After terminating thrombolytic infusion:* Restart heparin infusion without a loading dose or with a small loading dose when APTT or TT ≤1.5 times control

---

* Adapted, with permission, from Department of Health and Science Policy, Committee on Health and Science Policy (1995) p. 10.

[†] Duration of therapy. Streptokinase is recommended for 24-hour infusion in pulmonary embolism, 48–72 hours in deep venous thrombosis. Urokinase is recommended for 12-hour infusion in pulmonary embolism, 24–48 hours in deep venous thrombosis. tPA is recommended for a 2-hour infusion in pulmonary embolism at a total dose of 100 mg. APPT, activated partial thromboplastin time; TT, thrombin time.

PE with unstable circulation and in circumstances that prevent the use of thrombolytic therapy. Moser *et al.* (1987) have discussed the use of surgery in chronic recurrent pulmonary embolic disease and accompanying pulmonary hypertension.

Fluids and Inotropic/Vasoactive Drugs

There is controversy about how best to support the hemodynamic status of PE patients. Volume administration may have detrimental effects on hemodynamics (Belenkie *et al.*, 1989). We believe that volume administration should only be used when the patient is clearly hypovolemic. Fluid management should be guided by right heart catheterization and echocardiography.

Use of a vasoconstrictor is based on the assumption that right ventricular ischemia is the fundamental problem leading to shock and that vasopressors will increase coronary arterial blood flow. Norepinephrine, at 2 μg/min and adjusted to response, should be the drug of first choice when a vasoactive drug is needed for hypoperfusion. In animal models of sublethal PE, norepinephrine was shown to be superior to no therapy, to volume administration, and to isoproterenol (Molley *et al.*, 1984).

Isoproterenol is not an attractive choice in PE when there is a fixed mechanical obstruction to pulmonary flow. Inotropes (dopamine 5–10 μg/kg/min and dobutamine) may boost right ventricular function in some patients with pulmonary emboli and hypotension. Unfortunately, they will also increase myocardial oxygen demand. Vasodilators have been considered, but these also reduce systemic vascular resistance. Since the resultant hypotension may be fatal in the setting of massive PE, vasodilators should not be used.

Inferior vena cava filters are used both for prophylaxis and in selected therapeutic situations (Greenfield and Proctor, 1995) (see Chapter 10). In such situations filters prevent PE in carefully selected patients at risk of lethal embolism who have failed anticoagulation therapy or who have developed absolute contraindications to the use of these agents. The indications include:

- contraindication to anticoagulation,
- complications of anticoagulation,
- prophylaxis,
- failure of anticoagulation, and
- prior to lower extremity embolectomy.

The most aggressive extension of the indications for filter placement is found in trauma patients who are at high risk of venous thromboembolism, but are unable to receive anticoagulation therapy.

FUTURE CONSIDERATIONS

Modern medicine is focusing in on reducing the morbidity and mortality from DVT and PE. Even as this chapter is being written, and by the time you read it, many of the future predictions mentioned here may have already become reality. Progress is being made in the areas of prevention, more accurate diagnosis, and improved treatment.

It will soon become common practice that every patient admitted to hospital must have specific orders written for DVT prophylaxis. If no preventive measures are indicated, then this fact will need to be clearly stated. This approach has already reduced the mortality from PE. At their institution, Moser and colleagues (Timmins *et al.*, 1996) found that the autopsy incidence of PE, both incidental and clinically significant, had decreased from 16% to 2% over the past 20 years. They speculated that this decline may reflect the implementation, in the early 1980s, of a formal venous thromboembolism prophylaxis procedure.

The introduction of low-molecular-weight heparin (LMWH) has led to major advances in prevention and treatment. Table 9.1 includes proposed uses of LMWH, and in Europe many of these are available in clinical practice. At present, in the USA, LMWH (enoxaparin sodium) is indicated only for the prevention of DVT, which may lead to PE, following hip or knee replacement. It is easy to predict that indications will soon be broadened in the USA for a wider application for LMWH.

In the ICU, for DVT detection, a greater exploitation of the diagnostic capabilities of noninvasive ultrasound imaging will evolve. Will it become routinely used in every patient on admission and at 3–5 day intervals thereafter? A greater challenge lies in an early, accurate, and noninvasive test for PE. Development of radiolabeled monoclonal antibodies to thrombi, vascular imaging using spiral computed tomography, and magnetic resonance imaging may hold promise. Transesophageal echocardiography (TEE) allows high-resolution images of the main pulmonary artery and the proximal portions of the left and right pulmonary arteries. Patel *et al.* (1994) have described a group of 14 critically ill patients in whom TEE was performed for other reasons, but picked up the presence of pulmonary emboli. Pulmonary angioscopy, now used only for chronic PE, may have expanded use.

In the therapeutic arena, in addition to LMWH, criteria for the use of thrombolytic therapy will become less stringent and will allow its use in more cases. Thrombolytic therapy would be more widely used if we could accurately predict those patients at risk of complications. We await other therapeutic developments for those patients who are not candidates for heparin or thrombolytic therapy.

Initial therapy of DVT and pulmonary embolism is already leaving the hospital setting. Investigators have shown the effectiveness of LMWH in treating DVT on an outpatient basis. Two recent studies have shown that LMWH can be used with proximal DVT to treat patients at home (Koopman *et al.*, 1996; Levine *et al.*, 1996). We switch from heparin to coumadin earlier in treating PE and this leads to shorter hospital stays. Will hospital stay be even shorter when we begin the treatment of PE with LMWH? A pilot study by Meyer *et al.* (1995) has indicated that subcutaneous LMWH may be safe and effective treatment for submassive pulmonary embolism.

It will be a better day when we can think of and teach about DVT and PE as mainly historical problems and only as rare developments in day-to-day clinical practice. We have not yet reached this objective. The possibilities seem limitless for the young investigator wishing to study ways of decreasing morbidity from and improving patient survival after DVT and PE. In a recent editorial, the present state of knowledge about venous thromboembolism was characterized as the tip of the thromboembolism iceberg (Oudkerk *et al.*, 1993). DVT and PE challenge us to improve our diagnostic talents and therapeutic outcomes.

Acknowledgment

The author acknowledges the untiring technical support of Ms Jennifer Ross.

REFERENCES

Alpert, J.S., Smith, R., Carlson, J., *et al.* (1976) Mortality in patients treated for pulmonary embolism. *JAMA* **236**: 1477–1480.

Barnes, R.W., Nix, M.L., Barnes, C.L., *et al.* (1989) Perioperative asymptomatic venous thrombosis: Role of duplex scanning versus venography. *J Vasc Surg* **9**: 251–260.

Belenkie, I., Dani, R., Smith, E.R., Tyberg, J.V. (1989) Effects of volume loading during experimental acute pulmonary embolism. *Circulation* **80**: 178–188.

Benotti, J.R., Dalen, J.E. (1985) Pulmonary embolism. In: Rippe, J.M., Irwin, R.S., Alpert, J.F., *et al.* (eds) *Intensive Care Medicine*, p. 129. Boston: Little, Brown.

Bettman, M.A. (1987) Pulmonary angiography. In: Hirsch (ed.) *Venous Thrombosis and Pulmonary Embolism: Diagnostic Methods*, pp. 150–160, New York: Churchill Livingstone.

Cines, D.B., Kaywin, P., Bina, M., *et al.* (1980) Heparin-associated thrombocytopenia. *N Engl J Med* **303**: 788–795.

Adapted from Clagett, G.P., Anderson Jr, F.A., *et al.* (1995) Prevention of venous thromboembolism. *Chest* **108**: 312S–334S.

Come, P.C. (1992) Echocardiographic evaluation of pulmonary embolism and its response to therapeutic interventions. *Chest* **101**: 151S–162S.

Dalen, J.E., Alpert, J.S. (1975) Natural history of pulmonary embolism. *Prog Cardiovasc Dis* **17**: 257–270.

Department of Health and Science Policy, Committee on Health and Science Policy (1995) *Quick Reference Guide for Clinicians: Clinical Consensus Statement from the Fourth ACCP Consensus Conference on Antithrombotic Therapy*. Northbrook, IL: American College of Chest Physicians.

Dukes, G.E., Sanders, S.W., Russo, Jr. J., *et al.* (1984) Transaminase elevations in patients receiving bovine or procine heparin. *Ann Intern Med* **100**: 646–650.

Flinn, W.R., Sandager, G.P., Cerullo, L.J., *et al.* (1989) Duplex venous scanning for the prospective surveillance of perioperative venous thrombosis. *Arch Surg* **124**: 901–905.

Freiman, D.G., Suyemoto, J., Wessler, S. (1965) Frequency of pulmonary thromboembolism in man. *N Engl J Med* **272**: 1278–1280.

Geerts, W.H., Code, K.I., Jay, R.M., *et al.* (1994) A prospective study of venous thromboembolism after major trauma. *N Engl J Med* **331**: 1601–1606.

Goldhaber, S.Z. (1995) Contemporary pulmonary embolism thrombolysis. *Chest* **107**: 45S–51S.

Goldhaber, S.Z., Vaughan, D.E., Markis, J.E., *et al.* (1986) Acute pulmonary embolism treated with tissue plasminogen activator. *Lancet* **ii**: 886–889.

Goldhaber, S.Z., Kessler, C.M., Heit, J.A., *et al.* (1988) A randomized controlled trial of recombinant tissue plasminogen activator versus urokinase in the treatment of acute pulmonary embolism. *Lancet* **ii**: 2932 298.

Goldhaber, S.Z., Haire, W.D., Feldstein, M.L., *et al.* (1993) Alteplase versus heparin in acute pulmonary embolism: randomized trial assessing right ventricular function and pulmonary perfusion. *Lancet* **341**: 507–511.

Gottschalk, A., Sostman, H.D., Coleman, R.E., *et al*: (1993) Ventilation-perfusion scintigraphy in the PIOPED study. Part II. Evaluation of the scintigraphic criteria and interpretations. *J Nucl Med* **34**: 1119–1126.

Greenfield, L.J. and Proctor, M.C. (1995) Caval filters: indications and limitations. *Pulmon Perspect* **12**(1): 5–6.

Hirsch, D.R., Ingenito, E.P., Goldhaber, S.Z. (1995) Prevalence of deep venous thrombosis among patients in medical intensive care. *JAMA* **274**: 335–337.

Horattas, M.C., Wright, D.J., Fenton, A.H., *et al*. (1988) Changing concepts of deep venous thrombosis of the upper extremity – report of a series and review of the literature. *Surgery* **104**: 561–567.

Kierkegaard, A. (1980) Incidence of acute deep vein thrombosis in two districts. A phlebographic study. *Acta Chir Scand* **146**: 267–269.

Koopman, M.M.W., Prandoni, P., Piovella, F., *et al*. (1996) Treatment of venous thrombosis with intravenous unfractionated heparin administered in the hospital as compared with subcutaneous LMWH administered at home. *N Engl J Med* **334**: 682–687.

Leeper, K.V. Jr, Popovich, J., Adams, D. Jr., *et al*. (1988) Clinical manifestations of acute PE. Henry Ford Hospital experience: a five year review. *Henry Ford Hosp Med J* **36**: 29–34.

Levine, M., Gent, M., Hirsh, J., *et al*. (1996) A Comparison of LMWH administered primarily at home with unfractionated heparin administered in the hospital for proximal deep vein thrombosis. *N Engl J Med* **334**: 677–681.

Lund, O., Nielsen, T.T., Schifter, S., Roenne, K. (1986) Treatment of pulmonary embolism with full-dose heparin, streptokinase or embolectomy – results and indications. *Thorax Cardiovasc Surg* **34**: 240–246.

Magnani, H.N. (1993) Heparin induced thrombocytopenia: an overview of 230 patients treated with orgaran (Org 101072). *Thromb Hemost* **11**: 326–329.

Mattox, K.L., Feldtman, R.W., Beall, A.C. Jr, DeBakery, M.E. (1982) Pulmonary embolectomy for acute massive pulmonary embolism. *Ann Surg* **195**: 726–731.

McIntyre, K.M., Sasahara, A.A. (1971) The hemodynamic response to pulmonary embolism without prior cardiopulmonary disease. *Am J Cardiol* **28**: 288–294.

Mehra, M.R., Bode, F.R. (1997) Venous thrombosis and pulmonary embolism In: Civetta, J.M., Taylor, R.W., Kirby, R.R. (eds) *Critical Care*, 3rd edition, pp. 1887–1903. Philadelphia: Lippincott-Raven.

Meyer, G., Sors, H., Charbonnier, B., *et al*. (1992) Effects of intravenous urokinase versus alteplase on total pulmonary resistance in acute massive pulmonary embolism: a European muticenter double blind trial. *J Am Coll Cardiol* **19**: 239–45.

Meyer, G., Brenot, F., Pacouret, G., *et al*. (1995) Subcutaneous LMWH (Fragmin™) vs IV unfractionated heparin in the treatment of acute non-massive PE. An open randomized pilot study. *Thromb Haemost* **74**(6): 1432–1435.

Molloy, W.D., Lee, K.Y., Girling, L., Schick, G.U., Prewitt, R.M. (1984) Treatment of shock in a canine model of pulmonary embolism. *Am Rev Respir Dis* **130**: 870–874.

Moser, K.M., Paily, P.O., Peterson, K.L., *et al.* (1987) Thromboendarterectomy for chronic, major vessel thromboembolic pulmonary hypertension in 142 patients, immediate and long-term results. *Ann Intern Med* **107**: 560–564.

Oudkerk, M., Van Beek, E.J.R., Van Putten, W.L.J., Buller, H.R. (1993) Cost-effectiveness analysis of various strategies in diagnostic management of pulmonary embolism. *Arch Intern Med* **153**: 947–954.

Patel, J.J., Chandrasekaran, K., Maniet, A.R., Ross, J.J. (1994) Impact of the incidental diagnosis of clinically unsuspected central pulmonary artery embolism in treatment of critically ill patients. *Chest* **105**: 986–990.

Sasahara, A.A, Stein, M., Simon, M., *et al.* (1964) Pulmonary angiography in the diagnosis of thromboembolic disease. *N Engl J Med* **279**: 1075.

Schmidt, G.A. (1992) Pulmonary embolic disorders: thrombus, air, and fat. In: Hall, J.B., Schmidt, G.A., Wood, L.D.H. (eds) *Principles of Critical Care* pp. 1476–1492. New York: McGraw-Hill.

Sharma, G.V.R.K., Burleson, V.A., Sasahara, A.A., *et al.* (1980) Effect of thrombolytic therapy on pulmonary-capillary blood volume in patients with pulmonary embolism. *N Engl J Med* **303**: 842–845.

The PIOPED Investigators (1990) Value of ventilation/perfusion scan in acute pulmonary embolism: results of the PIOPED study. *JAMA* **263**: 2753–2759.

The Urokinase Pulmonary Embolism Trial. (1973) A national cooperative study. *Circulation* **47**: 1–108.

Timmins, W.N., Channick, R.N., Moser, K.M., *et al.* (1996) Decreasing incidence of pulmonary embolism as autopsy finding at UCSD Medical Center: 1972–1994. *Am J Resp Crit Care Med*, **153**: A94 [abstract].

Trottier, S.J., Veremakis, C., O'Brien, J., Auer, A.I., *et al.* (1995) Femoral deep vein thrombosis associated with central venous catheterizations: results from a prospective randomized trial. *Critical Care Med* **23**: 52–59.

Warkentin, T.E., Levine, M.N., Roberts, R.S., Gent, M., Horeswood, P., Kelton, J.G. (1993) Heparin induced thrombocytopenia is more common with infractionated heparin than with low molecular weight heparin. *Thromb Haemost* **69**: 911.

Weiss, M.E., Nyham, D., Peng, K., *et al.* (1989) Association of protamine IgE and IgG antibodies with life-threatening reactions to intravenous protamine. *N Engl J Med* **320**: 886–892.

10

Cava Filtering in Intensive Care

Jörg M. Neuerburg, Rolf W. Günther

INTRODUCTION

Despite an improved knowledge of its pathogenesis, diagnosis and therapy, acute pulmonary embolism remains a frequent and often fatal disease. Much attention has been given to the prevention of acute pulmonary embolism. Although the use of anticoagulants and other prophylactic measures have substantially reduced thromboembolic events, pulmonary embolism is a well-recognized postoperative complication. It is also a common finding in bedridden non-surgical patients secondary to medical disorders such as congestive heart failure, cerebrovascular accidents, systemic infections, chronic pulmonary disease and malignancies.

One of the most important aspects of pulmonary embolism is its prophylaxis, especially in intensive care patients, in whom bed rest and multimorbidity foster the occurrence of pulmonary embolism. Once pulmonary embolism has occurred, the treatment strategy usually includes heparinization for the haemodynamically stable patient, fibrinolysis and heparinization for major embolism and high-dose fibrinolysis in haemodynamically severely compromised patients.

Under particular circumstances, filters are used as a mechanical prophylaxis following a primary or recurrent event of pulmonary embolism.

OVERVIEW OF INFERIOR VENA CAVA INTERRUPTION

For several years, complete or partial interruption of the vena cava has been advocated for selected patients with pulmonary embolism. As the vast majority of significant pulmonary emboli arise from the lower extremities including the inferior vena cava (IVC), in most cases interruption of the IVC is sufficient. Only in rare cases is interruption of the superior vena cava necessary against emboli arising from the upper extremities.

Many approaches to the interruption of the IVC have been tried. Permanent ligation of the IVC was first suggested by Homans in 1944

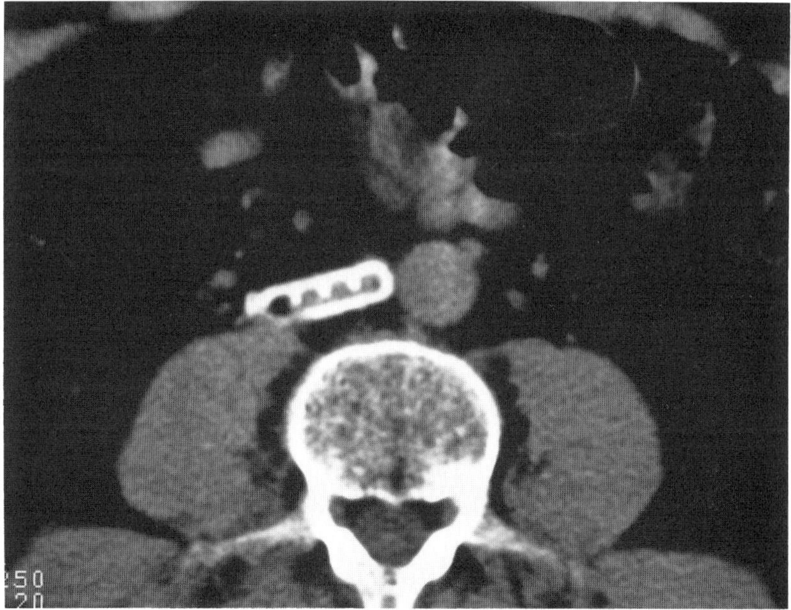

Figure 10.1. Partial caval interruption with an Adams–DeWeese clip. The posterior limb of the clip is smooth and the anterior limb serated. The cross-sectional area of the patent inferior vena cava is decreased.

(Homans, 1944). In the following years up until the late 1980s, complete or partial caval interruption (Figure 10.1) was performed surgically (Coleman, 1986). Several technical procedures designed to simplify caval interruption have been developed.

Devices evolved for transluminal insertion within the IVC lumen via either a jugular or femoral vein cut-down (Mobin-Uddin *et al.*, 1967; Greenfield *et al.*, 1973). In the following years these insertion techniques were modified to allow percutaneous introduction without a venous cut-down by either the jugular or femoral approach using local anaes-thesia (Coleman, 1986). To date, percutaneous access is the technique of choice and has replaced all other techniques of mechanical prevention. Various filters are currently in use, and these are discussed below.

TYPES OF INFERIOR VENA CAVA FILTER

New inventions are continually expanding the spectrum of caval filtration devices. Besides those filters being approved for clinical use, there are various filters under clinical evaluation and there is a large number of experimental devices in various stages of development.

The devices may be characterized by their properties:

- design (e.g. conical, non-conical; concentric, flat; self-centring, non-self-centring),
- material (e.g. stainless steel, Nitinol, Phynox),
- ferromagnetic features (e.g. ferromagnetic, non-ferromagnetic),
- profile of the introducer sheath (e.g. low profile, large profile), and
- retrievability (e.g. permanent non-retrievable, permanent retrievable, temporary).

Table 10.1   Percutaneous permanent non-retrievable caval filters

---

Anthéor filter (Medi-tech Boston Scientific Corporation, Watertown, MA, USA)
Characteristics: 9.5 Fr OD introducer sheath for ante- or retrograde insertion; self-centring within the IVC due to its geometry with two filtration levels

Bird's nest filter (Cook, Bloomington, IN, USA)
Characteristics: 14 Fr OD introducer sheath; not magnetic-resonance compatible; also suitable for megacavae

CARDIAL filter (Cardial S.A., Saint Etienne, France)
Characteristics: 12 Fr OD introducer sheath; cone-shaped filter

KEEPER filter (Cordis Europe, Roden, Holland)
Characteristics: 10.5 Fr OD introducer sheath; cone-shaped filter

Simon Nitinol filter (Nitinol Medical Technologies, Woburn, MA, USA; C.R. Bard, Karlsruhe, Germany)
Characteristics: 10 Fr OD introducer sheath; two filtration planes; made of the memory alloy NITINOL (nickel–titanium alloy)

Titanium Greenfield filter (Medi-tech Boston Scientific Corporation, Watertown, MA, USA)
Characteristics: 14.3 Fr OD introducer sheath; cone-shaped filter; successor of the 'gold standard' stainless steel Kimray Greenfield filter; retrievable, but not specially designed for this purpose

Vascor filter (Vascor, Toulon, France)
Characteristics: 9 Fr OD introducer sheath; cone-shaped filter; transjugular or transbrachial insertion

Vena-Tech LGM filter (B. Braun Celsa, Chasseneuil, France)
Characteristics: 12 Fr OD introducer sheath; cone-shaped filter with additional struts to maintain a central position

---

IVC, inferior vena cava; OD, outer diameter.

Table 10.2   Percutaneous permanent retrievable caval filters

DIL filter (Société Biomat, Igny, France)
Characteristics: 7 Fr OD introducer sheath; preformed memory coiled metal wire with a spring effect functioning like an internal clip by flattening the IVC; exact knowledge of caval diameter mandatory, as incomplete filter deployment may cause complications such as caval perforation, migration or caval thrombosis (Nägele *et al.*, 1995); filter retrieval up to 2 weeks after filter insertion

FCP 2002 filter (Promed, St Barthelemy, France)
Characteristics: 9 Fr OD introducer sheath; two different filter designs for femoral and jugular use; a thin string connected to the filter allows repositioning of the filter before final release or percutaneous retrieval within a time interval up to 10 days after insertion; the femoral filter is retrieved via the femoral and the jugular filter via the jugular approach; two filtration levels

Günther Tulip filter (Cook Europe, Bjaverskov, Denmark)
Characteristics: 10 Fr OD introducer sheath; cone-shaped filter; for filter retrieval, the filter is hooked up with a snare via a jugular approach; filter retrieval up to 2 weeks after filter insertion

OD, outer diameter.

Table 10.3   Percutaneous temporary caval filters

Anthéor filter (Medi-tech Boston Scientific Corporation, Watertown, MA, USA)
Characteristics: Atraumatic Phynox filter basket attached to an 8 Fr catheter; filter retrieval up to 2 weeks after filter insertion

LGT filter (B. Braun Celsa, Chasseneuil, France)
Characteristics: 10 Fr OD introducer sheath; cone-shaped Phynox filter attached to a guidewire; filter retrieval up to 2 weeks after filter insertion

PROLYSER filter (Cordis Europe, Roden, Holland)
Characteristics: plastic filter basket with an 8 Fr catheter; filter retrieval up to 2 weeks after filter insertion

Tempo filter (B. Braun Celsa, Chasseneuil, France)
Characteristics: 12 Fr OD introducer sheath; Phynox filter attached to a tethering catheter with silicone olive for subcutanous fixation; filter retrieval up to 6 weeks after filter insertion

Temporary Günther filter (Cook Europe, Bjaverskov, Denmark)
Characteristics: 6.5 Fr OD introducer catheter; stainless-steel filter basket attached to a 0.038-inch steel wire; filter retrieval up to 2 weeks after filter insertion

OD, outer diameter.

This list of devices (Tables 10.1–10.3) for percutaneous partial interruption of the vena cava is not complete; a selection of the most frequently employed IVC filters is shown in Figures 10.2 and 10.3.

CHOICE OF APPROPRIATE INFERIOR VENA CAVA FILTER

Permanent retrievable and permanent non-retrievable IVC filters (see Figure 10.2) as well as temporary IVC filters (see Figure 10.3), are available. Requirements for an appropriate caval filter are:

- high biocompatibility,
- low thrombogenicity,
- high effectiveness,
- high mechanical stability,
- high patency rate,
- low complication rate.

Furthermore, a filter should be easy to insert percutaneously through a small-calibre catheter (Neuerburg and Günther, 1994). However, as current data from clinical and experimental investigations of IVC filters are difficult to compare due to differing study designs, it is impossible to determine which device is optimal.

The choice of IVC filter type depends on the operator's familiarity with the device, the diameter of the IVC, the site of proposed filter deployment within the IVC, the access site, the patient's underlying disease and the availability of the device.

Most IVC filters are unsuitable for use in patients with a megacava (caval diameter >3 cm), a condition which may be observed in up to 5% of all cases (Prince *et al.*, 1983; Pais *et al.*, 1989). If cavography reveals a megacava, either bi-iliac insertion of two IVC filters (Ramchandani *et al.*, 1991) or insertion of a caval filter which is large enough and suitable for such a condition (e.g. bird's nest filter) may be considered.

In patients undergoing systemic fibrinolysis, the use of an atraumatic temporary filtration device is recommended to reduce the risk of retroperitoneal haemorrhage. With retrievable and non-retrievable permanent caval filters fixation of the device is achieved by hooks that grasp the wall of the IVC. Although fixation should be without penetration of the full thickness of the caval wall, there may be a potentially increased risk of retroperitoneal haemorrhage using this 'fishhook' filter fixation principle during systemic fibrinolysis. However, there are no reports in the literature about such cases.

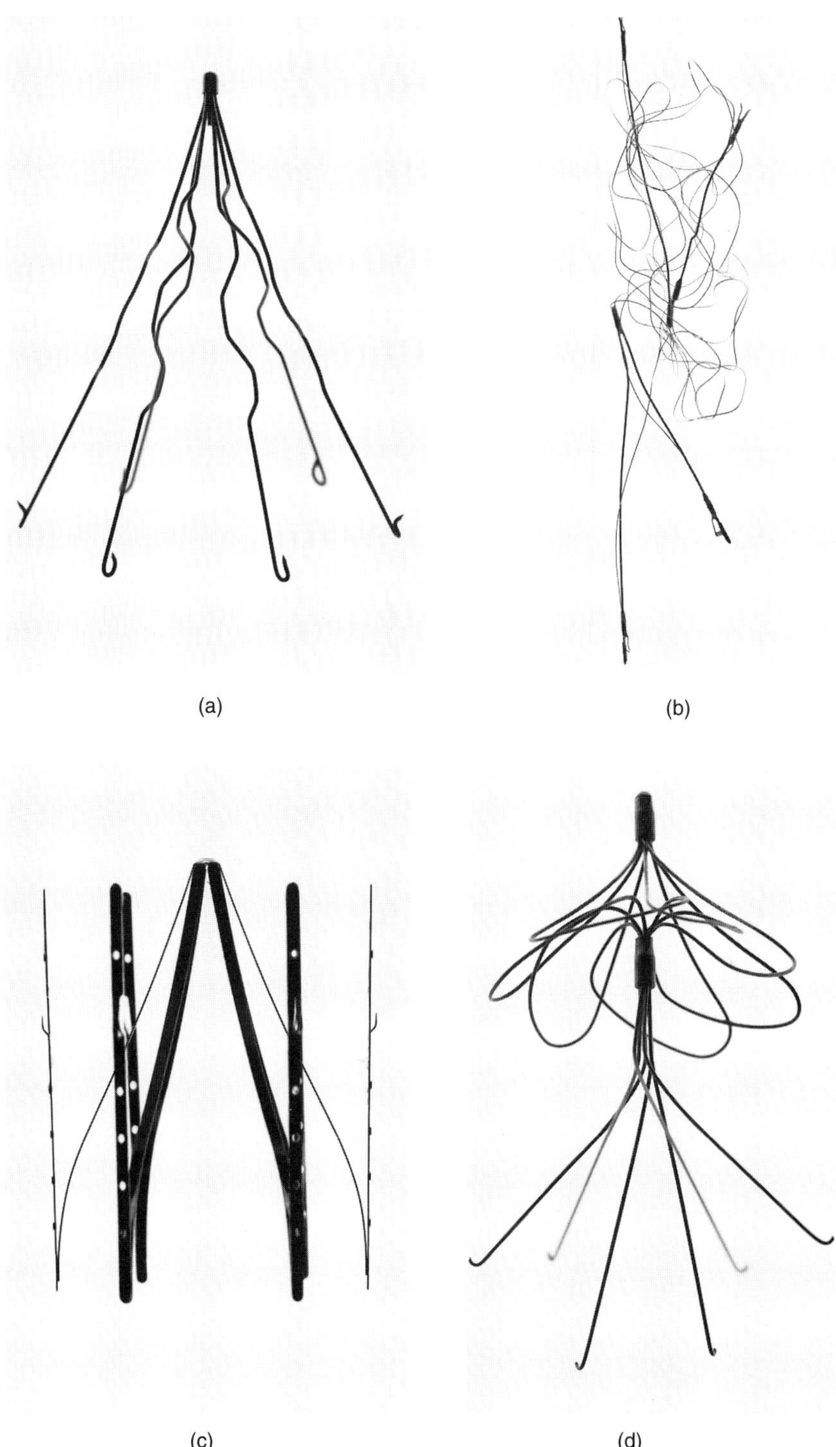

Figure 10.2 (Caption overleaf)

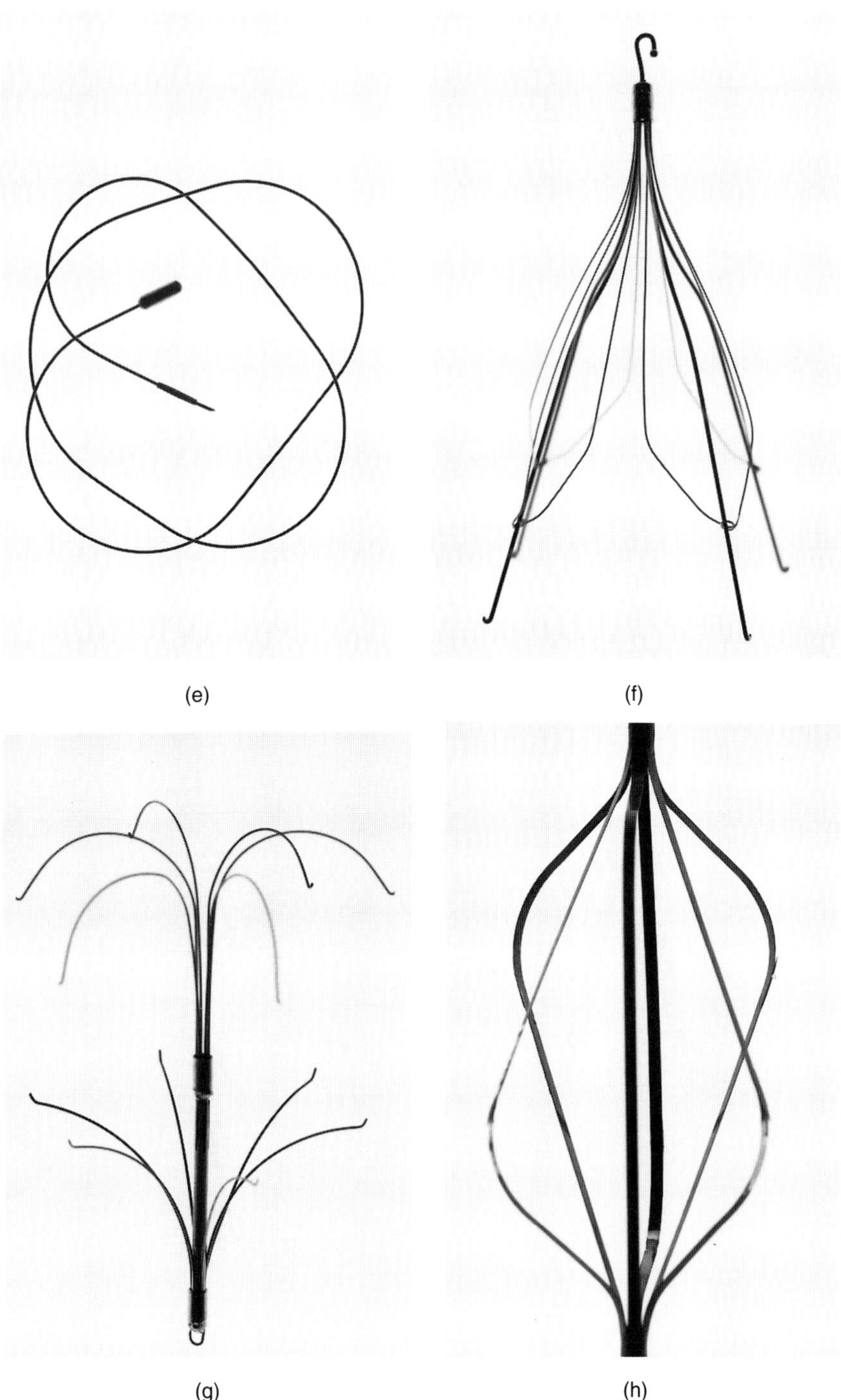

Figure 10.2 (Caption opposite)

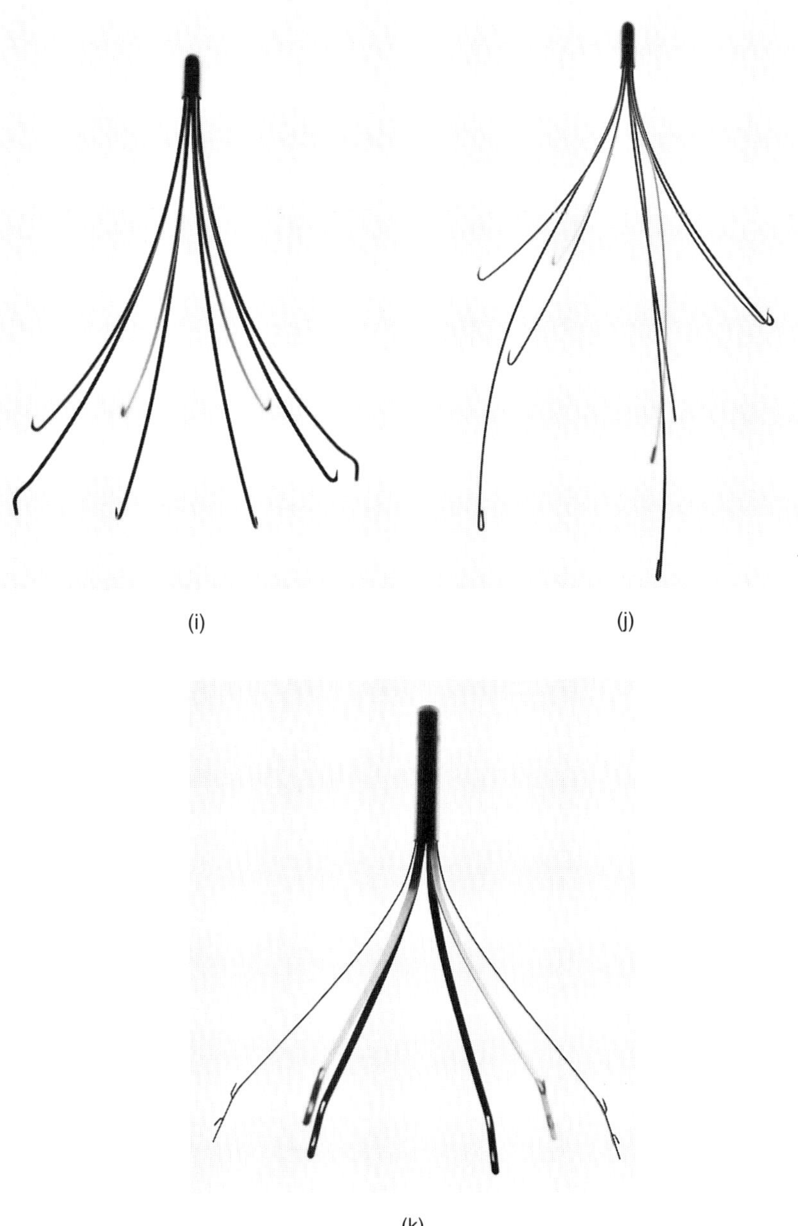

Figure 10.2. Selection of currently clinically applied percutaneous permanent inferior vena cava filters: (a) Titanium Greenfield; (b) Bird's nest; (c) Vena Tech LGM; (d) Simon nitinol; (e) DIL; (f) Tulip; (g) FCP 2002-FP; (h) Anthéor DC2; (i) CARDIAL; (j) Vascor; (k) KEEPER.

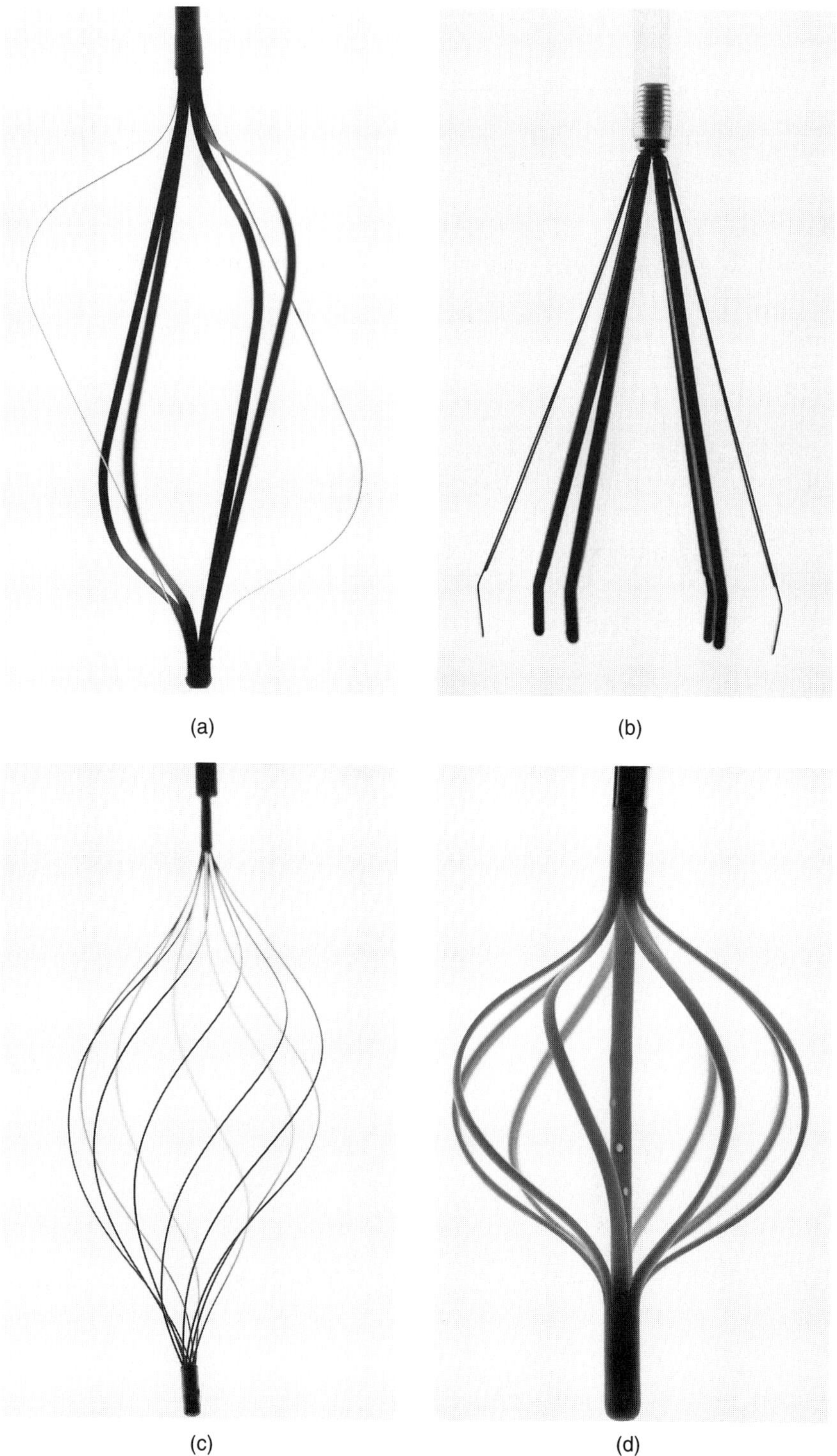

Figure 10.3 (Caption opposite)

Filters, which are designed for temporary use only are stabilized within the IVC atraumatically without any hooks. They are attached to a catheter or guidewire, which remains in place through the insertion vein. However, these filters must be removed after 10 days or moved to another place, otherwise they become incorporated in the caval wall. As the technical details of insertion vary considerably for different IVC filters, no details of the introduction technique are given here. The reader should refer to the manufacturer's operating instructions for the chosen device.

INDICATIONS FOR CAVAL FILTERS

Although significant complications associated with percutaneous filter insertion are rare, caval filters as a protection against pulmonary embolism should be reserved for a small group of patients as outlined below.

Before filter insertion the diagnosis of pulmonary embolism should be firmly established (see Chapter 9). The most important and reliable means for the diagnosis of pulmonary embolism are pulmonary angiography and/or lung scintigraphy. In patients with clinically suspected fulminant or massive pulmonary embolism the diagnosis may be confirmed initially by transoesophageal echocardiography or ultrasonography.

There are some absolute indications for caval filter placement (Table 10.4) and some controversial indications for caval interruption (Table 10.5).

Indications for *temporary filter placement* are not that well established. The most common indication for placement of a temporary caval filter is a short-term prophylaxis of pulmonary embolism during fibrinolysis in the presence of large caval or iliacal thrombi (Théry *et al.*, 1990; Neuerburg *et al.*, 1996a). All other indications for temporary caval filter placement are either anecdotal or controversial; placement of a temporary IVC filter or the temporary placement of a retrievable permanent IVC filter may be considered as a prophylactic measure prior to surgery when there is a displacing thrombi in patients with documented deep vein thrombosis (DVT), during pregnancy when there is DVT (Aburahma *et al.*, 1993), after pulmonary embolism and

Figure 10.3. Selection of various currently clinically applied percutaneous temporary inferior vena cava filters: (a) Anthéor; (b) LGT; (c) temporary Günther; (d) Prolyser.

Table 10.4 Absolute indications for inferior vena cava filter placement

- Recurrent pulmonary embolism despite adequate anticoagulation
- Pulmonary embolism (major event) when anticoagulation is contraindicated
- Prophylactic filter placement in patients at high risk of fatal pulmonary embolism (e.g. cor pulmonale, marginal respiratory reserve; occlusion of >50% of the pulmonary vascular bed) after one major event of pulmonary embolism
- Large free-floating or poorly adherent caval, iliac or femoral vein thrombi after one episode of pulmonary embolism or in patients at high risk of fatal pulmonary embolism (e.g. cor pulmonale; marginal respiratory reserve; occlusion of >50% of the pulmonary vascular bed)
- Prophylactic filter placement after successful pulmonary embolectomy
- Paradoxical embolism, i.e. passage of thrombi through an intracardiac or pulmonary arteriovenous shunt (e.g. atrial and/or ventricular septal defect, patent foramen ovale) with embolization of a systemic organ (Sabiston and Wolfe, 1990)

when there are short-term contraindications to anticoagulation therapy (Millward *et al.*, 1994).

There are no absolute *contraindications* for caval filter insertion. Due to filter thrombogenicity the indication for filter insertion should be very strict in patients with known hypercoagulopathy (e.g. protein C, protein S or AT III-deficiency, antiphospholipid syndrome).

In patients with thrombopathies or during systemic fibrinolysis, the use of an atraumatic temporary filtration device is recommended to reduce the risk of retroperitoneal haemorrhage (Théry *et al.*, 1990).

Pregnancy is not a principal contraindication for filter insertion, but if necessary the filter should be placed in the hepatic segment of the IVC in order to avoid compression of the filter by the enlarged uterus.

Table 10.5 Relative indications for inferior vena cava filter placement

- Free-floating emboli in the iliac and femoral veins, or in the inferior vena cava without previous pulmonary embolism
- Prophylactic filter placement instead of anticoagulation in tumour patients with deep venous thrombosis (Cohen *et al.*, 1992)
- Prophylactic filter placement in high-risk patients (e.g. cor pulmonale, occlusion of >50% of the pulmonary vascular bed) prior to pelvic surgery
- Prophylactic filter placement in multiple trauma patients, etc., with potential for a bedridden postoperative state and who have had documented deep vein thrombosis in the past (Leach *et al.*, 1994)
- Septic thromboembolism (Hoffman and Greenfield, 1986) (this indication is controversial in the literature; we consider septic emboli as a contraindication for caval filter placement)

The vast majority of IVC filters are non-ferromagnetic, thus enabling magnetic resonance imaging (MRI) even of the IVC (Teitelbaum *et al.*, 1990). However, immediately after insertion of a ferromagnetic device MRI may be risky. According to experimental studies it can be assumed that the device will be firmly fixed within the IVC approximately 4 weeks after insertion (Neuerburg *et al.*, 1993). Within a magnetic resonance scanner, the device tends to orientate parallel to the z-axis of the magnetic field, i.e. in most scanners the filter orients itself along the axis of the IVC (except in vertically oriented magnetic fields).

TECHNICAL CONSIDERATIONS

Selection of Insertion Route

Selection of the insertion route is based on the extent of DVT, the filter type chosen and the experience of the physician. In general, when the percutaneous technique is employed, an antegrade or retrograde approach via the right femoral (the most commonly chosen route of insertion) (Figure 10.4) or right internal jugular vein is used. Depending on the calibre and rigidity of the selected filter system, even a left femoral, left jugular (Figure 10.5) or an antecubital approach may be chosen. Cavography is mandatory prior to filter insertion in order to ascertain the size and the permeability of the vena cava, to assess caval abnormalities, such as a left-sided vena cava, and to localize the renal vein level.

It must be emphasized, that precise measurement of the caval diameter by biplanar cavography is mandatory prior to filter insertion, as proper fixation of most currently available caval filters may be compromised when the caval diameter exceeds 28–30 mm. Measurement of the caval diameter should be corrected for magnification. The size of the vena cava may change with respiratory movement.

The presence of thrombus above the femoral puncture site gives rise to a risk of dislodgement and pulmonary embolism secondary to catheter advancement. In such a case, a jugular approach would be favourable for filter insertion. To avoid the risk of transgression of the carotid artery using the jugular approach, sonographic guidance is recommended in order to localize the internal jugular vein and to document vein patency.

If documentation of pulmonary embolism is required prior to filter insertion, pulmonary digital subtraction angiography is performed using either a 5Fr pigtail catheter placed in the hepatic sement of the IVC or a selective pulmonary artery catheter, if necessary.

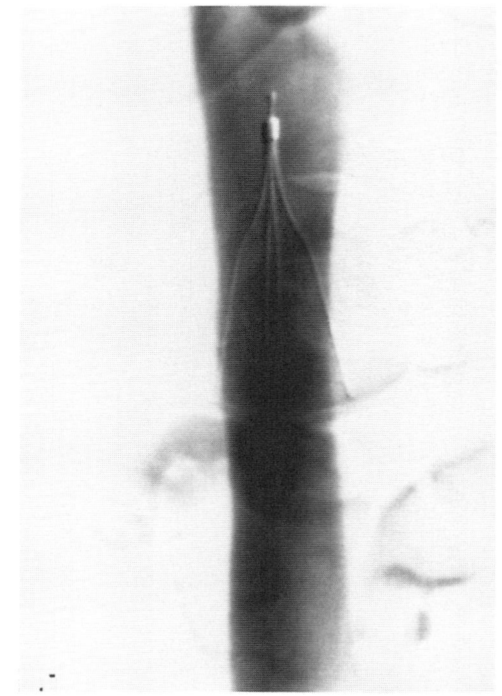

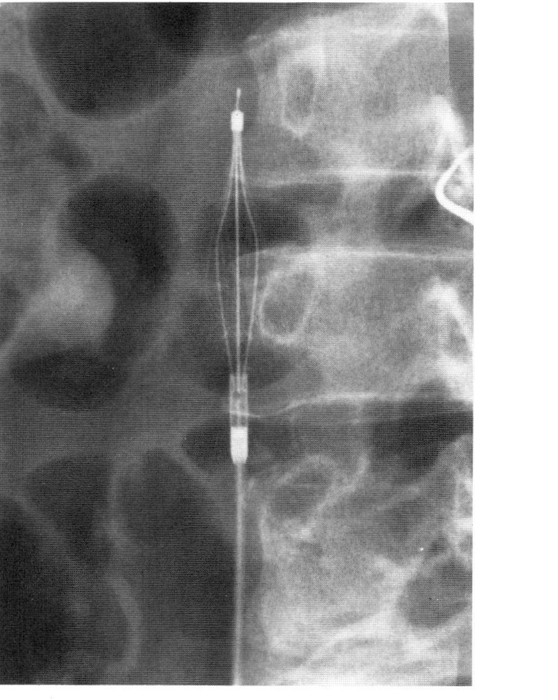

Figure 10.4. Percutaneous transfemoral insertion of a Tulip inferior vena cava filter: (a) the filter-introducer catheter with the filter attached is advanced through the sheath to the predetermined site; (b) proper filter placement is confirmed by cavography.

(a) 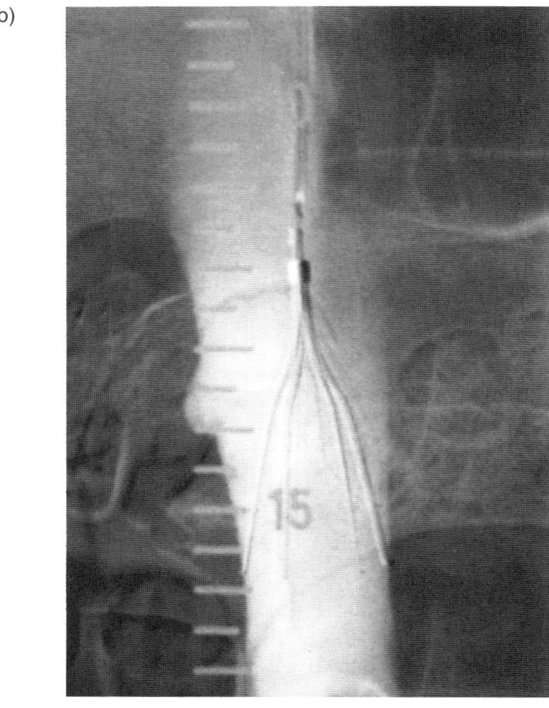

(b) 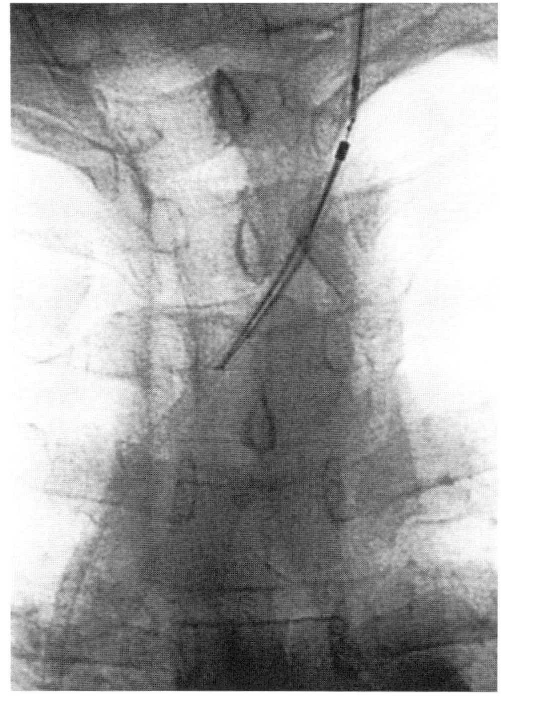

Figure 10.5. Percutaneous insertion of a Tulip inferior vena cava filter by left internal jugular vein puncture: (a) the filter-introducer catheter with the filter attached is advanced through the sheath and can be delineated within the vena brachiocephalica sinistra; (b) confirmation of the proper position for filter release is obtained by cavography prior to filter detachment.

When choosing a temporary filter system, selection of the appropriate insertion site is not easy. A major advantage of the femoral approach (Figure 10.6) is that a second permanent or retrievable IVC filter can be placed above a temporary filter prior to retrieval of the latter in case thrombus material has been caught in the temporary filter. The femoral approach, however, is not feasible in patients with advanced bilateral iliofemoral vein thrombosis or IVC thrombosis.

Although the antecubital or the jugular approach may be used without regard to the patency of the iliofemoral veins and the infrarenal IVC, the major disadvantage of this approach is the transcardiac passage of the filter system. If thrombi are captured in the temporary filter and the filter has to be removed to avoid incorporation in the caval wall, it might become necessary to withdraw the filter through the atrium, with the risk of thrombus dislodgement and secondary pulmonary embolism due to filter retrieval.

Implant Position

Most caval filters are deployed in an infrarenal position. Only in rare cases are caval filters inserted into the suprarenal segment of the IVC, the iliac veins or the superior vena cava.

Most filters are placed at a level of L 2/3. Optimally, the apex of cone-shaped filters should be located at the level of the lowest renal vein, because the venous inflow of the renal veins is purported to enhance natural lysis of entrapped thrombi. The vertical axis of the filter should be parallel to the longitudinal axis of the vena cava.

Only in some cases is suprarenal filter placement desirable (Stewart *et al.*, 1982; Brenner *et al.*, 1992, Greenfield *et al.*, 1992). Indications for suprarenal filter placement are listed in Table 10.6.

Indications for the use of superior vena cava filters are similar to those for IVC filters. The possibility of pulmonary embolism originating in the upper-extremity veins has to be considered, especially in patients with catheters and where medical instrumentation is being used to access the central venous system (Hoffman and Greenfield, 1986; Black *et al.*, 1993; Ascer *et al.*, 1996). Within the superior vena cava, filters are placed below the venous confluens of innominate veins. Using a cone-shaped device, the filter tip must be directed downwards (i.e. femoral filter set for a transjugular approach, and vice versa).

IVC Filter Retrieval

Although retrievable permanent filters are primarily designed for permanent use, in the case of accidental malpositioning or after

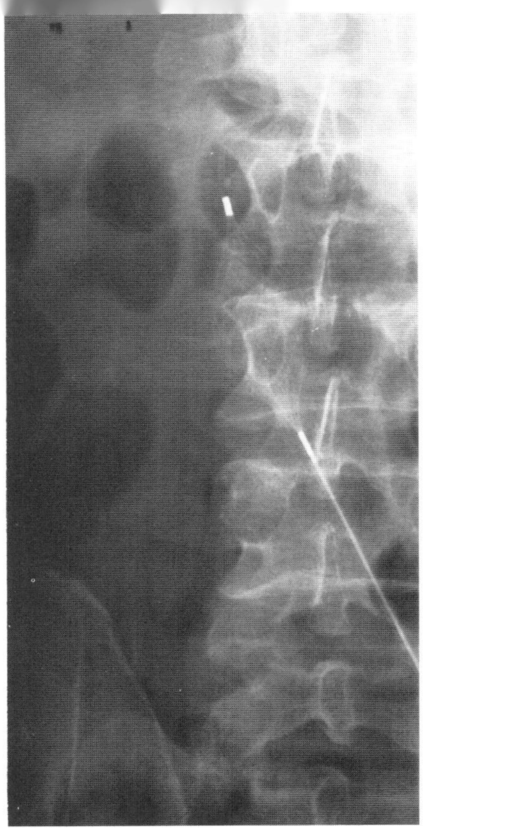

Figure 10.6. Transfemoral placement of a retrievable temporary Günther filter prior to thrombolysis. The filter basket can be delineated in the infrarenal inferior vena cava. (a) Plain film. (b) Cavography.

Table 10.6   Indications for suprarenal filter placement

- Inferior vena cava thrombi extending up to or above the level of the renal veins in unsuccessful anticoagulation therapy
- Renal vein thrombosis serving as a source of recurrent pulmonary embolism
- Recurrent pulmonary embolism despite adequate anticoagulation therapy, secondary to the presence of a large left ovarian vein
- Recurrent pulmonary embolism despite adequate anticoagulation therapy in patients with occlusion of the infrarenal inferior vena cava (collaterals as a source of pulmonary embolism)
- Pregnancy (alternative: infrarenal placement of a temporary IVC filter)

successful treatment of DVT retrieval of a permanent IVC filter may be recommended. Temporary filters are primarily designed for temporary protection against pulmonary embolism and have to be removed.

Clinical experience with retrievable (Darcy *et al.*, 1986; Neuerburg *et al.*, 1997) and temporary vena caval filters (Millward *et al.*, 1994; Nakagawa *et al.*, 1994; Zwaan *et al.*, 1995) and experimental in vivo data concerning the retrievability of Greenfield filters (Greenfield *et al.*, 1994) indicate that it is safe and acceptable to remove IVC filters up to 10 days (maximum 14 days) after insertion. Beyond this period, the filters become firmly fixed to the cava wall (Neuerburg *et al.*, 1993) and should be removed or their location changed if it is necessary that they remain in place for some more time.

Follow-up after Insertion of a Permanent IVC Filter

When the introducer sheath has been removed and haemostasis achieved, the patient is returned to the nursing unit or the intensive care unit. The patient is kept on bedrest for 10 days to avoid filter dislocation. Unless there is a contraindication, anticoagulation therapy should be continued to control the underlying thrombotic process. However, filter patency appears to be unrelated to anticoagulation therapy (Crochet *et al.*, 1993). Confirmation of filter position and filter patency is recommended at 24 hours and 10 days after filter insertion. For most filters, long-term anticoagulation therapy is not necessary.

Post-placement imaging

Abdominal plain films and ultrasound studies are usually sufficient for follow-up. Biplanar abdominal radiographs are useful in evaluating the position, configuration and integrity of IVC filters (Figure 10.6).

Ultrasound studies (especially colour-coded duplex ultrasound studies), venacavography, contrast-enhanced computed tomography (CT) and, for non-ferromagnetic devices, MRI may be used to evaluate the patency of the vena cava.

Colour-coded duplex sonography can be used to demonstrate caval patency and intraluminal thrombus. Especially in obese patients, sonography has limitations in imaging the IVC.

If ultrasound studies are inconclusive, venacavography and contrast-enhanced CT can be used to evaluate caval patency, assess caval penetration, and detect intraluminal thrombus. MRI may be used to evaluate caval patency after insertion of non-ferromagnetic IVC filters.

Follow-up after Insertion of a Temporary IVC Filter

In general, the introduction sheath of a temporary device is sutured to the patient's skin close to the puncture site. The filter itself is fixed within the sheath according to the operating instructions of the selected filter type. Patency of the introducer sheath is maintained by daily flushing with heparin solution. Unless there is a contraindication, anticoagulation therapy and/or thrombolysis is instituted as soon as possible. Anticoagulant and/or thrombolytic drugs can be given through the flushing port of the catheter. A plain abdominal radiograph is obtained every 2 days following filter placement to confirm that the filter is positioned correctly.

As soon as the patient is considered at low risk of further pulmonary embolism the filter should be removed. However, as stated above, retrieval of most currently available temporary devices should be performed by 10 days, up to a maximum of 14 days, after filter insertion in order to avoid ingrowth of the filter into the caval wall. The time interval for safe filter retrieval can be prolonged by slightly varying the position of the filter while it is still in place (there are exceptions to this, e.g. Tempofilter, B. Braun Celsa).

Prior to filter removal vena cavography is mandatory to confirm that there are no thrombi within the filter and IVC.

If small thrombi are present within the filter they may be retrieved by withdrawing them with the temporary filter into a large introducer sheath. If the filter is filled with thrombi, the filter can be cleaned by thrombolysis performed through the flushing port. Placement of a permanent IVC filter above the temporary one prior to filter removal is also possible.

RESULTS AND COMPLICATIONS

The most important criteria for evaluating caval filters are recurrence of pulmonary embolism, caval patency and complication rate.

In vitro studies have shown that filters are rather effective at capturing emboli (Neuerburg *et al.*, 1996b). The efficiency of IVC filters under clinical conditions, however, is more difficult to determine, since there have been no systematic follow-up studies using pulmonary angiography or ventilation–perfusion lung scanning. Thus, the clinical benefit for the patient is difficult to evaluate, and no prospective study has analysed this matter in depth. However, in many cases of recurrent major pulmonary embolism there is simply no means of preventing life-threatening embolism other than insertion of a mechanical barrier into the IVC.

The data reported in the literature confirm that IVC filters do not provide absolute protection against pulmonary embolism. In addition, IVC filters may even be the source of pulmonary embolism (McAuley *et al.*, 1984; Geisinger *et al.*, 1987; Murphy *et al.*, 1991). According to a follow-up study conducted by Ferris *et al.* (1993) on seven different designs of percutaneous permanent IVC filter (bird's nest types I and II; Amplatz; Nitinol; Titanium Greenfield, original design and modified hook design; LGM-Vena Tech), lethal recurrent pulmonary emboli despite filter insertion were proven at autopsy in 8 of the 320 patients studied.

The causes of recurrent pulmonary embolism despite filter insertion are:

- The development of collateral veins after complete caval occlusion.
- A large blind sac between the renal veins and an occluded IVC filter.
- Decreased IVC filter function (e.g. tilting, filter fractures, filter migration, incomplete opening of the filter).
- Propagation of a thrombus through the IVC filter (Geisinger *et al.*, 1987).
- Retraction of filter hooks from the caval wall due to organization and retraction of clots trapped within the IVC filter (Geisinger *et al.*, 1987).
- Pulmonary emboli arising from areas not protected by the filter (e.g. upper extremities, renal veins, hepatic veins, duplicated inferior vena cava, ovarian vein, right side of the heart).

Partial or complete filter occlusion with or without lower extremity venous stasis is not an uncommon finding in patients followed-up using imaging modalities (Ferris *et al.*, 1993). Caval patency is correlated with the time of follow-up. In a long-term follow-up study, Crochet *et al.* (1983) found a caval patency rate of 92% after 2 years, 80% after 4 years, and 70% after 6 years. Continuation of anticoagulation therapy does not seem to influence the patency rate.

Further complications associated with IVC filters include venous thrombosis at the puncture site, filter stress fractures, perforation of the caval wall and migration of the device or its components within the IVC to the heart and lungs (Figure 10.7). However, most complications are asymptomatic and do not require treatment (Ferris *et al.*, 1993).

Concerns about serious long-term complications arising in patients with a long life expectancy have led to the development of permanent filters that may be retrieved and temporary filters that must be removed. Temporary filters are mainly used for protection against pulmonary embolism during fibrinolysis in large caval or iliac thrombi. However, temporary filters do not appear to reduce the rate of IVC occlusion and insertion vein thrombosis to below that of permanent devices (Millward *et al.*, 1994; Nakagawa *et al.*, 1994). The major concern about the use of temporary filters is the possibility of thrombotic filter occlusion during treatment of pulmonary embolism, i.e.

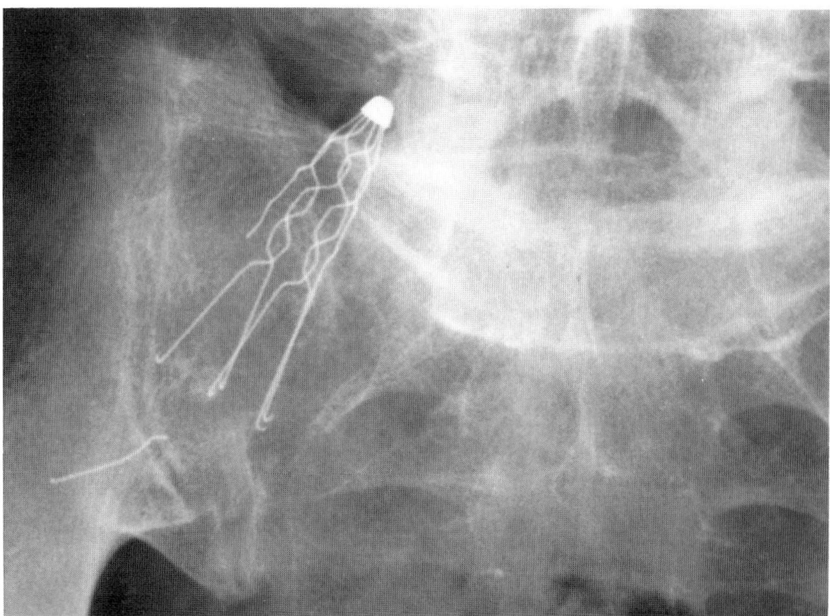

Figure 10.7.   Downward migration of an original Greenfield vena cava filter into the right iliac vein with fracture and dislocation of one filter strut.

when the filter fulfills the desired function, the problem starts again with filter removal.

To date, it has been difficult to make a reliable comparison of the reported clinical and experimental data on the various devices available for caval filtration. Many of the filters have not been in clinical use for long periods of time, and thus long-term follow-up data are not available for all devices. The study designs used in evaluating the compatibility and efficiency of filters are variable. In particular, the study populations investigated are not comparable, due to the wide range of 'traditional' and 'expanded' indications (Golueke *et al.*, 1988) for caval filter placement in various institutions. Even experimental studies are only partially reliable, as in vitro models are only an approximation of 'clinical reality'.

Caval filters are certainly a measure of last resort in the management of pulmonary embolism. Just as percutaneous filter insertion has replaced operative filter insertion, it is hoped that mechanical prevention of pulmonary embolism will be replaced by more efficient pharmacological prevention in the future. It must be borne in mind that percutaneous filter placement is only one of the various means available for managing venous thromboembolism.

REFERENCES

Aburahma, A.F., Robinson, P.A., Boland, J.P., Cochran, R.C., Conley, V.D., Snodgrass, K.R., Witsberger, T.A., Wood, D.J. (1993) Therapeutic and prophylactic vena caval interruption for pulmonary embolism: caval and venous insertion site patency. *Ann Vasc Surg* **7**: 561–568.

Ascer, E., Gennaro, M., Lorensen, E., Pollina, R.M. (1996) Superior vena caval Greenfield filters: indication, techniques, and results. *J Vasc Surg* **23**: 498–503.

Black, M.D., French, G.J., Rasuli, P., Bouchard, A.C. (1993) Upper extremity deep venous thrombosis. Underdiagnosed and potentially lethal. *Chest* **103**: 1887–1890.

Brenner, D.W., Brenner, C.J., Scott, J., Wehberg, K., Granger, J.P., Schellhammer, P.F. (1992) Suprarenal Greenfield filter placement to prevent pulmonary embolus in patients with vena caval tumor thrombi. *J Urol* **147**: 19–23.

Cohen, J.R., Grella, L., Citron, M. (1992) Greenfield filter instead of heparin as primary treatment for deep venous thrombosis or pulmonary embolism in patients with cancer. *Cancer* **70**: 1993–1996.

Coleman, C.C. (1986) Overview of interruption of the inferior vena cava. *Sem Intervent Radiol* **3**: 175–187.

Crochet, D.P., Stora, O., Ferry, D., Grossetete, R., Leurent, B., Brunel, P., Nguyen, J.M. (1993) Vena Tech-LGM filter: long-term results of a prospective study. *Radiology* **188**: 857–860.

Darcy, M.D., Cardella, J.F., Hunter, D.W., Smith, T.P., Castaneda-Zuniga, W.R., Lund, G., Amplatz, K. (1986) Experience with the Amplatz retrievable vena caval filter – work in progress. *Radiology* **161**: 611–614.

Ferris, E., McCowan, T.C., Carver, D.K., McFarland, D.R. (1993) Percutaneous inferior vena caval filters: follow-up of seven designs in 320 patients. *Radiology* **188**: 851–856.

Geisinger, M.A., Zelch, M.G., Risius, B. (1987) Recurrent pulmonary embolism after Greenfield filter placement. *Radiology* **165**: 383–384.

Golueke, P.J., Garrett, W.V., Thompson, J.E., Smith, B.L., Talkington, C.M. (1988) Interruption of the vena cava by means of the Greenfield filter: expanding the indications. *Surgery* **103**: 111–117.

Greenfield, L.J., McCurdy, J.R., Brown, P.P., Elkins, R.C. (1973) A new intracaval filter permitting continued flow and resolution of emboli. *Surgery* **73**: 599–606.

Greenfield, L.J., Cho, K.J., Proctor, M.C., Sobel, M., Shah, S., Wingo, J. (1992) Late results of suprarenal Greenfield vena cava filter placement. *Arch Surg* **127**: 969–973.

Greenfield, L.J., Proctor, M.C., James, E.A., Abrams, G.D., Moursi, M.M. (1994) Staging of fixation and retrievability of Greenfield filters. *J Vasc Surg* **20**: 744–750.

Hoffman, M.J., Greenfield, L.J. (1986) Central venous septic thrombosis managed by superior vena cava Greenfield filter and venous thrombectomy: a case report. *J Vasc Surg* **4**: 606–611.

Homans, J. (1944) Deep quiet venous thrombosis in the lower limb. *Surg Gynecol Obstet* **79**: 70–82.

Leach, T.A., Pastena, J.A., Swan, K.G., Tikellis, J.I., Blackwood, J.M., Odom, J.W. (1994) Surgical prophylaxis for pulmonary embolism. *Am Surg* **60**: 292–295.

McAuley, C.E., Webster, M.W., Jarret, F., Hirsch, S.A., Steed, D.L. (1984) The Greenfield intracaval filter as a source of recurrent pulmonary thromboembolism. *Surgery* **96**: 574–576.

Millward, S.F., Bormanis, J., Burbridge, B.E., Markman, S., Peterson, R.A. (1994) Preliminary clinical experience with the Gunther temporary inferior vena cava filter. *J Vasc Intervent Radiol* **5**: 863–868.

Mobin-Uddin, K., Smith, P.E., Martinez, L.O., Lombardo, C.R., Jude, J.R. (1967) A vena caval filter for the prevention of pulmonary embolus. *Surg Forum* **18**: 209–211.

Murphy, T.P., Dorfman, G.S., Yedlicka, J.W., McCowan, T.C., Vogelzang, R.L., Hunter, D.W., Carver, D.K., Pinsk, R., Castaneda-Zuniga, W., Ferris, E.J., Amplatz, K. (1991) LGM vena cava filter: objective evaluation of early results. *J Vasc Intervent Radiol* **2**: 107–115.

Nägele, M., König, C., Gorich, J., *et al.* (1995) DIL vena cava filter – Erste Erfahrungen bei 15 Patienten. *Fortschr Röntgenstr* **162**: 128–133.

Nakagawa, N., Cragg, A.H., Smith, T.P., Castaneda, F., Barnhart, W.H., DeJong, S.C. (1994) A retrievable nitinol vena cava filter: experimental and initial clinical results. *J Vasc Intervent Radiol* **5**: 507–512.

Neuerburg, J.M., Günther, R.W. (1994) Developments in inferior vena cava filters: a European viewpoint. *Sem Intervent Radiol* **11**: 349–357.

Neuerburg, J.M., Günther, R.W., Rassmussen, E., Vorwerk, D., Tonn, K., Handt, S., Küpper, W., Vagn Hansen, J. (1993) New retrievable percutaneous vena cava filter: experimental in vitro and in vivo evaluation. *Cardiovasc Intervent Radiol* **16**: 224–229.

Neuerburg, J.M., Vorwerk, D., Harlacher, R., Günther, R.W. (1996a) Ultrahochdosierte Urokinaselyse während Lungenembolieprophylaxe durch extrahierbaren Kavafilter. *Fortschr Röntgenstr* **165**: 76–79.

Neuerburg, J.M., Haupt-Pichler, A., Eilers, R., Siess, T., Buro, K., Pichler, C. V., Mottaghy, K., Günther, R.W. (1996b) Bestimmung der Effektivität perkutaner Kavafilter: Experimentelle Untersuchungen. *Fortschr Röntgenstr* **164**: 331–337.

Neuerburg, J.M., Günther, R.W., Vorwerk, D., Dondelinger, R.F., Jäger, H., Lackner, K.J., Schild, H.H., Plant, G.R., Joffre, F.G., Schneider, P.A. Janssen, J.H.A. (1997) Results of a multicenter study of the retrievable Tulip vena cava filter: early clinical experience. *Cardiovasc Intervent Radiol.* **20**: 10–16.

Pais, S.O., De Orchis, D.F., Mirvis, S.E. (1987) Superior vena caval placement of a Kimray–Greenfield filter. *Radiology* **165**: 385–386.

Prince, M.R., Novelline, R.A., Athanasoulis, C.A., Simon, M. (1983) The diameter of the inferior vena cava and its implications for the use of vena caval filters. *Radiology* **149**: 687–689.

Ramchandani, P., Zeit, R.M., Koolpe, H.A. (1991) Bilateral iliac vein filtration. An effective alternative to caval filtration in patients with megacava. *Arch Surg* **126**: 390–393.

Sabiston Jr, D.C., Wolfe, W.G. (1990) Pulmonary embolism. In Sabiston Jr, D.C., Spencer, F.C. (eds) *Surgery of the Chest* 5th edition, Vol. I, pp. 708–744. Philadelphia: W.B. Saunders.

Stewart, J.R., Peyton, J.W.R., Crute, S.C., Greenfield, L.J. (1982) Clinical results of suprarenal placement of the Greenfield vena cava filter. *Surgery* **92**: 1–4.

Teitelbaum, G.P., Ortega, H.V., Vinitski, S., Clark, R.A., Watanabe, A.T., Matsumoto, A.H., Rifkin, M.D., Barth, K.H. (1990) Optimization of gradient-echo imaging parameters for intracaval filters and trapped emboli. *Radiology* **174**: 1013–1019.

Théry, C., Asseman, P., Amrouni, N., Becquart, J., Pruvost, P., Lesenne, M., Legghe, R., Marache, P. (1990) Use of a new removable vena cava filter in order to prevent pulmonary embolism in patients submitted to thrombolysis. *Eur Heart J* **11**: 334–341.

Zwaan, M., Kagel, C., Marienhoff, N., Weiss, H.D., Grimm, W., Eberhard, I., Schwieder, G. (1995) Erste Erfahrungen mit temporären Vena-cava-Filtern. *Fortschr Röntgenstr* **163**: 171–176.

11

Clinical Studies in the Intensive Care Unit: Ethical and Legal Aspects

Erwin Deutsch

FACTUAL STARTING POINT

Clinical studies that are performed in the intensive care unit (ICU) take place on patients not probands. Two rules of the Revised Declaration of Helsinki by the World Medical Assembly as amended in Hong Kong 1989 limit experimentation on patients. The rules are:

> II.6
> The doctor can combine medical research with professional care, the objective being the acquisition of new medical knowledge, only to the extent that medical research is justified by its potential diagnostic or therapeutic value for the patient

> I.10
> When obtaining informed consent for the research project the doctor should be particularly cautious if the subject is in a dependant relationship to him or her or may consent under duress. In that case the informed consent should be obtained by a doctor who is not engaged in the investigation, and who is completely independent of this official relationship. (World Medical Association, 1975)

A patient in hospital, especially one in the ICU, is dependent on the hospital staff, especially the doctors. Therefore recruiting a patient to a clinical study requires another doctor not involved in the delivery of clinical care to obtain informed consent from the patient. Rule I.10 of the Revised Declaration of Helsinki assumes that there is bond between the doctor who provides professional care and the patient. Such a bond should not be used as means of obtaining the informed consent.

Rule II.6 of the Revised Declaration of Helsinki allows the combination of medical research and professional care, provided that the medical research is justified by its potential diagnostic or therapeutic value for the patient. This seems to disallow purely scientific research on patients by a doctor who also provides professional care.

The above-stated rules apply to all patients under professional care, but particularly to the patients in the ICU. Here the bond between the doctor and the patient is a strong one and his influence is even greater than in the normal ward or in the office.

RESEARCH ON PATIENTS UNABLE TO CONSENT

Rule I.11 of the Revised Declaration of Helsinki allows research on subjects unable to consent.

> In case of legal incompetence, informed consent should be obtained from the legal guardian in accordance with national legislation. Where physical or mental incapacity makes it impossible to obtain informed consent, or when the subject is a minor, permission from the responsible relative replaces that of the subject in accordance with national legislation.

The Revised Declaration of Helsinki does not mention research based on presumed consent. On the other hand, in Rule II.5 it is stated that if the doctor considers it essential not to obtain informed consent the specific reasons for this proposal should be stated in the experimental protocol for transmission to the independent committee. Thus it looks as if under certain circumstances research is allowed, if the ethics committee approves and the doctor has specific reasons not to tell the patient, maybe even in the case of an unconscious patient.

The final draft of the European Convention on Human Rights and Biomedicine (Council of Europe, 1996) addresses the protection of persons not able to consent to research with the following words:

> **Article 17.**
> 1. Research on a person without the capacity to consent as stipulated in Article 6 may be undertaken only if all the following conditions are met:
>
>   i.   The conditions laid down in Article 16, sub-paragraphs (i) to (iv), are fulfilled*;
>   ii. the results of the research have the potential to produce direct benefit to his or her health;
>   iii. research of comparable effectiveness cannot be carried out on individuals capable of giving consent;
>   iv. the necessary authorisation provided for under Article 6 has been given specifically and in writing; and
>   v.   the person concerned does not object.
>
> 2. Exceptionally and under protective conditions prescribed by law, where the research has not the potential to produce results of direct benefit to the health of the person concerned, such research may be authorised

* General conditions for research in patients.

subject to the conditions laid down in paragraph 1, sub-paragraphs (i), (iii), (iv) and (v) above, and to the following additional conditions:

i. The research has the aim of contributing, through significant improvement in the scientific understanding of the individual's condition, disease or disorder, to the ultimate attainment of results capable of conferring benefit to the person concerned or to other persons in the same age category or afflicted with the same disease or disorder or having the same condition.

ii. The research entails only minimal risk and minimal burden for the individual concerned.

(Council of Europe, 1996)

The draft of the European Convention on Human Rights and Biomedicine in another way allows medical experimentation on persons not able to consent. The approach of the draft is an abstract and a general one. There is no distinction between the three main groups of persons not able to consent to research, i.e. children, incompetent (especially old) adults and the unconscious. On the other hand, Articles 6 *et seq.* of the draft of the Convention on Human Rights and Biomedicine distinguishes under the heading 'Consent' between children, incompetent adults and persons who have a mental disorder, and gives rules concerning emergency situations and previously expressed wishes. But that chapter is devoted to medical treatment and not medical research. Article 16, on the other hand, refers generally to Article 6, but does not make use of the different types of incompetence, which may be distinguished at least when purely scientific research is concerned which does not have the potential to produce results of direct benefit to the health of the experimental subject. There is a great difference between research on conscious children and research on unconscious adults, for instance as far as the formation and use of a control group is concerned. Children, on the one hand, are represented by their parents, whose power to consent to clinical studies is restricted by the children's own interest. It would be a misuse of parental power to agree to a dangerous or unduly stressing study. The unconscious adult patient usually has no legal representative unless appointed by court. Therefore, one has to fall back on presumed consent.

GENERAL PREREQUISITES FOR CLINICAL STUDIES

Clinical studies in general have to meet the following conditions. Even if we distinguish between therapeutic and non-therapeutic research, on the one hand, and the formation of test and control groups or different arms of test groups of a study, on the other, there have to be some basic requirements:

- An acceptable level of risk for the patient.
- Informed consent.
- A research protocol that shows the scientific merit of the study.
- Inclusion and exclusion criteria.
- The number of experimental subjects used.
- The duration of the study.
- Specific reasons for termination of the study.
- The protection of privacy.
- Means and restriction of publication.
- The positive vote of an institutional review board or an ethics committee.

Naturally, there are specific rules, for instance prohibiting experimentation on prisoners or other people deprived of the freedom against their will, experimentation with the mentally handicapped or children, etc. These rules are to be found in different expressions in all the national and international guidelines, declarations, judgements, laws and conventions. Some examples are given in the following list:

- Prussian directive of 1900 (Anweisung an die Vorsteher der Kliniken usw., 1901).
- Case United States versus Rose, Trials of War Criminals before the Nuremberg Military Tribunals (United States versus Rose, 1947).
- Declaration of the World Medical Association: recommendations guiding doctors in clinical research (World Medical Association, 1975).
- Draft Convention on Human Rights and Biomedicine by the Council of Europe (Council of Europe, 1996).
- French statute of 1988 (Loi, 1988).
- German drug law of 1976 (Gesetz zur Neuregelung des Arzneimittelgesetzes, 1976).
- Good Clinical Practice guidelines by the European Commission (European Commission, 1991).

While all these requirements have to be fulfilled in a clinical study that takes place in the ICU, special problems are posed by the requirement for informed consent.

CONSENT TO CLINICAL STUDIES IN THE ICU

In the ICU there are 'normal patients', i.e. patients with all their faculties intact. However, they cannot be regarded as not willing probands, but as patients dependent on the doctor, the nurses and the other personnel in the ICU. From a strict legal point of view these patients are able to be informed and give their free consent. The local ethics committee will ask whether a doctor, not taking part in the treatment, is going to inform the patient and ask for the consent and whether there is any inappropriate pressure, even by friendly persuasion only. Generally speaking experimentation on these patients is not very different from clinical studies on non-ICU patients in the hospital.

More typically the patient in the ICU is unable to give free and timely informed consent. Sometimes these patients are unconscious, others are in different ways handicapped in receiving the information and weighing the pros and cons for the consent because they are semiconscious or heavily sedated. Here the problem of substituted consent arises. The following types of substituted consent should be considered.

Anticipated Consent

The patient is able to give his consent before becoming disabled for instance by anaesthesia. Two cases show the extent of the anticipated consent.

In Halushka versus the University of Saskatchewan (1965) a student had agreed for US $50 to participate in a research project. He had been told that a new drug would be tried out on him and that an intravenous catheter would be used. The drug turned out to be the general anaesthetic Fluoromar, and the catheter reached the heart, at which point he sustained a brief cardiac arrest followed rapidly by restoration of normal cardiac function. Although the court allowed anticipated consent even in scientific experimentation, the student won the case because the information had been imcomplete and his consent was therefore invalid.

In the case of Karp versus Cooley (1974) the patient had agreed to receive an artificial heart that was still in the experimental stage. During an operation it became necessary to install the experimental device. The patient died 2 days later having received a heart transplant in the interval. In this case the court held that the patient was able after full information to agree to the therapeutical experimentation that could have saved his life.

Consent by Proxy

In treatment it has become accepted practice that another person, especially the spouse or a near relative, is given the power of attorney in health care. In a German case in 1990 (Landgericht Göttingen, 1990) the patient had stipulated that, according to the intraoperative findings of the neurosurgeons, his wife should make the decision of whether to excise neural tissue or not. The operating team forgot to ask the wife of the patient and proceeded. Because of the mixed result of the surgery the patient sued and won the case. The same measure of informed consent by an empowered relative could be used in medical experimentation, at least if it is of therapeutic value.

Consent by Guardian

The legal representative of a child or a mentally handicapped adult is able to consent to experimental medical measures. Some statutes give the parents this right in a limited way, e.g. the German Drug Statute § 40 Abs. 4 AMG and the French statute of 1988. In the California case of Nielsen versus the Regents of the University of California (1975) a former member of the Institutional Review Board sued the university to prevent it from undertaking a purely scientific experiment on children. Healthy children were to be compared with children whose parents had already developed allergic reactions. All kinds of test were envisaged, especially the taking of blood, injections under the skin. The parents were to be paid US $300 for the participation of their children in the clinical trial. The court allowed the trial because it did not seem cruel for the children to participate.

Presumed Consent

Consent should be given in writing, orally, or at least implied (e.g. by participation). Intensive care, especially that of unconscious victims of traffic accidents, works on the principle of presumed consent. The presumption is that the patient would allow all medical interventions in his favour, unless otherwise stipulated. Presumed consent is sometimes invoked in clinical studies as well. The Hannover Ethics Committee has agreed to a clinically controlled study involving β-interferon in patients with severe burns. While the control group received the normal treatment for severe burns, the patients in the test group were given β-interferon additionally. Since all patients were unable to give a valid consent this was done under the presumption of consenting to promising medical measures. As far as the control group was concerned the participation did not create any danger for the patients. On the other hand, they did not receive the new treatment.

Deferred Consent

The ratification of a measure in a clinical study, that has been performed on the patient already, could be termed deferred consent. It is probably based on the assumption of presumed consent as well. In the late 1980s in Berlin there was a study of elderly patients who had suffered nearly fatal tachycardial symptoms. The clinically controlled study concerned about 300 patients, half of whom received a calcium antagonist while the reminder received a placebo. The patients were told subsequently that they had been included in the clinical study and were asked for their belated permission. If the permission was given, the study, at least retrospectively, had been performed with consent. If the permission had been withheld or the patient had died, all the doctors could do was to fall back on the idea of presumed consent.

The above examples show that in the cases which reach courts or ethics committees there are differences between a single-measure intervention, as in the Karp versus Cooley and the Halushka cases, and clinically controlled trials, as in the Hannover and Berlin cases. The clinically controlled studies prevent the doctor from adapting the medical measures for the purposes of the patient. On the other hand, the outcome is statistically more relevant. The more the discretion of the doctor is removed and objective criteria of the research protocol take over, the less there is reason for presumed consent, because patients will rarely contemplate taking part in a clinical study. But, on the other hand, they might think of an accident with grave consequences where an unproven method was indicated. Therefore it is easier to assume that they would have consented as far as the single measure is concerned. To ascertain the opinion of the patient the doctor should ask near relatives or other people who know the patient well. In questions of clinical studies for the benefit of the patients in the test group, the idea of necessity usually comes into play. If the patient were not enrolled in the study, he would miss a chance of becoming better. On this basis the presumed consent might be considered appropriate.

The other difference is that of the purely scientific experimentation as against the study that might directly benefit the health of the patient. A purely scientific enterprise was the basis of the case of Halushka versus the University of Saskatchewan (1965). The trying out of a totally new general anaesthetic on a proband is of purely scientific nature. But the proband gave his anticipated consent. A case of medical experimentation for the direct benefit of the patient can be found in Karp versus Cooley (1974). Here the use of an artificial heart was the last step in a desperate fight to save a person. The patient had already consented to it and, under these circumstances, what the doctors did was still unusual but justified.

If one draws a conclusion from the international and national rules, the researcher has to exclude purely scientific research with no direct possible benefit to the patient in cases where presumed consent or deferred consent are indicated. Even in a controlled clinical study where the control group receives only the standard treatment, one could still argue, although with less justification, that participating in the study somehow enhances the chances of the patient for recovery and he at least receives the standard treatment.

RESEARCH ON BRAIN-DEAD PERSONS

The discussion of whether brain-dead persons are dead or dying does not concern the researcher. If experimentation on brain-dead persons happens in the ICU, it will rarely be done as a clinical study. A few years ago the Göttingen Ethics Committee received such a proposal. The research protocol was drafted with the idea of testing all kinds of reflex of brain-dead persons awaiting explantation of at least one of their organs. Since it was not intended that the patients' relatives should be informed or asked for their permission and because of other reasons the Ethics Committee did not grant approval.

The recent Milhaud case in the Conseil d'Etat in France (Lebreton, 1994) concerned a single experiment on a brain-dead person. Here a forensic physician was called upon to testify in a murder trial. His expert testimony was intended to answer the question whether someone could have been killed with a certain mixture of different gases. To prove his point the doctor administered that mixture to a person who had been declared brain dead. The relatives of the patient had not been asked. The ethics committee had not been consulted. The case went up to the highest French administrative court where the principle that brain-dead persons are really dead was approved. Nevertheless, the court requires the doctor to obtain the permission of the ethics committee and to ask near relatives whether that experiment can be performed.

ICU STUDIES AND ETHICS COMMITTEES OR INSTITUTIONAL REVIEW BOARDS

ICU studies are not the normal fare of ethics committees or institutional review boards (IRB), in fact some members of these committees are somewhat apprehensive about reviewing a protocol from an ICU. They know that all kinds of problems will arise: the issue of the doctor–patient relationship, the issue of less competent or totally incompetent patients, the question of whether a control group is necessary, and the difference between therapeutic and purely scientific studies.

Normally, an ethics committee or IRB that tries to function well includes sitting members who are familiar with the routine in ICUs or running ICUs themselves. For an ethics committee or IRB it is absolutely necessary to have a clear picture of what is going on in an ICU and whether a clinical study can be performed under these circumstances. In this respect, the number of available persons is important; sometimes it is doubtful whether there will be enough participating patients to give a meaningful statistical answer. The ethics committee or IRB that is discussing the project should be the local one. This committee alone can judge whether the facilities of the hospital are sufficient for such a study. Advice from so-called 'international', 'European' or 'independent free' ethics committees are not helpful in this respect. They will not be able to judge the local conditions. This applies even to multicentre studies where different ICUs form part of the deliberations of the ethics committee. That the ethics committee must be involved in such studies is stated in the Revised Declaration of Helsinki, Rule II.5, which states that the doctor may consider it essential not to obtain informed consent. In this case a specific reason should be given in the protocol for transmission to the independent committee. The independent committee is the local ethics committee and the circumstances under which the doctors think it necessary not to obtain the informed consent can be therapeutic privilege or presumed, or deferred consent.

Rule II.5 of the Revised Declaration of Helsinki lets the ethics committee act as a kind of substitute for the patient. In doing this the ethics committee should insist that the doctor involves in the process of decision-making the next of kin of the patient. The relatives or persons with whom the patient has been living can provide information on what the patient's position would have been if he had faced the question. The presumed consent has to be tailored to the individual patient. The relatives cannot give the consent themselves, unless appointed as guardian. At least under continental European law, they are just people who can tell the doctor about the positions, beliefs and statements the patient has made or held previously. The ethics committee has to make certain that the patient's wishes can be identified and followed. Only in countries where the next-of-kin have become legal representatives of the unconscious patient can they give consent.

LIABILITY AND COMPENSATION

In nearly all countries in the world, if not specifically abolished by law, as in New Zealand, there is a liability for medical negligence (Palmer, 1979; Deutsch, 1980; Giesen, 1988). However, even in New Zealand punitive damages can be asked for (Green versus Matheson, 1989). Court cases brought because of negligent experimentation date back to 1767 (Slater versus Baker and Stapelton, 1767). Cases of liability for inclusion in clinical trials with no consent being given have arisen again and again in recent years in the USA (United States versus Stanley, 1987) and the Federal Republic of Germany (Bundesgerichtshof, 1956). Negligence not only provides for material damages, but also includes payment in compensation for pain and suffering. However, negligence implies that a standard of care has not been adhered to. This is hard to prove. Because medical experiments, particularly clinical studies, involve asking the participant to make a personal sacrifice for the good of mankind, there are many instances where compensation or some kind of third-party insurance, or even an objective liability, is provided for.

The French law of 1988 gives an example of an objective liability:

> Loi No. 88-1138 v.20.12.88 i.d.F. des Loi No. 90-86 v. 23.1.90
> Art. L. 209-7. Pour les recherches biomédicales sans bénéfice individuel direct, le promoteur assume, même sans faute, l'indemnisation des conséquences dommageables de la recherche pour la personne qui s'y prête, sans que puisse être opposé le fait d'un tiers ou le retrait volontaire de la personne qui avait initialement consenti à se prêter à la recherche.
>
> Pour les recherches biomédicales avec bénéfice individuel direct, le promoteur assume l'indemnisation des conséquences dommageables de la recherche pour la personne qui s'y prête, sauf preuve à sa charge que le dommage n'est pas imputable à sa faute ou à celle de tout intervenant, sans que puissent être opposé le fait d'un tiers ou le retrait volontaire de la personne qui avait initialement consenti à se prêter à la recherche.
>
> Pour toute recherche biomédicale, le promoteur souscrit une assurance garantissant sa responsabilité civile telle qu'elle résulte du présent article et celle de tout intervenant indépendamment de la nature des liens existant entre les intervenants et le promoteur. Les dispositions du présent article sont d'ordre public. (GazPal, Legislation 198, 605; J.O. v. 25.1.90)

The French law regulates all biomedical research, while the German Pharmaceutical Act of 1976 deals only with the testing of pharmaceuticals. Here, the experimental subject has been granted a third-party accident insurance which provides relief even if nobody is liable for the experimental accident. The German text is as follows:

§ 40 Abs. 1
Allgemeine Voraussetzungen

(1) Die klinische Prüfung eines Arzneimittels darf bei Menschen nur durchgeführt werden, wenn und solange

1. die Risiken, die mit ihr für die Person verbunden sind, bei der sie durchgeführt werden soll, gemessen an der voraussichtlichen Bedeutung des Arzneimittels für die Heilkunde ärztlich vertretbar sind,

2. die Person, bei der sie durchgeführt werden soll, ihre Einwilligung hierzu erteilt hat, nachdem sie durch einen Arzt über Wesen, Bedeutung und Tragweite der klinischen Prüfung aufgeklärt worden ist, und mit dieser Einwilligung zugleich erklärt, dass sie mit der im Rahmen der klinischen Prüfung erfolgenden Aufzeichnung von Krankheitsdaten und ihrer Weitergabe zur Überprüfung an den Auftraggeber, an die zuständige Überwachungsbehörde oder die zuständige Bundesoberbehörde einverstanden ist,

3. die Person, bei der sie durchgeführt werden soll, nicht auf gerichtliche oder behördliche Anordnung in einer Anstalt untergebracht ist,

4. sie von einem Arzt geleitet wird, der mindestens eine zweijährige Erfahrung in der klinischen Prüfung von Arzneimitteln nachweisen kann,

5. eine dem jeweiligen Stand der wissenschaftlichen Erkenntnisse entsprechende pharmakologisch-toxikologische Prüfung durchgeführt worden ist,

6. die Unterlagen über die pharmakologisch-toxikologische Prüfung, der dem jeweiligen Stand der wissenschaftlichen Erkenntnisse entsprechende Prüfplan mit Angabe von Prüfern und Prüforten und die Voten der Ethik-Kommissionen bei der zuständigen Bundesoberbehörde vorgelegt worden sind,

7. der Leiter der klinischen Prüfung durch einen für die pharmakologisch-toxikologische Prüfung verantwortlichen Wissenschaftler über die Ergebnisse der pharmakologisch-toxikologischen Prüfung und die voraussichtlich mit der klinischen Prüfung verbundenen Risiken informiert worden ist und

8. für den Fall, dass bei der Durchführung der klinischen Prüfung ein Mensch getötet oder der Körper oder die Gesundheit eines Menschen verletzt wird, eine Versicherung nach Maßgabe des Absatzes 3 besteht, die auch Leistungen gewährt, wenn kein anderer für den Schaden haftet.

(3) Die Versicherung nach Absatz 1 Nr. 8 muss zugunsten der von der klinischen Prüfung betroffenen Person bei einem im Geltungsbereich dieses Gesetzes zum Geschäftsbetrieb zugelassenen Versicherer genommen werden. Ihr Umfang muß in einem angemessenen Verhältnis zu den mit der klinischen Prüfung verbundenen Risiken stehen und für den Fall

des Todes oder der dauernden Erwerbsunfähigkeit mindestens eine Million Deutsche Mark betragen. Soweit aus der Versicherung geleistet wird, erlischt ein Anspruch auf Schadensersatz.

In other countries guidelines issued by associations of pharmaceutical industry are helpful. In Great Britain the Association of the British Pharmaceutical Industry obliges its members to provide compensation on an objective basis for patients taking part in a clinical trial. As in Germany, the guidelines of the British Association apply only to drug testing and not, like in France, to other biomedical research. There have been some problems in Great Britain with regard to pharmaceutical companies that sponsor drug trials shouldering their responsibility. Some ethics committees have now put specific questions to the companies and only after a satisfactory statement is obtained will ethical approval be given (Milne, 1991; Barton *et al.*, 1995). At present, the French and the German statutory provisions are the most satisfactory, if one disregards the limitation on drug trials in Germany. Whether the liability for presumed fault in cases of therapeutic experimentation or the strict liability for purely scientific experimentation is better than a third-party accident insurance will be decided after considerable time and the opportunity to compare the outcome of both systems. Because of the special circumstances of clinical research in the ICU there should be insurance coverage that does not apply only in cases of negligence, but applies also on an objective basis, be it liability insurance for strict liability or accident insurance directly granted to the experimental subject.

These differences in national law have to be taken into account when designing an international multicentre study. It is necessary to refer to the different legal rules of the countries concerned. This often creates difficulties in international acceptance of a study protocol.

COMMENTARY   Katherine Hall, *Dunedin*

The ethical issues at stake with intensive care research go beyond the more immediate concerns of developing new, effective and safe therapy for individual patients. Good research, particularly if it includes careful analysis of the effects of therapy on prognosis and outcome, can greatly aid decisions regarding the withholding and/or withdrawing of treatment, the effective allocation of resources, and minimizing risk/maximizing benefit for patients. These are all areas of great interest to medical ethics. The main problem for research in critical care medicine is the difficulty in obtaining informed consent. Even when the patient is competent and informed, there is always the possibility of coercion when the physician is also the researcher (as outlined in the preceding article). Frequently, only consent from surrogates (e.g. proxy consent), is obtainable and in some circumstances, such as cardiopulmonary resuscitation research, only retrospective or deferred consent can be obtained. Consent could be regarded as the *bête noire* of research; a threat to potentially extremely valuable advances. Research, however, is risky and it is, after all, the research subjects who bear the risks. How then can informed consent be applied to intensive care research in a way which takes into account the clinical realities without diminishing this protection, or denying the benefits of new therapies to the desperately ill?

When assessing the ethical validity of any research proposal, research ethics committees act in a paternalistic fashion, approving or disapproving a proposal on the behalf of future, potential research subjects. This paternalism, given that the *raison d'être* of ethics committees is to protect subjects from harm, could potentially weight decisions against research and researchers so heavily that approval for research could become extremely difficult to obtain. It is, however, balanced by three considerations: the nature and probabilities of benefits and risks to the subject (subject benefit/risk); the nature and probabilities of benefits; and risks to society, including future patients and efficiency of resource allocation (societal benefit/risk), and the use of informed consent.

The ideal research proposal would be one where there are large benefits and no risks to either the subjects or society, and where a high standard of informed consent is possible. In the real world, this is probably never the case. What tends to happen is that if one of these three parameters is deficient the research may be approved provided the other two are well upheld. The need for a subject to obtain personal therapeutic benefit may make the research ethically permissible even if the subject risks are high, provided the principle of informed consent is stringently upheld and the potential for society to benefit is great. An example is the willingness of acquired immune deficiency syndrome (AIDS) patients to participate in drug trials which have not undergone the usual stages of testing. Of more relevance to critical care medicine is the situation where good informed consent is not possible, but the subject benefit/risk and societal benefit/risk ratios are very good. Again, the research may be ethically permissible. An example would be an unconscious patient in severe respiratory failure from acute respiratory distress syndrome (ARDS), in whom the use of nitric oxide (with relatively low and known risks) is being considered. The deficiency in the patient's informed consent is offset by his or her potential to benefit from the therapy, and this provides the ethical justification for deeming proxy or deferred consent sufficient. If, however, the subject benefit/risk is less clear-cut, research may only be possible if the subject him or herself could give consent. Only in exceptional situations, however, would a research proposal be approved if two of the three parameters were poorly upheld. A theoretical example would be a case of plague where the survival of society is at stake; in these circumstances research may be permissible even if consent was not well upheld and the research was unlikely to benefit the subjects themselves.

Informed consent is an expression of the principle of autonomy, which contains the concepts of freedom of will, thought and action. For consent to be fully informed certain conditions are required: full and complete information, the capacity to comprehend that information, and the absence of any form of coercion. It is controversial whether fully informed consent is ever possible, even if the researchers were the subjects themselves. A cynic may suggest that a consent form is a *carte blanche* for researchers. A better way to regard informed consent is to consider it as an ideal which shapes the decision-making process, rather than as an all-or-nothing phenomenon. The conditions for informed consent may be upheld in any grade from poorly to completely. It is the degree to which this is upheld in relation to the subject benefit/risk and societal benefit–risk which is important. An example of this is the Halushka case cited in Professor Deutsch's article. The consent given in this case was deemed not sufficiently informed given the seriousness of the risk, regardless of any low probability, and hence was invalid. (The other legally pertinent point was that the subject had a permanent disability following his cardiac arrest.)

Review of the codes of conduct in research in Professor Deutsch's article reflect this balancing of the three parameters of informed consent, subject benefit/risk and societal benefit/risk. For example, the European Convention on Human Rights and Biomedicine only permits research on patients unable to consent for themselves if the research has direct therapeutic benefit for the subject, or potentially great societal benefit together with minimal risk for the subject. This is not to say that all controversy can be eliminated by such an analysis; the depth and degree of information required is often contentious. Recently in Australasian law there has been a movement away from the British standard of information being determined by 'the reasonable doctor' to that of the 'reasonable patient'. This is following the case of Rogers versus Whittaker in Australia where a woman lost the sight in her one functional eye from sympathetic ophthalmitis following an elective operation on her sightless eye (which was unsuccessful). The pertinent legal points are that the woman was not informed of the risk of sympathetic ophthalmitis and would not have consented to the operation if she had known there was a risk to her good eye, however small. How the 'reasonable patient' is exactly determined in clinical research is difficult to know, but it recognizes that concepts such as 'benefit' and 'risk' are in part defined by the patient, or at least given their relative weighting. As the Rogers versus Whittaker case shows, if the risks carry grave consequences, regardless of probability, a high standard of informed consent is likely to be necessary, particularly if a risk has great personal significance to a subject.

The gold standard of *fully* informed consent may not often be upheld in critical care research, but this does not mean that ethically valid research is not an achievable reality in this area of medicine. Informed consent is just one way of respecting the personhood of the patient – others such as truth-telling, maintaining confidentiality and communication with the patient and their family also are means of demonstrating such respect. This tends to be forgotten given the legal emphasis on informed consent. Care and consideration to these factors does not absolve a researcher from the need to obtain informed consent, but they do ensure that the spirit and not just the letter of the law is a part of research that takes place in critical care.

REFERENCES

Anweisung an die Vorsteher der Kliniken usw (1901) *v. 29.12.1900, Zentralblatt der gesamten Unterrichtsverwaltung in Preußen*, p. 188 f.

Barton, J.M., McMillan, M.S., Sawyer, L. (1995) The compensation of patients injured in clinical trials, *J Med Ethics* **21**: 166.

Bundesgerichtshof (1956) *BGHZ 20, 61; OLG Stuttgart VersR 1981*, p. 342

Council of Europe (1996) *Draft Convention for the Protection of the Human Rights and Dignity of the Human Being with Regard to the Application of Biology and Medicine: Convention on Human Rights and Biomedicine by the Council of Europe, 6 June.*

Deutsch, E. (1980) *Kunstfehler und medizinischer Behandlungsunfall in Neuseeland VersR 1980*, p. 201.

European Commission (1991) *Good Clinical Practice for Trials on Medical Products in the European Community.*

Gesetz zur Neuregelung des Arzneimittelrechts (1976) *v. 24.8.1976 BGBl. 1976 I 2445.*

Giesen. *International Medical Malpractice Law (1988) No. 1098 ff.*

Green vs Matheson (1989) *3 N.Z.L.R. 564.* Court of Appeals New Zealand.

Halushka vs the University of Saskatchewan (1965) *52 Western Weekly Reports 608.* Court of Appeals Saskatchewan.

Karp vs Cooley (1974) *493 F.2d 408.* Federal Court of Appeals.

Landgericht Göttingen (1990) *VersR 1990*, p. 1401.

Lebreton (1994), *Le droit, le medicine et la mort, Recueil Dalloz-Sirey 1994 Chronique 352.*

Loi (1988) *No. 88-1138 v. 20.12.1988, GazPal, Legislation 1988*, p. 605.

Milne (1991) Compensation for adverse consequences of medical intervention. In Goldberg (ed.) *Pharmaceutical Medicine and the Law*, p. 111.

Nielsen vs the Regents of the University of California (1975) Superior Court of California, December 8, 1975.

Palmer, G. (1979) *Compensation for Incapacity.*

Slater vs Baker and Stapelton (1767) *95 English Reports 1860.*

United States vs Rose (1947) *Trials of War Criminals before the Nuremberg Military Tribunals*, Vol. 2.

United States vs Stanley (1987) *107 S.Ct.3054; Fiorentino v. Wenger 227 N.E.2d 296.* New York Court of Appeals 1967.

Valenti vs Prudden (1977) *397 N.Y.S.2d 181.*

World Medical Association (1975) *Declaration of Helsinki: Recommendations Guiding Medical Doctors in Biomedical Research Involving Human Subjects adopted by the 18th World Medical Assembly as Revised by the 29th World Medical Assembly.* [Recent changes of the Revised Declaration of Helsinki did not concern these two rules.]